AAOHN CORE CURRICULUM FOR OCCUPATIONAL HEALTH NURSING

American Association of Occupational Health Nurses, Inc.

Edited by Mary K. Salazar, EdD, RN, COHN-S

Assistant Professor and Director,
Occupational Health Nursing Program
School of Nursing
University of Washington
Seattle, Washington

W. B. Saunders Company
A Division of Harcourt Brace & Company
Philadelphia London Toronto Montreal Sydney Tokyo

W. B. Saunders Company
A Division of Harcourt Brace & Company

The Curtis Center
Independence Square West
Philadelphia, Pennsylvania 19106-3399

Library of Congress Cataloging-in-Publication Data

Core curriculum for occupational health nursing / American Association
of Occupational Health Nurses; edited by Mary K. Salazar.—1st ed.

  p.   cm.

  ISBN 0–7216–6904–2

  1. Industrial nursing.   I. Salazar, Mary K.   II. American
Association of Occupational Health Nurses.
  [DNLM: 1. Occupational Health Nursing—education.   2. Health
Education.   3. Health Promotion.   WY18 C79676 1997]
RC966.C665   1997

610.73'46'0711—dc21

DNLM/DLC   97–7112

AAOHN CORE CURRICULUM FOR OCCUPATIONAL HEALTH NURSING   ISBN 0–7216–6904–2

Printed in the United States of America.

Last digit is the print number: 9   8   7   6   5   4   3   2   1

REVIEWERS

In their role as members of the AAOHN Professional Affairs Committee, the following individuals have provided oversight, reviewed two entire drafts of the document, and provided content input to the Managing Editor on this important association project. The association is grateful and appreciative of their invaluable contributions.

1995–96 AAOHN PROFESSIONAL AFFAIRS COMMITTEE

Elizabeth Lawhorn, MSN, RN, COHN-S, CCM, Chairman

Occupational Health Nurse Coordinator
Exxon Company, USA
Houston, Texas

Marilyn C. Benedict, BS, RN

Supervisor, Legal Operations
Eastman Kodak Company
Rochester, New York

Eleanor McCarthy Chamberlin, RN, COHN-S, CCM

Senior Occupational Health Nurse
Harris Corporation
Palm Bay, Florida

Debra Kay Olson, MPH, RN, COHN-S

Instructor
University of Minnesota
Minneapolis, Minnesota

Grace Rome, MA, BSN, RN, COHN-S

Occupational Health Consultant
Tucson, Arizona

Patricia Hyland Travers, SCM, MS, RN, COHN-S

Program Manager, Worldwide Health Strategy
Digital Equipment Corporation
Maynard, Massachusetts

CONTRIBUTORS

Jacqueline Agnew, PhD, MPH, COHN-S, FAAN,

Associate Professor & Director of
　　Occupational Health Nursing Program
Johns Hopkins School of Hygiene and
　　Public Health
Baltimore, Maryland

Mary C. Amann, MS, RN, COHN-S

Occupational Health Services Manager
AT&T
Chicago, Illinois

Kay Arendasky, MSN, CRNP

Associate Director, Occupational Health
　　Nursing Program
University of Pennsylvania, School of
　　Nursing
Philadelphia, Pennsylvania

Felicia J. Bayer, MSN, RN-C

Senior Occupational Health Specialist
Aluminum Company of America
Pittsburgh, Pennsylvania

Barbara J. Burgel, MS, RN, COHN-S, ANP

Clinical Professor
Adult Nurse Practitioner
Occupational Health Nursing Program
University of California School of Nursing
San Francisco, California

Kay N. Campbell, MEd, RNC, COHN-S

Manager, Health and Wellness Resources
Glaxo Wellcome, Inc.
Research Triangle Park, North Carolina

Eleanor McCarthy Chamberlin, RN, COHN-S, CCM

Senior Occupational Health Nurse
Harris Corporation
Palm Bay, Florida

Catherine L. Connon, MN, RN

Doctoral Student
University of Washington School of
　　Nursing
Seattle, Washington

Janet deCarteret, MN, RN, COHN-S

Occupational Health Nursing Consultant
Seattle, Washington

Deborah V. DiBenedetto, MBA, RN, COHN-S

Principal Consultant
Price Waterhouse LLP
New York City, New York

Mary E. Dirksen, MN, RN, COHN-S

Employee Health Nurse, Harborview
　　Medical Center
University of Washington
Seattle, Washington

Julia Faucett, PhD, RN

Associate Professor & Director of
　　Occupational Health Nursing Program
University of California, San Francisco
　　School of Nursing
San Francisco, California

Jeannie K. Hanna, MSN, RN, COHN-S

Manager, Corporate Occupational Health
Baxter Healthcare Corporation
Deerfield, Illinois

Marilyn L. Hau, MS, RNC, COHN-S, EMT-P, OHST

Corporate Manager, Health & Safety
McWhorter Technologies, Inc.
Carpentersville, Illinois

Winifred S. Hayes, PhD, MS, CRNP

President
Hayes, Inc.
Lansdale, Pennsylvania

Christina C. Johnson, BSN, RN, COHN-S

Health Services Specialist
BP Oil Company, Toledo Refinery
Oregon, Ohio

Diane K. Kjervik, JD, MS, RN, FAAN

Professor & Associate Dean for
　　Community Outreach and Practice
University of North Carolina-Chapel Hill,
　　School of Nursing
Chapel Hill, North Carolina

Diane J. Knoblauch, JD, MSN, RN, ANP
Attorney
Rohrbacher, Nicholson, & Light Co., LPA
Toledo, Ohio

Elizabeth Lawhorn, MSN, RN, COHN-S, CCM
Occupational Health Nurse Coordinator
Exxon Company, USA, Exxon Health
    Services
Houston, Texas

Jane A. Lipscomb, PhD, RN
Senior Scientist
National Institute for Occupational Safety
    and Health
Washington, DC

Kleia Luckner, JD, MSN, RN, CNM
Director, Program Development, Children's
    Medical Center & Women's Health
The Toledo Hospital
Toledo, Ohio

Sally L. Lusk, PhD, RN, FAAN
Professor & Director of Occupational
    Health Nursing Program
School of Nursing, University of Michigan
Ann Arbor, Michigan

Susan Martyn, JD
Professor
University of Toledo, College of Law
Toledo, Ohio

Mary E. Miller, MN, ARNP
Occupational Health Nurse Practitioner
Washington State Department of Labor and
    Industries,
Policy and Technical Services
Olympia, Washington

Karin Myerson, BSN, RN
Manager, Associate Health Services
Marriott International, Inc.
Washington, DC

Judith S. Ostendorf, MPH, RN, COHN-S, CCM
Clinical Instructor
University of North Carolina at Chapel
    Hill, School of Public Health
Chapel Hill, North Carolina

Jane E. Parker-Conrad, PhD, RN
Occupational Health Consultant
Conrad & Conrad Consultants
Knoxville, Tennessee

Merey Price, MSN, RN
Environmental Health and Safety Manager
Cray Research, A Silicon Graphics Company
Cheppewa Falls, Wisconsin

Jennifer B. Radford, MPH, RN, RHV, SCM, COHN, Adv. Dip. TCDHE, FRSH
Occupational Health Nursing Consultant
Woking, Surrey, United Kingdom

Genevieve B. Reed, MSN, RNC, COHN-S, OHNP
Occupational Health Nurse Consultant
Salisbury, North Carolina

Betsy Eddins Richards, MSN, RN, COHN-S
FNP Candidate, Duke University
Durham, North Carolina

Bonnie Rogers, DrPH, RN, COHN-S, FAAN
Associate Professor of Nursing and Public
    Health,
Director, Public Health Nursing and the
    Occupational Health Nursing Program
School of Public Health, University of
    North Carolina
Chapel Hill, North Carolina

Mary K. Salazar, EdD, RN, COHN-S
Assistant Professor & Director of
    Occupational Health Nursing Program
School of Nursing, University of Washington
Seattle, Washington

Sharon Tanberg, MA, RN, COHN-S
Safety & Health Manager
City of Seattle, Personnel Dept.
Seattle, Washington

Joy E. Wachs, PhD, RN, CS
Associate Professor
Johnson County Academic Health Center
East Tennessee State University
Mountain City, Tennessee

Ann Keenan Widtfeldt, MPH, BSN, RN, COHN-S, CCM
Health Services Administrator
Health Partners
Minneapolis, Minnesota

FOREWORD

The AAOHN Core Curriculum for Occupational Health Nursing has been developed to provide a framework for practice based on the profession's scope and standards of practice in occupational health nursing. The occupational health nursing specialty requires a broad base of knowledge and interdisciplinary perspective in occupational health with emphasis on illness and injury prevention and health promotion. In addition, while other nursing specialties focus primarily on the individual as the unit of care, occupational health nursing is population-focused. It is directed towards the provision of services and programs to work-forces, as well as to individual workers. The AAOHN Core Curriculum for Occupational Health Nursing provides the foundational content to address these elements.

The Core Curriculum resulted from careful deliberation and a detailed plan developed by the AAOHN Professional Affairs Committee. It is a product that extends the scope and standards of occupational health nursing practice defined and established by the American Association of Occupational Health Nurses, Inc. (AAOHN), the professional society for occupational health nurses.

Experts in occupational health nursing contributed in the development of the Core Curriculum, and commendations must be given to the chapter editors for their critical role and contributions, and to the Managing Editor who guided this resource to completion. The Core Curriculum is intended to be a comprehensive source of information in the field of occupational health nursing and should meet the needs of occupational health professionals in a variety of settings.

The Association is pleased to provide the Core Curriculum as a guide to assist occupational health nurses in their practice. It also serves as a guide in curricula development and educational program planning. Developing a Core Curriculum for Occupational Health Nursing has been a long-time goal of the Association. We hope you will find the first AAOHN Core Curriculum for Occupational Health Nursing to be a valuable resource.

Bonnie Rogers, President
AAOHN

Elizabeth Lawhorn, Chairman
Professional Affairs Committee.
AAOHN

PREFACE

The practice of occupational health nursing requires a broad base of knowledge in nursing, public health, and human relations. The focus of this specialty is the preservation and restoration of the health of workers and working populations. Occupational health nursing is an autonomous practice requiring independent decisions and creative solutions to complex occupational and environmental health and safety problems.

Occupational health nursing has experienced a remarkable period of growth and expansion since the 1970s. This expansion is reflected not only in the increasing numbers of occupational health nursing practitioners but also in the scope and breadth of professional practice. Occupational health nurses are assuming innovative roles and increasing responsibilities as they strive to respond to a changing and more complex work environment. The complexity of providing effective occupational health services has been compounded in recent years by a constantly changing social, economic, and political climate, by the many challenges precipitated by health care reform and managed care, and by rapid and multiple technological advances. Occupational health nurses are challenged to keep abreast of these and other changes in order to stay current in their knowledge of this continually evolving and ever-changing field.

This AAOHN Core Curriculum for Occupational Health Nursing is designed as a comprehensive resource and practical guide for occupational health nurses from a variety of backgrounds and with varying levels of preparation in this specialty. The book is structured into three major sections, namely, the foundations of occupational health nursing practice, strategies and approaches to practice, and issues related to professionalism in practice. The first section focuses on the theoretical and conceptual foundations that support this specialty. These include the traditions and the basic concepts that serve as the underpinnings of occupational safety and health practice, education, and research. A summary of the nursing, public and occupational health, and social sciences that provide the framework for practice are presented. Additional topics include principles of management and administration, a description of workers and working populations, legal and ethical issues, and political, economic, and business trends that shape and influence practice. The second section focuses on the practical application of occupational safety and health principles to occupational health nursing practice. It begins with an overview of the strategic processes that are essential to the development, implementation, and evaluation of a comprehensive health and safety program. The prevention and control of occupational health and safety hazards, health promotion, and the role of direct care in work settings are also presented. The section concludes with six examples of specific programs that are frequently offered in occupational settings. The final section highlights issues and activities that contribute to the growth of professionalism in occupational health nursing. Research and other professional activities which serve to advance the discipline are presented.

Clearly, this is an exciting time to be an occupational health nurse! Occupational health nursing promises to continue in its phenomenal growth and development over the coming years. The intention of this publication is to present state-of-the-art knowledge prepared by occupational health nursing experts that can serve as a guide in occupational health nurses' quest for excellence in practice. The inclusion of the resources and references identified in the various chapters can assist in identifying tools and knowledge that are specific to particular areas of interest. While the information in this text is comprehensive, it is recognized that it cannot possibly meet all of the needs of this constantly evolving area of practice. Thus, the reader is encouraged to apprise and inform the American Association of Occupational Health Nurses, Inc. (AAOHN) of unmet needs, so that the Association can continue to respond to and serve its members and occupational health nursing.

Mary K. Salazar
Managing Editor

ACKNOWLEDGMENTS

The development of this text is the result of the expertise and hard work of a large number of people who served as authors and reviewers. It has been my great pleasure and honor to work with each and every one of these individuals as we struggled through the ups and downs (the celebrations and frustrations) that are inevitable in a project of this scope and nature. The spirit of collaboration and negotiation as well as the commitment to excellence that characterized the many participants have resulted, I believe, in an outstanding contribution to occupational health nursing practice.

I wish to thank the chapter editors and contributors for their endurance and patience, and especially for their good-natured perseverance through the continual development of each of their chapters. I thank the reviewers whose wisdom and guidance served as major forces in shaping the final product. I thank the individuals from the American Association of Occupational Health Nurses who were always there to provide advice and counsel when I needed them. I thank Ann Schmidt for her assistance with the many logistical tasks related to this project. I also wish to extend my thanks to my family, especially my husband Jerry, for their ongoing support and encouragement through the duration of this project. And lastly, but importantly, I thank the members of the American Association of Occupational Health Nurses for the privilege of serving in the capacity of Managing Editor of this important association publication.

Mary K. Salazar
Managing Editor

CONTENTS

Chapter Editor: Sally L. Lusk, PhD, RN, FAAN
Contributors: Mary E. Miller, MN, ARNP
                   Catherine L. Connon, MN, RN
                   Mary E. Dirksen, MN, RN, COHN-S

4 *Legal and Ethical Issues*   59

Chapter Editor: Diane J. Knoblauch, JD, MSN, RN, ANP
Contributors: Deborah V. DiBenedetto, MBA, RN, COHN-S
                   Kleia Luckner, JD, MSN, CNM, RN,
                   Susan Martyn, JD, BA
                   Diane Kjervik, JD, MS, RN, FAAN

5 *Economic, Political, and Business Forces*   79

6 *Principles of Administration and Management*   95

7 *Scientific Foundations of Occupational Health Nursing Practice*   121

SECTION TWO:
STRATEGIES AND APPROACHES TO
OCCUPATIONAL HEALTH NURSING PRACTICE
149

Chapter Editor: Genevieve B. Reed, MSN, RNC, COHN-S, OHNP
Contributors: Barbara Burgel, MS, RN, COHN-S, ANP
                    Betsy Eddins Richards, MSN, RN, COHN-S

11 *Health Promotion and Adult Education* 233

Chapter Editor: Kay N. Campbell, MEd, RNC, COHN-S
Contributors: Judith S. Ostendorf, MPH, RN, COHN-S, CCM
                    Jeannie K. Hanna, MSN, RN, COHN-S

12 *Examples of Occupational Health and Safety Programs* 265

Chapter Editor: Janet deCarteret, MN, RN, COHN-S
Contributors: Barbara J. Burgel, MS, RN, COHN-S, ANP
                    Marilyn L. Hau, MS, RNC, COHN-S, EMT-P, OHST
                    Elizabeth Lawhorn, MSN, RN, COHN-S, CCM
                    Sharon Tanberg, MA, RN, COHN-S

Section One:
Foundations of
Occupational Health Nursing Practice

CHAPTER

1

Occupational Health Nursing Specialty Practice

MAJOR TOPICS

■ *Scope of practice*
■ *Standards of practice: overview*
■ *Clinical practice standards*
■ *Professional practice standards*

The American Association of Occupational Health Nurses (AAOHN) is the national professional association for occupational health nurses with regional, state, and local constituencies. AAOHN has developed a core curriculum utilizing the Scope of Practice and Standards of Occupational Health Nursing Practice as its framework. This specialty practice provides for the delivery of health care services to workers and worker populations. Through the promotion, protection, and restoration of workers' health within the context of a safe and healthy work environment, the profession promotes the integration of practice, education, and research, which constitutes a framework for excellence in professional practice. The nature of occupational health nursing practice is broad and autonomous, and the practice has evolved into a highly specialized field of nursing. The AAOHN Core Curriculum for Occupational Health Nursing delineates concepts and principles to support the knowledge base for occupational health nursing practice.

I

Scope of Practice

A. The American Association of Occupational Health Nurses (AAOHN), the professional organization for occupational health nurses, has the responsibility to define the scope of occupational health nursing practice and to develop and promulgate standards of practice in this specialty. (See Appendix A: AAOHN's Standards of Occupational Health Nursing Practice.)

1. Occupational health nursing is the specialty practice that provides for and delivers health care to workers and worker populations.
2. Occupational health nursing practice is research-based and is guided by the AAOHN Code of Ethics. (See Appendix B.)
3. Optimizing health, preventing illness and injury, and reducing health hazards is the foundational core for the practice base.
4. The framework that guides occupational health nursing practice is derived from a multidisciplinary base.

3

B. Essential components of this specialty practice include:
1. Health promotion and prevention principles: incorporation of primary, secondary, and tertiary prevention strategies to optimize the health and safety of the worker population
2. Worker and workplace health hazard assessment and surveillance: identification of health problems and health hazards and implementation of monitoring and surveillance strategies to mitigate health risk exposure, improve workers' health, and ensure safe working conditions
3. Injury and illness investigation, analysis, and prevention: examination of trends of work-related illnesses and injuries to develop preventive strategies
4. Primary care: health care delivery provided to workers at the worksite or in the community, including treatment, follow-up, referral for medical care, health monitoring, and emergency care
5. Case management: A process of coordinating an individual client's health care services to achieve optimal, quality care delivered in a cost-effective manner
6. Counseling: interventions and appropriate referrals aimed at helping workers clarify problems, deal with crises, and make informed decisions and choices
7. Management and administration: the overall setting of goals and planning for the organization, implementation, and evaluation of the work of the occupational health service
8. Legal/ethical monitoring: Process of assuring that the provision of occupational health nursing services is within the legal scope of nursing practice, that occupational health nurses are knowledgeable of the laws and regulations governing occupational health and safety, and that decision making is based on an ethical framework
9. Research: the development, dissemination, and utilization of knowledge to support practice
10. Community orientation: articulation with and utilization of appropriate community resources to provide services more efficiently and effectively to employees and the company (Rogers, 1994)

C. Occupational health nurses collaborate with workers, employers, and other professionals to:
1. Identify health needs
2. Prioritize interventions
3. Develop and implement interventions and programs
4. Evaluate care and service delivery

II

Standards of Practice

A. Standards provide guidance for professional practice and serve as a means to assure accountability of the profession to the public.

B. Standards of practice are dynamic and evolve over a period of time to reflect the changing scope of practice and development of new knowledge.

C. Practice standards consist of Standards of Clinical Nursing Practice and Professional Practice Standards, which are criteria-based and measurable.
1. Structure criteria describe organizational and resource measures for care delivery.
2. Process criteria describe nursing care actions.
3. Outcome criteria describe the end result of the care action.

D. Standard statements are listed below; however, the reader is referred to Appendix A, Standards of Occupational Health Nursing Practice (AAOHN, 1994), for fully detailed criteria for each standard.

1. *Clinical Practice Standards* describe components of care provided to all clients:
   a. Standard I: Assessment
      The occupational health nurse systematically assesses the health status of the client.
   b. Standard II: Diagnosis
      The occupational health nurse analyzes the data collected to formulate a nursing diagnosis.
   c. Standard III: Outcome Identification
      The occupational health nurse identifies expected outcomes specific to the client.
   d. Standard IV: Planning
      The occupational health nurse develops a plan of care that is comprehensive and formulates interventions for each level of prevention and for therapeutic modalities to achieve expected outcomes.
   e. Standard V: Implementation
      The occupational health nurse implements interventions to promote health, prevent illness and injury, and facilitate rehabilitation, guided by the plan of care.
   f. Standard VI: Evaluation
      The occupational health nurse systematically and continuously evaluates the client's responses to interventions and progress toward the achievement of expected outcomes.

2. *Professional Practice Standards* describe components of the professional role and behaviors nurses are expected to exhibit:
   a. Standard I: Professional Development/Evaluation
      The occupational health nurse assumes responsibility for professional development and continuing education and evaluates personal professional performance in relation to practice standards.
   b. Standard II: Quality Improvement/Quality Assurance
      The occupational health nurse monitors and evaluates the quality and effectiveness of occupational health practice.
   c. Standard III: Collaboration
      The occupational health nurse collaborates with employees, management, other health care providers, professionals, and community representatives in assessing, planning, implementing, and evaluating care and occupational health services.
   d. Standard IV: Research
      The occupational health nurse contributes to the scientific base in occupational health nursing through research, as appropriate, and uses research findings in practice.
   e. Standard V: Ethics
      The occupational health nurse uses an ethical framework as a guide for decision making in practice.
   f. Standard VI: Resource Management
      The occupational health nurse collaborates with management and worker groups such as unions to provide resources that support an occupational health program that meets the needs of the worker population.

BIBLIOGRAPHY

American Association of Occupational Health Nurses (1994). *AAOHN standards of occupational health nursing practice.* Atlanta: AAOHN Publications

Rogers, B. (1994). *Occupational health nursing: Concepts and practice.* Philadelphia: W.B. Saunders

2

Occupational Health and Safety and Occupational Health Nursing: An Overview

MAJOR TOPICS

- *Occupational health and safety goals*
- *Categories of hazards*
- *Measuring occupational injuries and illnesses*
- *Historical overview*
- *Government and occupational health*
- *Occupational health nursing*
- *Characteristics of occupational health nursing practice*
- *Future challenges and opportunities*

The primary focus of occupational health nursing practice is on preventing work-related illnesses and injuries and promoting health and safety among worker populations. Achieving these goals requires a clear understanding of the basic terminology used in the field and a knowledge of the principles that underlie occupational health and safety practice, education, and research. This chapter is intended to introduce the reader to the traditions and concepts inherent to this specialty area and to provide an historical overview of the development of occupational health and occupational health nursing.

Introduction and Overview

I

The Primary Focus

The mission of occupational health and safety is "to assure so far as possible every working man and woman in the Nation safe and healthful working conditions" (United States Congress, Occupational Safety and Health Act, 1970).

A. Because the majority of Americans are directly or indirectly affected by hazards in the workplace, occupational health and safety should be considered an integral part of all health services.

B. The occupational environment is complex and multidimensional; the recognition of occupational hazards requires an appreciation of the social, cultural, political, and economic context of work; examples of factors that affect the work environment are as follows:

1. Social: the meaning of work, the social milieu of the worker, and the structure of work
2. Cultural: beliefs, attitudes, and values related to work
3. Political: the prevalent ideology in a society, the distribution of power, and government support for health and safety of workers
4. Economic: level of unemployment, competition, wage regulation, and nature of local economy

C. Occupational health and safety affect not only the worker but also the worker's family and significant others, the worker's community, and the larger society.

D. Occupational health as a specialty within public health is a population-based practice.

E. Occupational health sciences are in an early stage of development; much remains to be known about the effect of the work environment on the health and safety of worker populations.

II

Professional Goals

Professionals from multiple disciplines work cooperatively to achieve the goals of occupational health and safety:

A. Occupational health nurses' central mission is to promote and maintain the health and safety of workers through a systematic process of assessment, planning, intervention, and evaluation.

B. Occupational physicians focus on the prevention, detection, and treatment of work-related diseases and injuries.

C. Industrial hygienists recognize, evaluate, and control toxic exposures and hazards in the work environment.

D. Safety engineers and other safety professionals focus on the prevention of occupational injuries and the maintenance or creation of safe workplaces and safe work practices.

E. Other professionals include:

1. Epidemiologists, who study and describe the natural history of occupational diseases and injuries in population groups
2. Toxicologists, who study and describe the toxic properties of agents used in work applications to which workers may be exposed
3. Industrial engineers, who design the tools, equipment, and machines used in manufacturing and other work applications
4. Ergonomists, who study, design, and promote the healthy interface of humans, their tools, and their work
5. Health educators, who promote workers' healthy lifestyles and work practices
6. Environmental engineers, who concentrate on environmental controls to limit environmental pollution and achieve a healthy environment

III

The Practice

Occupational health nursing "is the specialty practice that provides for and delivers health care services to workers and worker populations" (American Association of Occupational Health Nurses [AAOHN], 1994, pp. 2–3).

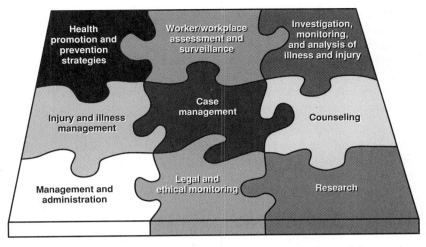

FIGURE 2-1 *Essential Elements of Occupational Health Services*
(Adaptation of original unpublished drawing by B. Rogers. Reprinted with permission)

A. Occupational health nurses focus on the "promotion, protection, and restoration of workers' health within the context of a safe and healthy work environment" (p. 2).

B. Autonomy and independent nursing judgments characterize the practice of occupational health nursing.

C. With a research-based foundation, occupational health nursing's theoretical, conceptual, and factual framework is multidisciplinary.

D. "Occupational health nurses are advocates for workers" and "encourage and enable individuals to make informed decisions about health care concerns" (p. 2).

E. Through collaborative practice with other occupational health and safety professionals, occupational health nurses are "key to the coordination of [a] holistic approach to [the] delivery of quality, comprehensive occupational health services" (p. 2).

F. Occupational health nurses are professionally accountable to workers (their primary responsibility), employers, their own profession, and themselves.

G. The essential elements of occupational health and safety services (Figure 2-1) are defined by the Standards of Occupational Health Nursing Practice as described in the previous chapter.

IV

Workplace Hazards

Categories of workplace hazards affecting worker health and safety:

A. Physical hazards:
   1. Physical hazards are agents within the work environment that may cause tissue damage or other physical harm (Rogers, 1994).
   2. Physical hazards include radiation, temperature extremes, noise, electric and magnetic fields, lasers, microwaves, and vibration.

3. Health effects may be acute or chronic, depending on the dose and the body part affected. Examples:
   a. Acute: acoustic trauma from excessive noise; heat stress or stroke; skin rashes; eye injuries from infrared radiation; skin burns, cuts, or contusions
   b. Chronic: Noise-induced hearing loss (NIHL); multiple myeloma and leukemias from exposure to ionizing radiation; teratogenic or genetic effects induced by certain types of radiation

B. Chemical hazards:
1. Various forms of either synthetic or naturally occurring chemicals in the work environment may be potentially toxic or irritating to the body system through inhalation, skin absorption, ingestion, or accidental injection.
2. Chemical hazards include solutions, mists, vapors, aerosols, gases, medications, particulate matter (fumes and dust), solvents, metals, oils, synthetic textiles, pesticides, explosives, and pharmaceuticals.
3. Health effects may be acute or chronic and can affect the pulmonary, reproductive, urologic, cardiovascular, neurologic, and immune systems. Examples:
   a. Acute: respiratory irritation due to smoke; poisoning from accidental ingestion; metal-fume fever; chemical burns; contact dermatitis and other dermatoses
   b. Chronic: cancers (e.g., mesothelioma, bronchogenic and gastrointestinal carcinomas); pleural disease; occupational asthma; hypersensitivity pneumonitis; birth defects; neurological disorders

C. Biological hazards:
1. Biological agents such as viruses, bacteria, fungi, mold, or parasites may cause infectious disease via direct contact with infected individuals/animals, contaminated body fluids, or contaminated objects/surfaces (Rogers, 1994).
2. Workers in certain occupations (e.g., health care, biologic research, animal handling) have a high incidence of infectious disease.
3. Health effects may be acute or chronic, depending on the nature of the organism. Examples:
   a. Acute: self-limiting infections such as colds and influenzas; measles; skin and parasitic infections.
   b. Chronic: tuberculosis; chronic hepatitis B; human immunodeficiency virus (HIV) infection, progressing to acquired immunodeficiency syndrome (AIDS).

D. Mechanical hazards:
1. Mechanical agents may cause stress on the musculoskeletal or other body systems.
2. Hazards include inadequate work-station and tool design, frequent repetition of a limited movement, repeated awkward movements with hand-held tools, local vibrations.
3. Health effects may be acute or chronic; they may result in a permanently disabling health effect. Examples:
   a. Acute: neckstrain and other muscular fatigue from forceful exertion or awkward positioning; visual fatigue
   b. Chronic: Raynaud's syndrome from use of vibrating power tools; carpal tunnel syndrome and other work-related musculoskeletal disorders; back injury

E. Psychosocial hazards:
1. Psychosocial hazards are often related to the nature of the job, the job content, the organizational structure and culture, insufficient training and education regarding job requirements, and the physical conditions in the workplace; leadership and management styles can also contribute to psychosocial hazards.
2. Psychosocial hazards include interpersonal conflict, unsafe working conditions, overtime, sexual harassment, racial inequality, role conflict, shift work, limited autonomy, poorly defined expectations and work instructions, and absent or limited job reward.
3. Health effects may be acute or chronic, including temporary and permanent disabilities; the occurrence of accidents and injuries may be a secondary effect of these hazards. Examples:
   a. Acute: increased heart rate; increased blood pressure; sleep disturbances; fatigue; depression; substance abuse; worksite violence
   b. Chronic: hypertension; alcoholism; coronary artery disease; mental illness; gastrointestinal disorder

V

Work-Related Injuries and Illnesses

A. Occupational Safety and Health Administration (OSHA) definitions:
1. An *occupational injury* is any injury, such as a cut, fracture, sprain, or amputation, that results from a single incident in the work environment.
2. An *occupational illness* is any abnormal condition or disorder, other than one resulting from an occupational injury, caused by exposure to environmental factors associated with employment.

B. Facts about occupational injuries and illnesses:
1. Occupational injuries are more likely to be reported than are workplace illnesses; in 1994, of 6.8 million nonfatal injuries and illnesses, nearly 6.3 million were injuries (U.S. Department of Labor [USDL], 1995).
2. The majority of workplace illnesses are disorders associated with repeated trauma (USDL, 1995).
3. Injury rates tend to be higher for mid-size organizations (50 to 249 workers) than for smaller or larger organizations (USDL, 1995).
4. An average of 18 work-related fatalities occur each day (USDL, 1995).
   a. Men, the self-employed, and older workers are the workers most at risk.
   b. Highway accidents and homicides are the leading causes of fatal work injuries.
5. In 1994, eight industries accounted for nearly 30% of reported injuries (USDL, 1995): eating and drinking places, hospitals, trucking and courier services, grocery stores, nursing and personal care facilities, motor vehicle and equipment manufacturing, department stores, hotels and motels.

C. Examples of sources of information about occupational injury and illness:
1. U.S. Department of Labor, Bureau of Labor Statistics
2. National Safety Council
3. Workers' compensation records
4. State and federal occupational safety and health administrations (OSHAs)
5. National Institute for Occupational Safety and Health

D. Challenges in defining the extent of occupational injury and illness (Levy & Wegman, 1995):
1. Occupational illnesses and injuries tend to be underreported.
   a. Health problems may not be recognized as work-related.
   b. There may be disincentives for reporting problems (i.e., fear of being dismissed, pressure to achieve a "perfect" safety record).
2. The occupational origin of an illness or injury may not be recognized; thus, the problem may be misdiagnosed.
3. Because the association of a health problem with work may be equivocal, health care providers may not report it as an occupational problem.

E. Implications of occupational illness and injury rate measurement (see Chapter 7, Epidemiology, for a description of rates):
1. Changes in rates can serve as a measure of the effectiveness of worksite prevention programs.
2. Measures of rates can serve as an indicator of areas that should be targeted for interventions.

History of Occupational and Environmental Health
VI

The History of Work

As the nature of work changed through the ages, so did the concerns for occupational health and safety.

A. The Middle Ages (about 500–1500 A.D.)
1. This period was characterized by a growing number of trades, crafts, and artisans.
2. Some manufacturing was done in guild shops in towns; most was done in homes in rural areas.
3. With the increase in occupations came competition, increased production needs, and an escalation in occupational hazards.
4. The expanded use of metals, chemicals, and minerals also increased potential and actual effects on health.

B. Prior to the industrial revolution
1. Georgius Agricola (1494–1555 A.D.) described the ailments of miners, such as joint, lung, and eye problems.
2. Paracelsus (1493–1541 A.D.) wrote about the poisonous effects of metals and differentiated their acute and chronic effects on workers' health.
3. Bernardino Ramazzini (1633–1714 A.D.), the "father of occupational medicine":
   a. Wrote *De Morbis Artifactum Diatriba,* a book that describes the diseases of tradespeople
   b. Stressed that one should be able to work "without acquiring a wretched disease"
   c. Encouraged doctors to ask, "What is your occupation?" as part of their assessments

C. The industrial revolution (18th and 19th centuries)
1. Home-based hand manufacturing shifted to large-scale factory production.
2. As families and communities moved to cities, the result was urban overcrowding and unsanitary housing.
3. Production was accomplished with power-driven machinery.
4. Child labor and/or slavery were routine.

5. Jobs became more specialized, and work was monotonous.
6. The first nurses were hired by companies in the late 19th century to provide home care to workers and their families. (See section IX, Occupational Health Nursing History.)

D. The industrial revolution in America
1. Economic and social conditions
   a. American economic life shifted from agriculture to industry.
   b. Urban areas suffered from overcrowding and unsanitary conditions.
   c. Trends toward division of labor, ownership of production, and capitalism emerged.
   d. Rising death rates from accidents were attributed in part to hazardous working conditions, such as working with unprotected machinery.
   e. The economic and social conditions prevalent in the early 20th century led to a proliferation of "industrial" nurses.
2. American business and occupational health and safety
   a. During the early 1900s, businesses focused interventions on the workers' health and safety practices rather than workplace exposures.
      1) Ignorance of the English language, inexperience, and carelessness were identified as primary causes of accidents.
      2) Methods used to prevent worker accidents included educating workers in both personal and work-related safety practices.
   b. The New Deal in 1933 brought labor militancy and occupational health reform, resulting in advocacy for workplace safety and health.
   c. In 1934, the Division of Labor Standards (DLS) was established; the DLS worked with other organizations to develop safety codes and standards, to disseminate information about chemical hazards, and to improve factory inspections.
   d. After World War II, an increasingly conservative business and political era was accompanied by rising conflict between labor and management.
3. Labor militancy and strikes were used as strategies to improve working conditions.
   a. Labor unions began to influence workers' health, safety, and compensation.
   b. Labor leaders began to encourage injured employees to sue for damages as a strategy to promote better working conditions (Bale, 1987).
   c. Only about 15% of workers in the United States belong to labor unions; however, their influence extends beyond workplaces where their members are employed (Levy & Wegman, 1995).
4. Alice Hamilton (1869–1970) "matriarch of American occupational health":
   a. Was the first American physician to devote her life to industrial medicine
   b. Studied human effects of toxins used in industry such as lead, arsenic, carbon monoxide, and solvents
   c. Published *Industrial Poisons in the United States* (1925) and *Exploring Dangerous Trades* (1943); served as editor of *The Journal of Industrial Hygiene*

E. More recent developments in occupational health and safety in America
1. Environmental and occupational campaigns gained legitimacy as a result of activism in the 1960s.
   a. Initially, the environmental movement took little interest in workers' problems.
   b. Occupational health and safety approaches included advocacy for comprehensive protection of workers that included strategies to deal with plant safety and other health hazards.

2. After 1970, a wellness/health promotion movement began to grow.
   a. Wellness programs were intended to reduce costs by enhancing aware-ness of self-care, decreasing absenteeism, improving worker morale, and increasing productivity.
   b. Critics complained that this movement shifted blame from work and the environment to the individual worker (thus repeaing a trend from earlier years).
   c. This movement also resulted in concern about discrimination against populations at risk (i.e., smokers, obese workers, hypertensives).
3. Although the benefits of health promotion continue to be debated, programs continue to grow in favorable business climates.

VII

The History of Workers' Compensation

A. Prior to the passage of workers' compensation laws, employers could seek shel-ter from injury claims under three common legal defenses.
1. *Assumption of risk* assumed that workers were aware of and accepted the risk incident to their job.
2. The *fellow servant rule* assumed that if a fellow worker contributed to an in-jury, that fellow worker should be responsible for compensation.
3. *Contributory negligence* argued that the employer was not held liable if the em-ployee contributed in any way to an injury.

B. Passage of workers' compensation laws
1. The first workers' compensation laws were created in 1911.
2. Between 1911 and 1921, 25 states had enacted workers' compensation laws.
3. By 1932, 48 states and territories had enacted workers' compensation laws of some kind; only four states had no compensation acts.
4. By 1950, all states had workers' compensation laws; the last statute was enact-ed in Mississippi in 1948.

C. Under these new compensation laws, workers gave up the right to sue in ex-change for the guarantee of prompt and reasonable income, health benefits, and rehabilitation during disability arising out of an occupational injury or disease.

VIII

Government and Occupational Health and Safety

A. The U.S. Public Health Service (PHS) was established in 1912.
1. PHS sought leadership in scientific investigations and analyses.
2. As part of this effort, PHS measured the effects of toxins on individual workers.
3. The 1970 Occupational Safety and Health Act established the National Insti-tute for Occupational Safety and Health (NIOSH) as an institute within U.S. Public Health Service.
   a. NIOSH was originally a part of Health Services and Mental Health Ad-ministration.
   b. In 1973, the Health Services and Mental Health Administration was divid-ed into three agencies, one of which was the Center for Disease Control (CDC, now known as the Center for Disease Control and Prevention); NIOSH is currently part of the CDC.

B. United States Department of Labor (USDL) (formerly called the U.S. Depart-ment of Commerce and Labor)

1. USDL was "created in the interest of the welfare of all wage earners of the United States" (from William B. Wilson, first USDL secretary, 1913–1921).
2. USDL advocated for government regulation related to occupational health and safety.
3. After World War I, with a strengthening of business, an antilabor sentiment prevailed; thus, reform related to occupational health and safety lost its momentum.
4. The 1970 Occupational Safety and Health Act established the Occupational Safety and Health Administration as an agency within the Department of Labor.

C. International Agencies and Occupational Health (See Appendix E for additional information.)
1. The World Health Organization (WHO) was established in 1948 to further international cooperation to improve health conditions.
   a. The purpose of WHO is "to promote the attainment of the highest level of health by all people in the world" (WHO, 1994).
   b. Following the 1994 Declaration on Occupational Health for All, WHO developed a global strategy on occupational health (WHO, 1995).
   c. In 1990, WHO created a global network of Occupational Health Collaborating Centers.
2. The International Labor Organization (ILO) was established in 1919 to protect the life and health of working men and women and to control occupational hazards; its services include:
   a. Policy and advisory guidance through its International Program for the Improvement of Working Conditions and Environment
   b. Provision of information through its International Occupational Safety and Health Information Center in Geneva, Switzerland (known as CIS in European communities)
3. The European Commission has developed directives aimed at harmonizing national occupational health and safety laws in member countries in the European Union.
4. The International Commission on Occupational Health (ICOH) is an international scientific society established in 1906; it is recognized by the United Nations as a nongovernmental organization (NGO).
   a. The purpose of ICOH is to foster the scientific progress, knowledge, and development of occupational health in the international community.
   b. ICOH has a close working relationship with WHO, ILO, and other United Nations agencies.
   c. Since 1969, ICOH's Scientific Committee on Occupational Health Nursing has produced nine reports for occupational health nurses internationally.

D. Occupational health and safety problems in developing countries that lack government support for occupational health services include:
1. Poor general working conditions
2. Inadequate wages
3. Inadequate or no workers' compensation
4. Inadequate health and safety legislation and nonenforcement of existing laws
5. Exploitation of the labor force
6. Environmental pollution and degradation
7. Lack of access to occupational health and safety expertise
8. Hazardous industries, operations, equipment, machinery, and products often imported from developed countries.

Nursing and Occupational Health and Safety
$\overline{\text{IX}}$

Occupational Health Nursing History

A. Occupational health nursing traces its roots to 19th-century Great Britain and the United States (McGrath, 1946; AAIN, 1976).
  1. Key figures in occupational health nursing:
     a. Philippa Flowerday worked for the J.J. Coleman Company in England in 1878, visiting workers and their families.
     b. In 1888, Betty Moulder, believed to be the first American occupational health nurse, was hired by a group of coal mining companies in Drifton, Pennsylvania.
     c. In 1895, Ada Mayo Stewart was hired by Fletcher D. Proctor, president of the Vermont Marble Company; in 1896, she became the superintendent of the company-built hospital in Proctor.
  2. Department stores were among the first companies to hire industrial nurses.
  3. The employment of nurses began to grow in mining and manufacturing companies as well.

B. Several events contributed to the development of the profession:
  1. In 1909, the Milwaukee Visiting Nurse Association placed a nurse in a plant to offer public health services in order to demonstrate the economic value of the service.
  2. For the most part, industrial nurses remained visiting nurses until workers' compensation laws were instituted, at which time first-aid stations were opened in plants.
  3. In 1916, Florence Wright, in an address to the National Safety Council, described the valuable work done by the industrial nurse as follows:
     a. Promotes pleasant industrial relations
     b. Reduces time lost through accident and illness
     c. Minimizes the results of accidents by providing first aid and subsequent care under the direction of the surgeon
     d. Searches out the causes of illness and accident through cooperation with employers and outside agencies in the community and the home
     e. Makes possible healthy, happy, thrifty home life in the families of those visited, preventing waste of life and health and increasing the efficiency of each member
  4. In 1916, Ella Phillips Crandall described the roles of occupational health nurses as follows:
     a. First aid and dispensary service
     b. Hospital duty
     c. Making rounds in plant for observation of employees and inspection of plant
     d. Consultation—chiefly for women
     e. Teaching health and hygiene classes
     f. Making home visits to provide nursing and social services, including domestic education in food economics, cookery, and budget-making
     g. Keeping records of occupational diseases and injuries, relationship of employment to disease and mortality

C. Occupational health nursing organizations have defined the profession and established its professional foundations (Table 2-1).

TABLE 2-1

Historical Development of Occupational Health Nursing Organizations

- 1913: The first industrial nurse registry was opened in Boston for the purpose of supplying factory emergency room nurses.

- 1915: The Boston Industrial Nurses' Club was formed, the forerunner of the New England Association of Industrial Nurses.

- 1916: The Factory Nurses' Conference was formed; it admitted only graduate, state-registered nurses who belonged to the American Nurses' Association.

- 1917: Boston University's College of Business Administration offered the first industrial nurse educational course.

- 1922: The Factory Nurses' Conference changed its name to the American Association of Industrial Nurses (AAIN) in order to more closely identify with the industrial physician's group.

- 1933: The AAIN merged with the New England Association of Industrial Nurses.

- 1938: The first annual joint conference of industrial nurses' associations of New England, New Jersey, New York, and Philadelphia met in New York City.

- 1942: On April 19, at the conference in Philadelphia, the American Association of Industrial Nurses became a national organization; Catherine R. Dempsey was its first president.

- 1943: The first annual meeting of the new AAIN was held in New York City.

- 1944: AAIN prepared an "Outline of Basic College Courses for Industrial Nurses" and distributed it to colleges and universities in the United States.

- 1944: *Industrial Nursing* became the official publication of AAIN.

- 1949: Publishing of *Industrial Nursing* halted due to increased publishing costs; a newsletter was substituted.

- 1953: *Industrial Nurses Journal* was re-established; it won several awards in the years that followed.

- 1964: AAIN copyrighted its publication as the *American Association of Industrial Nurses Journal, The Journal of Occupational Health Nursing.*

- 1966: A committee consisting of members from AAIN, the American Industrial Hygiene Association, the Industrial Medical Association, and the American Academy of Occupational Medicine was formed to study the formation of an American Board of Certification for Occupational Health Nurses.

- 1969: The name of the journal was changed to *Occupational Health Nursing,* the Official Journal of the American Association of Industrial Nurses.

- 1971: The American Board of Occupational Health Nurses (ABOHN) was established as a separate organization whose purpose was the certification of occupational health nurses.

- 1977: To better reflect the broader scope of practice, the name AAIN, Inc. was changed to the American Association of Occupational Health Nurses, Inc. (AAOHN).

- 1983: The official headquarters of AAOHN moved from New York City to Atlanta, Georgia.

- 1986: The journal became known as the *AAOHN Journal,* the Official Journal of the American Association of Occupational Health Nurses.

- 1988: Occupational Health Nursing celebrated its centennial year.

- 1992: AAOHN celebrated its 50th anniversary with 12,500 members.

- 1997: AAOHN *Core Curriculum for Occupational Health Nursing* published.

1. In 1943, at its first annual meeting in New York City, the American Association of Industrial Nursing (AAIN) described its purposes and objectives:
   a. To develop sound standards of education and practice in industrial nursing.
   b. To cooperate with physicians, management, safety professionals, and other allied groups in conserving the health of industrial workers.
   c. To promote mutual understanding of the goals of occupational health and safety programs among these groups.
   d. To interpret the objectives and ideals of industrial nurses to the professional and lay world.
   e. To bring industrial nursing participation into the plans for the advancement of industrial and community health.
2. The official publication of AAIN was originally called *Industrial Nursing.*
3. In 1971, the American Board for Occupational Health Nurses (ABOHN) was established; its purpose is to certify occupational health nurses.
4. In 1977, the American Association of Industrial Nurses' name was changed to the American Association of Occupational Health Nurses (AAOHN) to reflect the broader scope of practice of its members.
5. In 1986, the journal became known as the *AAOHN Journal,* the Official Journal of the American Association of Occupational Health Nurses.

X

Work Settings and Roles of Occupational Health Nurses

A. Practice settings for occupational health nurses are widely varied. The type of employment opportunities for occupational health nurses include the following:
1. Industrial or business settings
   a. Occupational health nurses are generally employed in settings with over 250 employees.
   b. Firms with higher occupational injury and illness rates are more likely to employ occupational health nurses.
   c. The most common employer-based sites include manufacturing, services, and the transportation, communication and utility industries.
2. Insurers and third-party administrators (TPA)
   a. Occupational health nurses monitor and manage the work-related injury and illness cases for whom insurers and TPAs provide workers' compensation insurance coverage.
   b. Insurers and TPAs provide occupational health and safety consultation to their clients; consultation support may include:
      • Employee and supervisor training
      • Program and regulatory compliance audits
      • Health screening and surveillance
      • Management support
      • Case management protocol development
      • Injury and illness trend analysis
3. Government agencies
   a. Government agencies employ occupational health nurses as consultants, analysts, program developers, and compliance officers as well as providers of occupational health services.

      b. The focus of these agencies is on public health rather than individual client care.

      c. Agencies may be federal (e.g., U.S. Public Health Service, the Occupational Safety and Health Administration (OSHA), the National Institute for Occupational Safety and Health (NIOSH); state agencies (e.g., state OSHAs, state health departments); and city or county health departments.

4. Health care facilities

      a. Occupational health nurses manage and administer occupational health and safety services to workers in these facilities.

      b. Health care facilities include hospital-affiliated clinics and programs, independent clinics and practices, for-profit clinics (multiple sites), clinics based within health maintenance organizations (HMOs), contract clinics at employer locations, and rehabilitation clinics and facilities.

5. Utilization review and case management firms

      a. Occupational health nurses may work directly with employees and employers and/or through insurers and third-party administrators or in managed care settings.

      b. They monitor and manage the health care and return-to-work programming necessitated by work-related injuries and illnesses on an individual employee-client basis.

      c. The ultimate objectives are cost-effective, quality health care and facilitation of returning employees to work.

      d. A utilization review and case management firm may be a single-nurse company (a self-employed nurse) or a large multimillion-dollar firm.

6. Consulting firms

      a. Consulting firms employ occupational health nurses to provide occupational health and safety services to client employers.

      b. Consulting services encompass evaluation and audit activities, training, trend analysis, program and system development, and management support.

      c. Consulting firms may include:

        • Independent environmental and occupational health and safety consulting firms

        • Financially oriented consulting firms, such as insurance or accounting consulting firms

B. Functional roles of the registered nurse who specializes in occupational health nursing can be categorized as follows (AAOHN, unpublished document):

1. Clinician: provides direct client care within the scope of the applicable states' nurse practice act

      a. The clinician assesses workers' health needs, makes nursing diagnoses, plans and implements care, and evaluates the impact of interventions.

      b. Health services are directed at preventing health problems and restoring and maintaining health.

2. Case manager: coordinates health care services for an individual worker from the onset of an injury or illness to a safe return to work or an optimal alternative

      a. The case manager assesses, plans, implements, coordinates, monitors, and evaluates all aspects of a case management program (see Chapter 12 for example of such a program).

      b. Services are focused on achieving quality care that is delivered in a cost-effective manner.

3. Occupational health nurse (single-nurse service): assesses the health and safety needs of the worker population and the health and safety of the worksite
   a. The occupational health nurse develops, interprets, and administers occupational health and safety services.
   b. Programs are designed to address the needs identified in the assessment.
4. Health promotion specialist: manages a multilevel, wide-ranging health promotion program that supports the corporate business objectives
   a. The health promotion specialist plans, implements, and evaluates health promotion programs with input from multiple sources, including management, occupational health and safety staff, and employees.
   b. Programs are designed to meet specific needs of an organization as determined through an analysis of appropriate health and safety data.
5. Manager/Administrator: directs, administers, and evaluates occupational health services that are consistent with the organization's goals and objectives (see Chapter 6).
   a. The occupational health nurse manager develops, administers, and maintains the policies of the occupational health and safety program.
   b. Management services may be directed at a clinic, program/division, product line, or other activities.
6. Nurse practitioner: assesses the health status of workers through health histories, physical assessments, and diagnostic tests
   a. The nurse practitioner interprets data to determine needs and problems and to plan appropriate therapeutic interventions.
   b. Services range from pre-placement physical examinations to comprehensive primary care for workers and their families.
   c. The nurse practitioner has additional specialized preparation that meets the state requirements for advanced nursing practice.
7. Corporate director: serves as a corporate manager and policy maker within an organization
   a. The corporate director plans, administers, and evaluates the organization's occupational health and safety programs and oversees occupational health nursing services.
   b. Services are provided under the direction of the corporate director by an interdisciplinary team that may include occupational health nurses, occupational physicians, industrial hygienists, safety specialists, and other occupational health and safety professionals.
8. Consultant: serves as an advisor for evaluating and developing occupational health and safety services
   a. The occupational health nurse consultant performs needs assessments and analyses of occupational health and safety programs.
   b. Services include administration as well as education and/or research in occupational health and safety.
9. Educator: develops, implements and evaluates curricula and clinical experiences appropriate for the professional educational development of occupational health nurses
   a. The educator teaches and administers graduate programs, continuing professional education, and/or staff development.
   b. The educator uses and/or conducts occupational health and safety research to support and enhance occupational health nursing educational programs.

C. Occupational health nurses who have received specialized education and/or training have expanded their roles to some nontraditional areas.

1. Occupational health nurses may provide risk management services.
   a. Responsibilities include the anticipation and control of potential causes of human and financial loss related to occupational health and safety.
   b. Risk managers help manage insurance coverage for workers' compensation and other health and disability-related insurance products.
2. Occupational health nurses may be responsible for managing occupational safety as well as health.
   a. Regulatory compliance is a key part of this function.
   b. Functional activities may include some tasks that are usually performed by industrial hygienists and/or safety professionals.
3. Occupational health nurses may serve as counselors for workers with either occupational or nonoccupational health problems.
   a. The occupational health nurse counselor addresses the worker's psychosocial needs, wellness/health-promotion concerns, and other health problems.
   b. The counseling role ranges from one of many roles for the occupational health nurse in a single-nurse unit to a specialty role for nurses who work in employee assistance programs (see Chapter 11 for description of these programs).

D. An increasing number of occupational health nurses are self-employed, working as independent contractors in many of these functional roles.

XI

Future Opportunities and Challenges

A. Globally, workplaces and workforces are changing as a result of demographic, social, and technological changes.
1. Changes in the United States:
   a. The demographics of the country and, consequently, the workforce are changing (see Chapter 3).
   b. Managed care is replacing "free choice" as the predominant system for the delivery of health care in this country; employers have a major role in the provision of health care packages for employees (see Chapter 5).
   c. The information, technology, and service industries are expanding; at the same time, the manufacturing industry is shrinking as a result of closures of companies and increased automation.
   d. Increasingly, businesses are choosing to use part-time and temporary workers and to outsource work as cost-cutting measures (see Chapters 3 and 5).
   e. Technology is affecting communication patterns and the nature of work for many Americans.
   f. An increasing number of people are choosing to work out of their homes, resulting in a transfer of occupational hazards to the home setting.
2. Emigration and the development of multinational corporations have increased the likelihood that occupational health nurses will be working with an ethnically and racially pluralistic workforce.
   a. Culturally based norms, beliefs, and behaviors affect work ethics, practices, and health-related values.
   b. Multilingual workforces are increasingly common, creating communication challenges.

B. Implications for occupational health nurses
1. Health and safety services provided must be adjusted to accommodate a changing workforce and their changing needs.
2. Occupational health nurses have a professional responsibility to keep abreast of changes in the field by reading professional literature and by participating in continuing education and other forms of professional development.
3. Increasing opportunities exist for global and international practice, teaching, and research.
4. Occupational health nurses should participate in an effort to ensure that industries exported to developing countries incorporate adequate occupational and environmental safeguards.
5. Continual expansion of the occupational health nurses' functional roles, especially those relating to direct clinical interventions and management/administrative responsibilities, is creating additional opportunities to affect the health and safety of working populations.

BIBLIOGRAPHY

American Association of Industrial Nurses, Inc. (AAIN). (1976). *The nurse on industry.* New York: Author.

American Association of Occupational Health Nurses (AAOHN). (1994.) *Standards of occupational health nursing practice.* Atlanta: AAOHN Publications.

Andrews, J. M. (1932). *Labor problems and labor legislation.* New York: American Association for Labor Legislation.

Bale, A. (1987). America's first compensation crisis. In D. Rosner & G. Markowitz (Eds.). *Dying for work.* Indianapolis: Indiana University Press.

Breasted, J. H. (1930). *The Edwin Smith papyrus.* Chicago: University of Chicago Press.

Brown, M. L. (1981). *Occupational health nursing.* New York: Springer Publishing Company.

Colombo statement on occupational health in developing countries (1985). *Journal of Occupational Health and Safety,* Australia and New Zealand, *2,* 437–441.

Crandall, E. P. (1916). Industrial welfare nursing. *The Public Nurse, 32*(8), 32–47.

Davey, C. (1928). Industrial nursing. *American Journal of Nursing, 28*(12), 1191–1194.

Fielding, E., & Piserchia, P. V. (1989). Frequency of worksite health promotion activities. *American Journal of Public Health, 79*(1), 16–20.

Hamilton, A. (1943). *Exploring the dangerous trades.* Boston, MA: Little, Brown and Company.

Hamilton, A. (1925). *Industrial poisons in the United States.*

Kahl, F. R. (1947). Trends in industrial nursing. *Industrial Nursing, 6*(4), 9–15.

Lauck, W. J., & Sydenstricker, E. *Conditions of labor in American industries.* New York: Funk and Wagnall.

Leake, C. D. (1952). *The Old Egyptian medical papyri.* Lawrence, KS: University of Kansas Press.

Lehtinen, S., & Mikheev, M. (1994). *WHO Worker's Health Programme & Collaborating Centers in Occupational Health.* Geneva: World Health Organizataion.

Levy, B. S., & Wegman, D. (1995). *Occupational health: Recognizing and preventing work-related disease* (3rd ed.). Boston: Little, Brown and Company.

Markowitz, G., & Rosner, D. (1986). More than economism: The politics of workers' safety and health, 1932–1947. *The Milbank Quarterly, 64*(3), 331–354.

McGrath, D. J. (1946). *Nursing in commerce and industry.* New York: The Commonwealth Fund.

Murray, R. (1987). Man and his work. In P. A. D. Raffle, W. R. Lee, R. I. McCallum, & L. R. Murray (Eds.). *Hunter's diseases of occupations.* Boston, MA: Little, Brown and Co.

Olson, D. K., & Stovin, D. (1992). *Occupational health nursing in Canada: Its social foundation and future. Canadian Journal of Public Health/Revue Canadienne de Santé Publique, 83*(6), 452–455.

Parker-Conrad, J. (1988). A century of practice: Occupational health nursing. *AAOHN Journal, 36*(4), 156–161.

Phillips, E., & Radford, J. (1989). Occupational health nursing in developing countries. In J. Radford (Ed.), *Recent advances in nursing (26): Occupational health nursing.* Edinburgh: Churchill Livingstone.

Pursell, C. (1995). *The machine in America.* Baltimore: The Johns Hopkins University Press.

Rogers, B. (1994). *Occupational health nursing: Concepts and practice.* Philadelphia: W.B. Saunders.

Rogers, B. (1988). Perspectives in occupational health nursing. *AAOHN Journal, 36*(4), 151–155.

Rosner, D., & Markowitz, G. (1985). Research or advocacy: Federal occupational safety and health policies during the New Deal. *Journal of Social History, 18,* 365–381.

Rossi, K. (1987). Occupational health nursing worldwide. *AAOHN Journal, 35*(11), 505–509.

Rossi, K., & Heikkinen, M. R. (1989). A view of occupational health nursing practices: Current trends and future prospects. In: J. Radford (Ed.), *Recent advances in nursing (26): Occupational health nursing.* Edinburgh: Churchill Livingstone.

Sellers, C. (1991). The Public Health Service's Office of Industrial Hygiene and the transformation of industrial medicine. *Bulletin of the History of Medicine, 65*(1), 42–73.

Stein, J. (1985). Industry's new bottom line on health care costs: Is less better? *Hastings Center Report, 15*(5), 14–18.

United States Congress, S. 2193. (1970). Occupational Safety and Health Act of 1970, Public Law 91-596. Washington DC: U.S. Government Printing Office.

United States Department of Labor (1995). Bureau of Labor Statistics, new 1994–2005 employment projections (Bulletin 95-485, December 1995). Washington DC: U.S. Government Printing Office.

U.S. Department of Health, Education and Welfare. (1964). *50 years of occupational health.* Washington DC: Public Health Service, Division of Occupational Health, Publication No. 1171.

Wald, L. (1912). The doctor and the nurse in industrial establishments. *American Journal of Nursing, 12,* 403–408.

World Health Organization (WHO) (1994). *Declaration on occupational health for all.* Geneva: Author.

World Health Organization (WHO) (1995). *Global strategy on occupational health for all—the way to health at work.* Geneva: Author.

Wright, F. S. (1919). *Industrial nursing.* New York: Macmillan.

Wright, F. S. (1916). The visiting nurse in industrial welfare work. *The Public Health Nurse Quarterly,* 73–79.

3

Workers and Worker Populations

MAJOR TOPICS

- *Demographic trends*
- *Social trends*
- *Technological trends*
- *Female workers*
- *Aging workforce*
- *Children in the workforce*
- *Contingent workers*
- *Labor unions*
- *Disabled workers*
- *Agricultural workers*
- *Construction workers*
- *Health care workers*
- *International workers*

Workers and workplaces are affected by changes and trends that occur in the larger society. It is essential that occupational health nurses be knowledgeable about the potential effects that these changes have on the workforce. This chapter provides an overview of current demographic, social, and technological trends; it then presents a description of some of the many worker populations that characterize the modern workplace.

Demographic, Social, and Technological Trends Affecting Work

I

Demographic and Social Trends

A. Supportive and explanatory data

1. Population and workforce changes

   a. Assuming no change in immigration laws and fertility rates, the United States population will increase by 25% from 1993 to 2020 (Jarratt, Coates, Mahaffie, & Hines, 1994).

   b. From 1994 to 2005, the size of the labor force is expected to increase by 16 million, a slower increase than that for the previous 11-year period (U.S. Department of Labor, Bureau of Labor Statistics [USDL, BLS], 1995a).

   c. The workforce will include an increase in the proportion of women workers, an increase in the average age of workers, and continued, though variable, growth of all multiethnic groups.

2. Society is placing a higher priority on family relationships, leisure time, and recreational activities.

   a. Many white-collar workers are unwilling to continue to work long hours, and many blue-collar workers are opposed to overtime (Lewin, 1995).

   b. Work and career goals may have a diminished importance (Lewin, 1995; Stone, 1995).

   c. Many professional-level workers are unwilling to accept transfer due to its effects on their families (Capell, 1995).

   d. Flex-time and job sharing are work options increasingly used to assist workers in handling competing demands of work and family (Scott, 1995; Olmsted and Smith, 1994).

3. Workers may arrive at work more fatigued due to long commutes (Burke, 1995).

4. Virtual offices, or offices without walls, are increasingly used as telecommuting options to reduce office costs and commuting time (Tanzillo, 1995; Ditlea, 1995; McNerney & Dennis, 1995; Brimsek & Bender, 1995; Burke, 1995).

5. Health care benefits provided at worksites are undergoing rapid changes.

   a. Health care options are increasingly being restricted with implementation of managed care systems (Burke & Jain, 1995).

   b. Workers are increasingly being required to pay more out-of-pocket expenses and may have reduced choice of providers (Service, 1995; Burke & Jain, 1995).

6. Stress and psychological problems are increasingly seen as common problems, and the workplace is the greatest single source of stress (Dear, 1995).

   a. Layoffs and corporate downsizing are occurring with greater frequency (Lambert, 1995; NIOSH, 1996).

   b. The organization of work is a major contributor to workplace stress (NIOSH, 1996); work organization refers to any or all of the following:
- Scheduling of work (work-rest schedules, number of hours of work, shift work)
- Job design (complexity of tasks, skill and effort required, and degree of worker control)
- Interpersonal aspects of work (relationships with supervisors and co-workers)
- Career concerns (job security and growth opportunities)
- Management style (participatory versus autocratic)
- Organizational characteristics (climate, culture, and communications)

   c. Longer hours, compressed workweeks, shift work, reduced job security, and part-time and temporary work are realities of the modern workplace (NIOSH, 1996).

   d. The shift from manufacturing to service continues with service sector jobs now employing 70% of workers (NIOSH, 1996); because service sector jobs require more interaction with people, they are more likely to involve stress, confrontation, and violence.

7. Violence in the workplace is on the increase; it is often associated with situations involving disputes and problem resolution (Dear, 1995; Stone, 1995).

a. Security of workers is an increasing problem due to worksite burglaries, robberies, assaults, and homicides; armed robberies are a growing concern, especially in small retail and manufacturing businesses.

b. Homicide is the number one cause of worksite death for women and the second most common cause for men (Dear, 1995; Crime: Death on the Job, 1994).

c. Workplace violence is classified according to the following (Kraus & McArthur, 1996):
  - Business disputes (between co-workers)
  - Disputes with customers
  - Disputes involving a relative of the victim
  - Incidents involving police or security guards in the line of duty
  - Incidents in which death occurs during a robbery or crime (accounts for 80% of workplace homicides)

d. Health care workers are at particularly high risk for violent situations due to the prevalence of handguns, the decrease in care for the mentally ill, and the increasing use of hospitals for care of disturbed persons (Dear, 1995).

e. Women and older workers are at highest risk for assault in the workplace (Kraus & McArthur, 1996).

B. Implications for occupational health nurses

1. Occupational health nurses will need to take into account the changing population and workforce when designing and implementing worksite programs.

2. Changes in health care benefits may influence the type of services available to workers from their primary providers; this then may influence the choice of services provided at worksites.

3. Workers may need assistance in handling conflicting demands.

4. Workers who are transferred will benefit from assistance with family concerns (Capell, 1995).

5. Occupational health nurses may have less opportunity for face-to-face communication with workers; thus they will have to develop less personal methods of communication with offsite workers.

6. Occupational health nurses need to be alert to the potentially dangerous effects of fatigue on worksite health and safety.

7. Programs are needed to aid worksites in identifying and preventing potentially dangerous and/or explosive personal reactions due to stress or mental illness (American Psychological Association, 1995; Stone, 1995; Harvey & Cosier, 1995).

8. Appropriate violence prevention and control measures should be developed for the work setting (See Table 3-1).

9. Guidelines for Preventing Workplace Violence for Health Care Workers (USDL, 1996) can be used to design engineering and administrative controls as well as post-incident response and evaluation.

II

Technological Trends

A. Explanatory and supportive data

1. The service sector is the most rapidly growing job sector in the United States.

   a. Of the top ten fastest growing industries, nine are in health services, business services, or social services (USDL, BLS, 1995a).

TABLE 3-1

Examples of Violence Prevention and Control Measures

Engineering Controls and Workplace Adaptations	Administrative and Work Practice Controls
• Security systems for use by staff: panic buttons, handheld noise devices, cellular phones	• Conduct periodic workplace safety and security analyses
• Metal detectors at high-risk doorways	• Establish a zero-tolerance violence policy
• Closed circuit video recording in high-risk areas	• Establish a trained response team to respond to emergencies
• Curved mirrors in hallway intersections and secluded areas	• Ensure adequate and qualified staffing at all times
• Bullet-resistant, shatterproof glass in reception, triage, and admitting areas	• Provide management and administrative support during emergencies
• Furniture arrangement to avoid entrapment of staff	• Control access to areas other than waiting rooms or lobbies
• Limitation or elimination of items that can be used as weapons	• Prohibit employees from working alone in high-risk areas
• Two exits provided whenever possible	• Use adequate numbers of properly trained security personnel
• Bright lighting indoors, outdoors, and in parking areas	• Provide security escort to parking lots
• Lockable, secure restrooms for staff, separate from visitor facilities	• Develop specific policies and procedures for off-site workers' safety
• Locks on rarely used doors, in accordance with local fire codes	• Train workers in de-escalation and personal protection techniques
• Vehicles used in the field maintained in good working condition	

Source: Adapted from: USDL, OSHA, (1996).

b. From 1994 to 2005, nearly all job growth will be in the service-producing sector; manufacturing's share of total jobs will decline (USDL, BLS, 1995a).

c. The fastest rate of increase and the greatest job growth are in the professional specialty occupations; faster-than-average growth will occur for executive, administrative, managerial, technical support, marketing, and sales roles (USDL, BLS, 1995a).

d. Although there will continue to be new jobs based on all levels of education from 1994 to 2005, the largest growth (29%) will occur in occupations requiring a master's degree, and the smallest growth (5%) will occur in those requiring moderate (1 to 12 months) on-the-job training.

2. Equipment using increasingly high technology will be used in all work settings.

a. Advances in technology have increased the speed of production and the subsequent demands on workers.

b. Automation (robots, robotic systems, and automated machinery) eliminates certain types of jobs so that fewer workers are responsible for complex systems (Levy & Wegman, 1995).

B. Implications for occupational health nurses

1. New technologies will present new hazards that will need to be considered in occupational disease surveillance and prevention.

2. Occupational stress related to job ambiguity, role uncertainty, and job insecurity may become increasingly apparent as technological changes in worksites are implemented.

Changes/Trends in Work and Work Force
III

Females in the Workforce
An increasing proportion of workers are female.

A. Supportive and explanatory data
1. Demographics
    a. In 1992, 58% of women age 16 and older were in the labor force, up from 51% in 1977 (U.S. Department of Labor, Women's Bureau [USDLWB], 1994).
    b. The proportion of female workers increased from 42.5% in 1980 to 45.6% in 1991 (USDLWB, 1994).
    c. Among white, black, Hispanic, and Asian males and females, Hispanic women had the lowest rate of participation of any group in the labor force in 1992; this trend is expected to continue through 2005 (USDLWB, 1994).
    d. Overall in 1992, 67.2% of women with children participated in the labor force; this rate dropped to 58.0% for women with children under six years of age (USDLWB, 1994).
    e. Marital status affects labor force participation; the proportions of working women are as follows (USDLWB, 1994):
        • 64.7% of women who have never married
        • 59.3% of married women with spouses
        • 74.0% of divorced women
        • Only 18.8% of widowed women
    f. "Women accounted for 62% of the total labor force growth between 1980 and 1991" (USDLWB, 1994).
    g. Seventy-one percent of working mothers with children at home reported they worked to support the family (USDLWB, 1994).
2. Social factors
    a. Women are disproportionately represented in the lower-paying service sector occupations; job segregation by gender continues.
    b. "Of the 20 leading occupations of women, 11 are known as traditionally 'female' jobs. . . ." (USDLWB, 1994).
    c. Women have greater responsibilities for care of dependents, both children and elderly; more women are single custodial parents than men.
    d. Women have higher health care utilization rates than men; women assume greater responsibility for their health and seek more preventive services (Verbrugge & Wingard, 1987).
3. Work-related factors
    a. Females are often shorter, lighter in weight, with less physical strength than males; as a result, they may be more at risk for certain types of injuries.
    b. Higher rates of work-related musculoskeletal disorders have been reported in females as compared to males; risk factors may include differences in stature and physiology and the nature of jobs performed by women.
    c. Lung cancer rates are increasing faster in females than in males.
    d. Worksite exposures that present reproductive hazards are a serious consideration for female workers. (Note: Reproductive hazards are also a serious consideration for male workers.)
    e. Stress is the number one problem for working women, identified by almost 60% of working women (Dear, 1995).

B. Implications for occupational health nurses
1. Worksite programs should address the specific needs/problems of females. These programs may include education, support groups, referral to community resources, and other strategies that promote health and safety.
   a. Programs on prenatal care, women's health, and menopause concerns should be increased.
   b. Programs for early detection of breast, uterine, and ovarian cancer should be offered.
   c. Support for caregiver roles assumed outside of work may be required.
   d. Worksite day care for children and dependent adults may be needed.
   e. Women should be targeted for smoking cessation programs in view of their increasing smoking rates.
2. Worksite adjustments will need to be made to accommodate biological characteristics of female workers.
   a Work stations should be adjusted to accommodate females' stature.
   b Ergonomic programs should be targeted to females to prevent work-related musculoskeletal disorders.
   c. Surveillance for potential reproductive hazards should be conducted.
   d. Personal protective equipment that fits females should be provided.

IV

Minorities in the Workforce

An increasing proportion of the population consists of minority groups. Minority populations in the U.S. are defined as blacks (African-American), Hispanics, Asian and Pacific Islanders, and American Indians and Alaskan Natives (USDHHS, 1991).

A. Supportive and explanatory data
1. Demographic and social factors
   a. Because of immigration and the growth of resident minority populations, the United States is becoming increasingly a multiracial, multiethnic society.
   b. By 2013, Hispanics will replace African-Americans as the largest minority group (Jarratt et al., 1994).
   c. By 2020, minorities will constitute 36% of the population (Jarratt et al., 1994).
   d. Due to limited opportunities and, in some cases, language and cultural barriers, some minority groups may have poorer education outcomes and lower household incomes (Jarratt et al., 1994); low socioeconomic status is related to higher rates of illness and premature death.
   e. "Excess deaths," defined as the number of deaths occurring in relation to the number expected based on the death rate for the white population, occur in minority populations (USDHHS, 1991).
   f. Leading causes of death differ by minority group; for example, hypertension is more common among African-Americans, diabetes among Native Americans, and chronic liver disease among Hispanics.
2. Employment factors
   a. "Minorities (in the year 2000) will be a larger share of new entrants into the labor force" (Johnson & Packer, 1987).
   b. "Immigrants will represent the largest share of the increase in the population and the workforce since the First World War" (Johnson & Packer, 1987).
   c. Educational, linguistic, and cultural barriers can lead to underrepresentation in certain jobs that require a high level of education (Jarratt et al., 1994).

    d. An increasing proportion of jobs are projected to require advanced education; thus groups with less education will be at a disadvantage in the job market.

    e. Changes in labor force composition include continued growth in women's participation, a decline in men's, and continued growth by all racial groups (white, black, Hispanic, Asian, and other) (USDLBLS, 1994).

    f. Hispanic men will compose the largest share of the nonwhite workforce in 2005 (6.4%); African-American women will be the second largest share (5.6%) (USDLBLS, 1994).

    g. The African-American labor force is projected to grow more rapidly than the overall labor force (USDLBLS, 1994).

B. Implications for occupational health nurses

    1. Because of the increasing number of minority workers, occupational health nurses will need to have greater knowledge of and make greater use of multicultural approaches.

    2. Occupational health nurses will need increased knowledge of diseases that are common in certain minorities.

    3. For workers with fewer educational opportunities, remedial programs offered at the worksite will present avenues to learn new skills and knowledge.

    4. In order to assure participation, worksite safety and health programs will need to consider the special needs of workers who are non–English speaking or who have low literacy levels.

$\overline{V}$

Age of Workers

    The average age of the workforce is increasing.

A. Supportive and explanatory data

    1. Demographic and social factors

        a. The U.S. population is growing older; in 1990 the median age was 32.8; it is projected to climb to 35.7 years of age by the year 2000 and to 38 by the year 2020 (Jarratt et al., 1994).

        b. The numbers and proportion of older adults in the population is increasing; by 2020, 16.6% of the U.S. population may be over 65 years of age (Jarratt et al., 1994).

        c. With greater longevity and healthier lives, retirees at age 65 can look forward to as much as 30 more productive years (Fyock, 1990).

        d. More older workers are returning to or remaining in the work force.

        e. "In 1995 there were 3.4 workers per retired person and in the year 2030 there will be only 2.0 workers per retired person" (Jones, 1995).

        f. A study of retired men found that almost one-third returned to work, typically within the first year of retirement, with two-thirds of these taking full-time jobs (Mergenhagen, 1994).

        g. Savings for retirement for middle-aged workers who suffer a reduction in salary or disruption of employment will be seriously affected.

        h. "Baby-boomers," the population of workers born between 1946 and 1964, indicate interest in early retirement, but may not be able to afford it (Mergenhagen, 1994).

        i. The incidence and prevalence of musculoskeletal problems and chronic diseases increase with age.

2. Employment and work-related factors
   a. U.S. law has changed so that there is no longer a mandatory retirement age for workers in nearly all job categories.
   b. The middle-aged and older worker is more likely to have responsibilities for a dependent elderly parent or spouse.
   c. Some older workers would like to work, but they think no work is available to them; the needs for money and life satisfaction are the chief reasons cited for wanting to work (McNaught, Barth, & Henderson, 1989).
   d. A study of available middle-aged nonworkers found that most considered themselves involuntarily retired (McNaught et al., 1989); many may embark on second and third careers after age 65 (Fyock, 1990).
   e. The retiring workforce represents an important worker pool (Herz, 1995).
   f. Middle-aged and older workers may experience increased musculoskeletal problems and decreased vision, hearing, and agility.

B. Implications for occupational health nurses
   1. Occupational health nurses should consider the following strategies to address the special needs/problems of older workers:
      a. Programs to prevent and treat musculoskeletal disorders related to poor ergonomics
      b. Increased light at worksite to improve visibility for workers, as their light requirements increase with age
      c. Increased attention to assure adequate hearing ability
      d. Increased support for caregiver roles assumed outside of work
      e. Promotion of worksite or community day care facilities for dependent adults
      f. Increased programs focusing on the illnesses more common in middle age, such as cardiovascular disease and cancer
      g. Increased programs to prepare workers for retirement
   2. Interactions with older workers should allow for possible decreases in their differences in ability to hear, process information, and handle new technology (Table 3-2).

TABLE 3-2

Recommendations for Training Programs for Older Workers

Training programs for older workers should:

- Allow self-paced learning
- Use training materials with high-contrast colors and bold typeface
- Avoid posting training materials above eye level
- Speak clearly and distinctly during training sessions
- Use adult learning principles to train older adults on new skills
- Provide a friendly, supportive environment
- Eliminate jargon from the worksite, or at least explain it from the start
- Use multiple training methodologies
- Use older workers to teach other older adults
- Group older workers in the learning process
- Build upon valuable life experiences
- Link learning with rewards
- Give older learners something in writing to help reinforce learning

Source: Adapted from Fyock (1990), pp. 105–110.

3. Disease prevention programs may become increasingly important to employers as a means of decreasing health care costs, including the costs of supplemental health care insurance.
4. As corporations attempt to improve their profit picture by reducing employment of mid level middle-aged workers, programs will be needed to assist workers with job and career transitions.
5. Occupational health nurses should ensure that wellness programs take into consideration the needs and interests of older workers.
6. Health promotion by mail has been successful in reducing health care costs of retirees and decreasing health risk behaviors; this approach represents an opportunity for occupational health nurses to implement a cost-savings program (Lusk, 1995).

VI

Children in the Workforce

Children represent a significant portion of the workforce; the number of working children has been increasing.

A. Supportive and explanatory data
  1. Demographics
     a. Children and adolescents under the age of 18 are legally considered minors and are regulated differently than adults in the worksite for certain activities.
     b. The minimum age for youth employment is 14 years, except for certain agricultural jobs in which 12- and 13-year-olds are permitted to work; children working on family farms are exempt from regulations.
     c. It is estimated that 5.5 million children between the ages of 12 to 17 years are employed, with approximately 676,000 more working in a variety of undocumented settings (National Safe Workplace Institute, 1992).
     d. The percentage of 16- and 17-year-olds working at some point during the school year ranges between 50% and 80%, with most working from 16 to 21 hours per week (Parker, Carl, French & Martin, 1994a; Government Accounting Office [GAO], 1991).
     e. Most minors are employed in retail trade, primarily restaurants and grocery stores, and in service industries (Miller, 1995).
     f. Low-income and minority children are less likely to be employed and, when employed, work in more hazardous jobs than high-income youths (GAO, 1991).
  2. Injury and illness data
     a. Occupational injuries experienced by children, including disabilities and fatalities, have been increasing in numbers and severity (GAO, 1991; Richter & Jacobs, 1991).
     b. Although most adolescents work part-time, their injury rate may actually be more than three times greater than for adults, based on the number of hours worked or exposure time on the job (Miller, 1995).
     c. The National Institute for Occupational Safety and Health (NIOSH, 1995) estimates that 70 adolescents die from injuries at work each year, and nearly 200,000 suffer nonfatal injuries, a substantial number of which require hospitalization.
     d. The occupational fatality rate for 16- and 17-year-olds is 5.1 per 100,000 full-time workers, similar to that found in adults (6.0 per 100,000 full-time workers) (Castillo, Landen & Layne, 1994).

    e. The youngest workers (under 16 years of age) have been found to have a higher proportion of injury claims in agricultural work than in other industries (Heyer, Franklin, Rivara, Parker & Haug, 1992; Layne, Castillo, Stout & Cutlip, 1994; Miller, 1995).

3. Work-related factors
   a. Most occupational injuries occur in restaurants, grocery stores, service jobs, agriculture, construction, and manufacturing (Banco et al., 1992; Belville, Pollack, Godbold, & Landrigan, 1993; Miller, 1995; Parker, Clay, Mandel, Gunderson & Salkowicz, 1991).
   b. Many nonfatal injuries involve working with knives, cooking and working around cooking appliances, fall hazards, and hazardous manual lifting (NIOSH, 1995).
   c. Most fatal occupational injuries to minors involve working in and around motor vehicles, operating tractors and other heavy equipment, working near electrical hazards, and working in jobs with a high risk of homicide (Castillo & Jenkins, 1994; NIOSH, 1995).
   d. Industries that are known to hire youths, such as grocery stores, restaurants, and services, are also known to have a high risk for worksite violence (Castillo et. al., 1994; Jenkins, Kisner, Fosbroke, Layne, Stout, Castillo, et al., 1993).
   e. Little research has been done that evaluates children for acute, chronic, or latent effects on their health from exposure to toxic chemicals, such as pesticides, or to physical hazards, such as noise.
   f. Specific federal and state child labor laws regulate youth employment and establish the permitted hours of work, prohibited work activities, and administrative requirements.

4. Social factors
   a. The failure to prevent work-related injuries and provide adequate protection to children in the worksite is a serious public health problem.
   b. Children who work have two jobs—education and employment—but typically their work is not connected to their educational needs and goals.
   c. Causes of the increase in the number of children working include social pressure, acceptance of child employment, adult unemployment, lower wages, growing poverty, relaxation in law enforcement, and increasing immigration.
   d. The health and safety problems of child workers typically fall outside the scope of pediatric public health programs, as well as of modern occupational health and safety efforts, which focus primarily on adult workers.
   e. The number of hours worked by teens may affect academic performance and participation in peer and family activities and increase the risk of drug and alcohol use (Greenberg & Steinberg, 1986; Carskadon, 1990b).
   f. In addition to possible lost work time, work-related injuries contribute to missed school time (Parker, Carl, French & Martin, 1994b).

5. Unique health considerations
   a. Injury is the major cause of death among children of all ages (National Safety Council, 1993).
   b. Children and adolescents are not just small adults; they differ in physical development, maturity, experience, and judgment, and these differences put them at greater risk of injury on the job.

    c. Risk-taking behavior is a typical characteristic of adolescents as they explore their capabilities, but they often fail to perceive their limitations and vulnerability.

    d. In a work setting, teens may not recognize that a hazard exists or may not feel capable of speaking up to an adult supervisor refusing to do a task that is inappropriate or dangerous, especially if they desire to be treated more like adults than children.

    e. Adolescents have a physiological need for more sleep than adults; longer and later work hours may lead to sleep deprivation and thus to increased levels of stress, anxiety, and depression (Carskadon, 1990a; Steinberg & Dornbusch, 1991).

    f. The worksite is an adult setting, and the special learning and supervisory needs of young workers are not always recognized by employers and adult co-workers.

B. Implications for occupational health nurses

  1. Advocacy

    a. Programs should be developed to:
- Address special learning needs and limitations of working adolescents
- Address risks of injury related to specific jobs and tasks
- Extend programs to the front-line supervisors and adult co-workers who directly interact with the young workers

    b. Parents should be encouraged to take an active role in their children's employment decisions.

    c. The development of jobs for youths that provide both educational opportunities and a balanced schedule allowing participation in family and peer activities should be promoted.

    d. Students should be involved in the development and delivery of health and safety training programs in order to enhance their own investment in the prevention of injury.

    e. Work practices should be modified to accommodate the particular abilities, skill levels, and developmental needs of adolescents.

    f. Appropriate supervision of adolescent workers should be provided, and only age-appropriate tasks should be assigned.

  2. Education and outreach

    a. Public health professionals should be educated regarding the risk of injury for young workers.

    b. Worksite health and safety education and training programs should be age-appropriate (i.e., hazard communication, injury and illness prevention, safe task performance).

    c. Information on teenagers' rights and responsibilities in the worksite should be provided in all high schools.

    d. Farm families should be involved in educational and prevention activities to increase awareness of the risk of injury in the home and farm work environment.

  3. Research

    a. Current research should consider the special needs of adolescents in the workplace.

    b. Intervention research projects should be developed that evaluate the effectiveness of training activities for adolescents.

VII

Contingent Workers

The use of contingent workers is markedly increasing; they may be floaters, regular part-time workers, formal intermittents, limited duration hires, informal intermittents, casuals, contract labor service workers, independent contractors, leased workers, or temporary help service workers (Mayall, 1995).

A. Supportive and explanatory data
1. Demographics
   a. "In 1988, contingent workers were about a quarter of the workforce. By 2000, they are expected to be half of it" (Morrow, 1993).
   b. "The number of people employed full time by Fortune 500 companies has shrunk from 19% of the work force two decades ago to less than 10% today" (Castro, 1993).
   c. Wage differentials between temporary and permanent work are much larger for blue-collar workers, but nearly zero for those in professional or managerial positions (Segal & Sullivan, 1995).
   d. The model selected for utilizing contingent workers is influenced by
      • Volume, periodicity, and duration of work
      • Skill required for the work
      • Labor supply
      • Cost of hiring, benefits, job security
      • Legislation and unions (Mayall, 1995)
   e. The number of part-time female workers is increasing dramatically; from 1980 to 1991 there was a 16% increase in female part-time workers and only a 3% increase in male part-time workers (USDLWB, 1994).
   f. All types of workers may be employed as temporary workers. e.g., doctors and nurses, bank officers, attorneys, and corporate executives (Castro, 1993).
   g. The trend among large corporations is to outsource their occupational health services, with the following results:
      • Occupational health nursing positions may be eliminated.
      • Nurses with inadequate occupational health and safety preparation may deliver worksite services.
   h. Contingent workers, as compared to noncontingent workers, are:
      • More likely to be female and black
      • More than twice as likely to be aged 16–24 than noncontingent workers and thus more likely to be enrolled in school (USDL, BLS, 1995b)
2. Work-related factors (Lenz, 1994)
   a. "Co-employment" is the term used to describe ". . . a relationship between two or more employers in which each has actual or potential legal rights and duties with respect to the same employee or group of employees" (Lenz, 1994, p. 13).
   b. Co-employment influences civil rights, workers' compensation, labor relations and practices, workers' benefits, reasonable accommodation for the disabled, worksite safety, and job training.
      1) Liability is generally determined by the employer's relationship with or actions toward the worker.
      2) Workers' compensation and unemployment insurance laws related to co-employment vary by state in terms of single or joint responsibility.

      3) Generally, health and pension benefits, if any, are provided by the staffing agency; although few workers receive these benefits now, they may increase as work assignments become more long-term.

      4) Both the staffing agency and the worksite employer can be held liable for infringements of civil rights (Lenz, 1994).

  c. The Americans with Disabilities Act (ADA) requires reasonable accommodation on the part of the staffing agency and the worksite, but it is not clear regarding specific responsibilities, making cooperation essential.

  d. Under ADA, staffing companies have the right to ask relevant health questions prior to considering a worker for a specific job assignment.

  e. Worksite employers, rather than staffing agencies, are required to maintain OSHA records of workers' illnesses and injuries and to provide worksite safety programs; however, staffing agencies are responsible for workers' compensation.

  f. A greater use of staffing agencies is expected in the future.

  g. The increased use of contingent workers is estimated to account for about one-half of the decline in permanent jobs in manufacturing (Segal & Sullivan, 1995).

  h. Temporary workers may be less willing to report illnesses or injuries due to fear that doing so may interfere with the possibility of being hired as a permanent employee (Morris, 1995).

  i. Use of temporary employees offers a business the opportunity to more carefully screen and evaluate potential employees (Segal & Sullivan, 1995).

3. Health considerations

  a. Contingent workers are less likely to have health insurance than noncontingent workers, and for those who do have coverage, it is less likely to have been provided by their employers (USDL, BLS, 1995b).

  b. The lack of job security may increase a contingent workers' stress.

  c. Contingent workers may be less willing to report illness or injuries if they fear that doing so may interfere with the possibility of their being hired as regular workers (Morris, 1995).

  d. Assignment to hazardous work without adequate training increases temporary workers' risk of illness and injury (Castro, 1993).

  e. Tensions may exist between contingent workers and regular workers in a given job site (Caudron, 1994).

  f. The lack of an emotional and psychological attachment to a place of employment may have a negative effect on a worker's health.

B. Implications for occupational health nurses

1. Occupational health nurses in some organizations will be serving an increasing number of temporary workers.

2. Because temporary workers are less likely to have health insurance, they will be constrained in their follow-up of recommendations for preventive care or for ongoing treatment of chronic problems.

3. Occupational health nurses must be familiar with state and federal laws governing worksite and staffing agency obligations regarding civil rights, disabilities, safety education, and job training.

4. Occupational health nurses may be involved in negotiating arrangements between the staffing agency and the worksite employer regarding selection criteria, care of injured workers, disability adjustments, and safety education.

5. Because the majority of temporary workers are female, all implications for female workers apply to this group as well. (See III. B)

6. Stress reduction programs may be particularly important in worksites with large numbers of contingent workers.

7. Temporary workers may need extra help in assessment of jobs for hazards and direction regarding job training and job safety.

8. As corporations outsource their health care services, more occupational health nurses may experience the challenges of being temporary workers; occupational health nurses may need to move into entrepreneurial roles to sell their services to industry.

VIII

Workers in Labor Unions

A decreasing proportion of workers are represented by labor unions.

A. Supportive and explanatory data

1. In contrast with other developed countries, American unions have seen a decline in membership from a high of 35% of workers to less than 16%; if this trend continues, only about 5% of workers will be unionized by 2000 (Groenveld, 1995).

2. After ten years of decline in union membership in the United States, 1993 saw a slight increase in membership, largely due to an increase in female members (Johnson, 1995).

3. Union membership has increased among government workers, in administrative, professional, and technical occupations, and in the service industry, while declining in the manufacturing setting (Johnson, 1995).

4. Union membership varies by type of employer; it includes (Johnson, 1995):
   - 38% of government workers
   - 33% of communication and public utilities
   - 29% percent of transportation
   - 19% of construction workers

5. Factors contributing to the decline in union membership include (Zieger, 1994):
   - International competition
   - More diversified and specialized production techniques
   - Deregulation of industries
   - Increased use of part-time and temporary workers
   - Failure of unions to focus on recruitment
   - Disenchantment with union leadership
   - Lack of enforcement of labor laws

B. Implications for occupational health nurses

1. In worksites without union contracts, occupational health nurses may serve as the primary advocate for the promotion of occupational health and safety programs and activities.

2. In worksites without unions, occupational health nurses may have the primary responsibility for ensuring that workers are informed and knowledgeable about health and safety hazards in the workplace.

3. Occupational health nurses need to involve worker representation in program planning and implementation, whether they are from the union or other work team structures.

IX

Disabled Workers

There are increased numbers of disabled workers with needs for accommodations.

A. Supportive and explanatory data

1. Terms and definitions regarding disabilities from the Americans with Disabilities Act (ADA) (See Chapter 4 for more information about the ADA.)

   a. Disability: "1) a physical or mental impairment that substantially limits one or more of the major life activities of such individual; 2) a record of such an impairment, or; 3) being regarded as having such an impairment" (ADA, 1990).

   b. Physical or mental impairment: "Any physiological disorder, or condition, cosmetic disfigurement, or anatomical loss affecting one or more body systems (specified); or, any mental or psychological disorder such as mental retardation, organic brain syndrome, emotional or mental illness, and specific learning disabilities" (ADA, 1990)

   c. Qualified individual with a disability: An individual with a disability who, with or without reasonable accommodation, can perform the essential functions of the job (ADA, 1990)

   d. Reasonable accommodation: a) modification of work processes or existing facilities used by workers such that they be readily accessible to and usable by individuals with disabilities; b) [reasonable accommodation] may include job restructuring, modified work schedules, modified equipment, job reassignment, and training (ADA, 1990)

   e. Work disability: "A person has a work disability if they are of working age and are limited in ability to work" (Kraus & Stoddard, 1991)

   f. It is important to distinguish between work disability and work-related disability; not all work disabilities are work-related.

2. Demographics and social factors

   a. In 1993, 16.7 million persons, 10.1% of the working age population, had work disabilities (U.S. Bureau of the Census, 1995).

   b. In 1988, 55.6% of all work disabilities were severe (Kraus & Stoddard, 1991).

   c. Work disability increases with age, as follows (U.S. Bureau of the Census, 1995):
      - 4.5% of persons 16–24 years of age
      - 6.8% of persons 25–34 years of age
      - 9.2% of persons 35–44 years of age
      - 13.2% of persons 45–54 years of age
      - 23% of persons 55–65 years of age

   d. In 1993, more males had work disabilities than females, and more African-Americans had work disabilities than Caucasians (U.S. Bureau of the Census, 1995).

   e. Educational level is inversely associated with work disability, as follows (Kraus & Stoddard, 1991):
      - Less than 12 years of education, 17.7%
      - Completed high school, 8.8%
      - Four or more years of college, 3.8%

3. Work-related factors

   a. From 1990 to 1993, the number of disabling injuries occurring on the job has decreased from 3.9 million to 3.2 million (U.S. Bureau of the Census, 1995).

      b. The unemployment rate for persons with work disabilities is estimated at 14.2%, while the unemployment rate for persons without work disabilities is less than half of that (approximately 5.8%) (Kraus & Stoddard, 1991).

      c. By 1993, more disabling injuries occurred to persons employed in service, trade, manufacturing, and construction industry groups (U.S. Bureau of the Census, 1995).

      d. Women with disabilities are concentrated in the service and retail sectors, and men in service and manufacturing sectors (Kraus & Stoddard, 1991).

B. Implications for occupational health nurses

    1. Increased attention will need to be given in the worksite to specific needs of disabled workers (Harber & Fedoruk, 1994; West, 1995).

    2. Worksite adjustments will be needed to accommodate physical limitations of disabled or functionally impaired workers; these include (Pruitt, 1995):
- Modification of equipment
- Installation of mechanical aids
- Job restructuring
- Work schedule modifications
- Additional training or conditioning for the worker

    3. Job requirements, including job tasks, will need to be clearly defined.

    4. Case management is a strategy to ensure attainment of timely health services and supportive worksite accommodations for workers with disabilities or functional impairment (Martin, 1995).

    5. Program efforts need to be directed at preventing work-related disabling conditions or functional impairments.

    6. Comprehensive surveillance programs, including hazard and health surveillance, should be incorporated into existing health monitoring systems (Baker & Matte, 1992).

Worker Populations with Special Needs

Agricultural Workers

A. Supportive and explanatory data

    1. Characteristics of the population

      a. About 2.9% of the labor force worked in farm occupations in 1992 (USDLBLS, 1994).

      b. Farm workers are classified into three categories:
- Resident farm workers
- Nonresident farm workers
- Migrant farm workers who travel north and south for seasonal harvesting

      c. All three categories of farm workers often include their children as workers.

      d. Migrant workers are subject to all hazards described for resident farm workers, plus those associated with frequent moves, poor housing, poverty, social and cultural isolation, lack of health insurance, and work-related musculoskeletal disorders due to postures required for harvesting (Smith, 1986).

      e. The majority of nonresident farm workers are local persons with lower levels of education, wages, and often, only seasonal work with no benefits;

the nonresident farm worker is one of the lowest paid and least protected workers in the United States (Beale, 1990).

   f. Nonresident farm workers may experience the same problems as migrant workers except for the frequent moves.

   g. All farm workers, including resident farm workers, are likely to be under-insured for health care.

2. Illnesses and injuries

   a. Due to underreporting and lack of an established monitoring or surveillance system, no complete and accurate data base exists regarding agricultural injuries and illnesses (Cordes & Rea, 1991a).

   b. Although farm workers are a small proportion of the labor force, their rate of injury is higher than any other occupational group (National Safety Council, 1993).

   c. In 1992, 140,000 agricultural work injuries and 1,200 agricultural work-related deaths occurred in workers 14 years of age or older.
   - Approximately one-half of the injuries and deaths involved farm residents.
   - One-half involved nonresidents working on farms or in other industries classified as agricultural (fishing, agricultural services, and forestry, excluding logging) (National Safety Council, 1993).

3. Causes of injury and illness

   a. Farm machinery is the most common cause of injury and death in children and adolescents (Merchant, 1991). Causes include the following:
   - Rollovers of tractors or harvesting equipment that causes crushing or amputation injuries; one-half of deaths are caused by tractors.
   - Power-take off equipment (machinery with a long powered rotating shaft) that can twist the worker around the shaft causing suffocation, scalping, and avulsion injuries;
   - Machinery running in enclosed spaces that can cause carbon monoxide poisoning (Wright, 1993).

   b. Farm machinery may cause noise-induced hearing loss (NIHL).
   - NIHL may occur at an earlier age and be more severe among farmworkers (Thelin, Joseph, Davis, Baker & Hosokawa, 1983; Wright, 1993).
   - Approximately 25% of the male farmworkers in one study had a hearing loss affecting communication by age 30, and 50% by age 50 (Karlovich, Wiley, Tweed, & Jansen, 1988).
   - Hearing loss has been documented in high school students involved in farm work, suggesting that the hearing loss seen in adult farmers may begin in childhood (Broste, Hanson, Strand, & Stueland, 1989).
   - Noise-induced hearing loss can be prevented through engineering changes to equipment to reduce the noise levels and by workers' use of hearing protection (Lusk, Ronis, & Kerr, 1995).

   c. Safety features in farm equipment
   - New equipment may have built-in safety features; however, much of the machinery in use is older.
   - Even new machines may be altered to circumvent safety features that are perceived as interfering with efficiency.

   d. Agricultural workers are exposed to a number of hazardous materials (Table 3-3).

   e. Exposures can be prevented through proper work practices and use of personal protective equipment.

TABLE 3-3

Hazards to Agricultural Workers

Hazardous Substance	Health Effects
Anhydrous ammonia fertilizer	Contact with it can cause irritation, burns, or asphyxiation (Wright, 1993).
Insecticides and herbicides	Used to increase crop productivity, they can cause coma and death; both insecticides and herbicides have been associated with increased incidence of cancers (Blair & Zahn, 1991; Wright 1993).
Fungal spores and moldy grains	These cause "farmer's lung," a chronic debilitating condition (Wright, 1993).
Nitrogen oxides	These oxides, found in silos, can cause chemical pneumonitis and pulmonary edema (Wright, 1993).
Methane gases	Gases formed in manure holding tanks and livestock confinement buildings can cause asphyxiation (Wright, 1993).
Extreme heat and cold	Due to their outside work, agricultural workers may suffer heat exhaustion or frostbite. Because of their extensive exposure to the sun, they have higher rates of skin cancer and melanoma (Brown, 1991; Blair & Zahn, 1991).
Occupational infections	These infections, acquired from working with soil, animals, and their wastes, affect thousands of farm workers each year, causing disability (Kligman, Peate, & Cordes, 1991).

---

    4. National Institute for Occupational Safety and Health (NIOSH) Agricultural Initiative, developed in 1990, is a comprehensive research-based intervention program to reduce injury and disease among agricultural workers and their families.
      a. The Agricultural Initiative is designed to:
        • Assign nurses to rural areas to talk about prevention and to distribute information about injury and illness prevention to farmers.
        • Assess incidence of injury and illness
        • Provide cancer screening and assess cancer rates
        • Evaluate farms for safety hazards and determine the incidence of illness among farm family members
        • Award academic grants to establish new centers and to support applied research (Cordes and Rea, 1991b, p. 548)
      b. An Occupational Health Nurse in Agricultural Communities (OHNAC) program was initiated with thirty-one nurses in rural hospitals, clinics, and health departments in ten states to provide surveillance of illnesses and injuries related to agricultural work (Connon, Freund, and Ehlers, 1993).

B. Implications for occupational health nurses
    1. Agricultural workers generally do not receive services focused on their occupational health and safety needs.
    2. There is an opportunity and need for collaboration between community health services and occupational health nursing to meet the needs of agricultural workers, including the following:

    a. Improved record keeping and a national monitoring and surveillance system for agricultural occupational illnesses and injuries

    b. Input regarding occupational health and safety illnesses and injuries into federally sponsored programs, such as migrant worker programs

    c. Improving farm families' understanding of and ability to appropriately respond to hazards that may result in their children's illness and injury

3. NIOSH's OHNAC program begins to address the needs of agricultural workers, but it is available to only a small proportion of agricultural workers.

4. Although the role of the agricultural health nurse has been described (Randolph and Migliozzi, 1993), studies are needed to determine the effectiveness of interventions to prevent agricultural illnesses and injuries.

5. Intervention programs may include engineering improvement in equipment, advocacy for legislation related to agricultural safety and health, and education of agricultural workers (Cordes and Rea, 1991a).

6. Nurses not trained in occupational health nursing nonetheless need information regarding agricultural hazards in order to assess and treat rural residents.

XI

Construction Workers

A. Supportive and explanatory data

  1. Characteristics of population

    a. There are approximately 5 million workers in the construction trades in the United States, representing 4.3% of all nonfarm workers (U.S. Bureau of the Census, 1992).

    b. Construction workers are a diverse and mobile population, comprising numerous specialists and skilled and semiskilled workers on job sites that are varied and changeable (Lusk, Ronis & Hogan, in press).

    c. Subcontractors and laborers may work for several different employers on several different job locations in the space of only a few days (Lusk, 1993).

    d. According to trade association executives, the construction industry has ". . . one of the worst histories for attracting women and minorities . . ." (Dunbar, 1992, page 12).

    e. Workers in the skilled and semiskilled trades tend to identify more with their trade rather than with the employer and are often self-supervised.

    f. Approximately one-fifth of all construction workers are self-employed (U.S. Bureau of the Census, 1992).

    g. A high proportion of construction workers are without health insurance (Ringen, Pollak, Finklen, Melius, & Englund, 1995).

  2. Work characteristics

    a. A significant portion of the work is done outdoors, and indoor activities occur in relatively small spaces.

    b. Employment may be seasonal, and workers and subcontractors may work for more than one employer at one time.

    c. Job sites are temporary; workers may work on several different job sites in a single day.

    d. The variability of the job sites, job conditions, tools used, and patterns of employment inhibit the use of environmental and engineering controls to reduce hazards (Lusk, 1993).

    e. Better general safety practices exist among unionized workers than among nonunionized workers (Dedobbeleer, Champaign, & German, 1990).

3. Injury and illness data
   a. In 1993, national injury and illness rates for the construction industry were 12.2 cases per hundred workers, a rate higher than that for mining (6.8), and agricultural, forestry, and fishing (11.2) (U.S. Bureau of the Census, 1995).
   b. Because injury rates are calculated with numbers of workers rather than hours worked as the denominator, the rates of construction worker fatalities is underestimated because many construction workers are employed part-time.
   c. "In two decades, the rates of lost-time injuries and lost work time per injury have remained fairly constant" (Ringen, Englund, Welch, Weeks, & Segal, 1995, p. 445).
   d. Fatalities and injuries in the construction industry are often a result of falls.
   e. Because of the large amount of time spent outdoors, construction workers are at increased risk from effects of heat, cold, and sun exposure.
   f. Construction health hazards have been characterized as ranging "from A to Z" (Table 3-4).
   g. Exposure to hazardous materials may spread to family members when construction workers carry home toxic substances on their clothing and tools.
   h. Some believe that construction workers are not afforded the same level of protection from health hazards as their counterparts in general industry (Rekus, 1994).
      • Standards for hearing conservation programs are less stringent for construction than for manufacturers even though construction workers are exposed to excessive noise in many of their job sites.
      • No requirement exists for periodic noise monitoring, dosimetry, periodic audiometric testing, or worker education.
      • Beginning in 1991, U.S. legislators began to seriously consider extension of more stringent standards to the construction industry (Dumas, 1991).
   i. "Many hazardous exposures result from inadequacies in access to information, measurement technology, and personal protective equipment" (Ringen, Englund, & Seegal, 1995, p. 165).
   j. OSHA has issued three regulations for the construction industry:
      • Hazardous Waste Operations and Emergency Response Standard (29CFR1926.65)
      • Process Safety Management of Highly Hazardous Chemicals Standard (29CFR1926.64)
      • Lead Exposure and Construction: Interim Final Rule (29CFR1926.62)

B. Implications for occupational health nurses
   1. Construction workers are underserved by occupational health and safety programs; therefore, there is a need for development of programs to reach this segment of the worker population.
   2. Programs should focus on the major hazards of the construction industry: falls, machinery, chemicals, and noise.
   3. Because construction workers work for multiple employers, there may be entrepreneurial nursing opportunities for provision of occupational health and safety services.
   4. Because of the strong identification with the trade, trade union groups represent potential avenues for provision of occupational health and safety services to construction workers.

TABLE 3-4

Construction Hazards A to Z

Hazardous Substance	Sources of Exposure
Asbestos	Pipe insulation, asbestos concrete building materials, roofing felts
Beryllium	Work with beryllium-copper alloys
Carbon monoxide	Gasoline-powered engines and power tools
Diesel emissions	Portable power tools, heavy equipment
Electromagnetic radiation	X-radiography, UV from welding, RF
Formaldehyde	Plywood, particleboard, carpeting
Gasoline	Operating and refueling equipment
Heat stress	Roofing, carpentry
Insect bites	Ticks or other insects
J-Band radio energy	Construction around radar sites
Ketones	Adhesives, glues, mastics
Lead	Fumes from hot work on painted structural elements
Metal fumes	Welding, cutting, and burning metal
Noise	Heavy equipment, portable power tools
Overexertion	Materials handling, lifting
Polynuclear aromatics	Combustion products
Q-switched lasers	Surveying, sewer pipe alignment
Repetitive trauma	Laying carpet, rebar tying
Styrene	Plastic materials
Tar	Roofing materials, coatings and lining for underground tanks and pipelines
Urethane paints	Decomposition products, including hydrogen cyanide
Vibration	Pneumatic tools
Welding fumes	Lead, copper, cadmium, iron, chrome, nickel
Xylene	Paints, glues, adhesives, mastics
Zinc	Fumes from cutting galvanized metals

Source: Rekus (1994), p. 104.

XII

Health Care Workers (HCW)

A. Supportive and explanatory data
1. Demographics / Trends
   a. The health care industry is the largest employer in the United States, contributing 15% of the nation's gross domestic product (USDL, BLS, 1989).
   b. By 2005, the number of people employed in the health care industry will exceed 12 million (USDLBLS, 1994).
   c. The health care workforce is a diverse population that includes workers from all socioeconomic strata and with varying levels of education and English language skills.

    d. The hospital-based workforce, numbering over 4 million, is the single largest group of workers in the United States (USDL, 1994).

    e. The trend toward shifting the delivery site of health care services from hospitals and institutions to community clinics and provider offices is expected to continue.

    f. Home and residential care services are expected to remain among the fastest growing occupations through at least the year 2005 (USDL, 1994).

2. Work environment

    a. Occupational injury and illness incidence rates per 100 full-time equivalents (FTE) of HCWs in 1993 are as follows (National Safety Council, 1995):
- Nursing and personal care facilities: 17.3 per 100 FTEs
- Hospital incidence rates: 11.8 per 100 FTEs
- Workers providing residential care: 10.4 per 100 FTEs

    b. The health care industry provides little health and safety attention to its workers; hospital-based settings in particular have very few comprehensive health promotion programs (Felton, 1990; Rogers, 1994).

    c. HCWs who provide home care are exposed to all the hazards traditionally associated with acute care settings in addition to hazards unique to residential environments (Smith & White, 1993).

    d. Workers in health care settings are routinely exposed to a number of biological hazards, including (Table 3-5):
- Blood-borne pathogens (BBP)
- Airborne pathogens
- Vaccine-preventable communicable diseases

    e. Health care workers are exposed to chemical hazards, such as:
- Anesthetic gases
- Chemotherapeutic and antineoplastic agents
- Disinfectants, detergents
- Sterilizing agents
- Solvents
- Latex
- Tissue fixatives and reagents

    f. HCWs are regularly exposed to multiple physical and environmental hazards (Table 3-6).

    g. Psychological and emotional hazards result from (Table 3-7):
- Dealing directly with human suffering
- Ethical dilemmas regarding client care decisions
- Work overloads, staff shortages, hectic work schedules
- Job insecurity
- Verbal and physical aggression
- Working rotating or nighttime shifts

B. Implications for occupational health nurses

1. Collaborative relationships should be developed to facilitate the prevention, control, and abatement of occupational hazards and thus contribute to risk reduction.

2. Comprehensive worker health services should be available to all health care workers including those who work off-site, those who provide home care services, and night shift workers.

TABLE 3-5

Biological Occupational Hazards of Health Care Workers

Biologic (Infectious) Agent(s)	Major Source(s) of Exposure
Hepatitis A, E	Feces
Hepatitis B (HBV), Hepatitis C (HCV)	Blood and body fluids
Hepatitis D (found only in patients with HBV)	Blood and blood products
Human immunodeficiency virus (HIV)	Blood and body fluids
Cytomegalovirus (CMV)	Blood and body fluids
Rubeola (hard measles, red measles, 10-day)	Respiratory secretions (direct contact, droplet)
Mumps	Saliva (droplet, direct contact)
Rubella (German measles, 3-day)	Respiratory secretions (direct/indirect contact, droplet, airborne); virus shed in urine and stool
Influenza	Respiratory secretions, airborne droplet
Varicella zoster virus (VZV):	Indirect contact with freshly soiled articles (both types)
Chickenpox	Respiratory secretions (direct contact, airborne)
Shingles	Secretions of lesions, saliva
Herpes simplex virus (HSV)	Secretions of lesions, saliva
Tuberculosis (pulmonary)	Airborne droplet
Salmonella, Shigella, Campylobacter	Feces
Respiratory syncytial virus (RSV)	Respiratory secretions (direct/indirect, droplet)
Pertussis	Airborne droplets, respiratory secretions
Scabies	Direct skin contact with infected lesions
Methicillin resistant staph aureus (MRSA)	Contact with purulent lesion, airborne (rare)
Fungal infection: dermatitis, parenychia	Frequently moist skin; direct contact

Source: Adapted from Benenson (1995); DiBenedetto (1995).

3. Occupational health nurses will increasingly be responsible for the health and safety of employees in satellite clinics that are affiliated with a larger health care organization.
4. Worker health services for home care workers need to be expanded to include assessments of the client's living environment.
5. A crisis plan for handling violent incidents should be developed (Table 3-1).
6. Attention to the health and safety concerns of workers of childbearing age, particularly with respect to reproductive hazards, will be needed.

TABLE 3-6

Physical/Environmental Hazards in Health Care Settings

- Needle-sticks are the most frequently reported injury among HCWs.

- Over one-half of all reported back injuries occur within the health care field.

- Radiation: • Ionizing radiation has cumulative detrimental effects to all living tissue, including fetal tissue.

        • Nonionizing radiation poses thermal and light hazards to skin and eyes.

- Workers in health care are at greater risk for violent incidents than in other industries.

- Noise levels in housekeeping, dietary, laboratories, engineering, laundry, some nursing units, and other departments are frequently recorded at 80 dBA or higher.

- Ergonomic hazards in health care include cluttered hallways, patient rooms crowded with equipment, wet floors, maneuvering multiple pieces of equipment, awkward patient transfers, and the fast pace of emergent situations.

- Verbal and physical aggression is increasing in health care work environments.

- Lasers, a type of electromagnetic radiation increasingly used in health care settings, pose a risk of tissue trauma, particularly to vulnerable tissue, such as the eye.

TABLE 3-7

Adverse Effects of Psychological Stress in Health Care Workers

- Higher incidence of depression than the general population

- Higher incidence of chemical substance addiction than the general population

- Career burnout

- Psychological and physical effects of shiftwork:
  - Chronic fatigue
  - Alterations in mood and personality
  - Strained interpersonal relationships; decreased socialization
  - Disorders of sleeping, eating, and elimination
  - Decreased alertness; higher rates of accidents
  - Increased rates of subfecundity and adverse reproductive outcomes among workers who rotate shifts

- Altered work performance due to anxiety related to actual or potential exposures to biological, chemical, or other occupational hazards

XIII

International Workers

A. Supportive and explanatory data
  1. Demographics/Trends
    a. More than 60 million international workers are employed by over 100,000 U.S. business concerns abroad (Marquardt & Engel, 1993).
    b. At least 220,000 U.S. nationals were working abroad in 1991 (figure based on Internal Revenue Service tax forms) (Bryce, 1995).
    c. Ninety percent of U.S. expatriates are male; the percentage of female expatriates is increasing.
    d. New capitalistic countries and developing nations are enthusiastically re-

cruiting business enterprises and skilled labor from the United States and other developed nations.
  e. The numbers of Americans and foreign nationals working in U.S. concerns abroad is increasing due to:
  • The globalization of the marketplace
  • Economic and regulatory incentives
  • Trade reforms
2. The international workplace
  a. Approximately 80% of U.S. companies with expatriate workers provide pre-departure orientation regarding health issues; of these, only 42% offer orientation to all expatriate workers (Solomon, 1994).
  b. Health systems abroad vary widely and some may not be able to offer the quality or quantity of services to which U.S. workers are accustomed.
  c. Local business, cultural, and social norms abroad may differ significantly from those in the U.S. workplace; a lack of understanding of norms may lead to interpersonal conflict and workplace stress, among expatriate workers.
  d. Economic and environmental regulatory incentives that bring multinational companies to foreign locations may contribute to unsafe, unhealthy, and repressive working conditions for local workers (Ballinger, 1995; Coats, 1995; Levy, 1995).
  e. Occupational health in developing countries is generally poorly funded and has inadequately trained occupational health professionals (Levy, 1996).
  f. A number of member countries in the European Union have adopted occupational health and safety regulations that are more advanced than those in the United States.
  g. Many developing countries continue to use the labor of children, despite local and international prohibitions against this practice.
  h. Hazardous industries relocated in developing and newly industrialized countries, are often without adequate worker health and safety precautions (Johanning, Goldberg, & Kim, 1994; LaDou, 1992; Levy & Rest, 1996).
  i. While international guidelines for selected toxicants exist, efforts to develop international uniform occupational exposure limits have been unsuccessful; political and social forces increasingly influence scientific decisions about exposure limits (Levy & Rest, 1996).
  j. The most common health threat abroad is contamination of water supplies and food, particularly outside of urban centers in developing countries (Palchak & Schmidt, 1996; Russi, 1993).

B. Implications for occupational health nurses
1. The breadth and depth of pre-departure orientation related to health issues of U.S. nationals planning to work abroad will need to be increased. (See Chapter 12 for example of an international travel program.)
2. U.S. nationals who are dispatched to work abroad need appropriate vaccinations against infectious agents endemic to the destination country.
3. Contingency plans for accessing local emergency services and for emergency evacuation should be developed.
4. Occupational health and safety programs need to be sensitive to regional management practices and cultural norms.
5. Occupational health nurses should be advocates for ethical practices related to child labor, women's health, and other workplace health and safety issues.

Acknowledgment: The primary author of this chapter wishes to acknowledge the assistance of Dara Ganoczy, graduate student research assistant, in identifying literary sources used in the preparation of this chapter.

BIBLIOGRAPHY

Americans with Disabilities Act of 1990. Public Law 101-336. 42 USC, 12101–12134.

American Psychological Association. (1995, May–June). Society: Violence in the workplace. *The Futurist, 29*, 51–52.

Atkinson, C. L., Markowitz, L. E., Adams, N. C., & Seastrom, G. R. (1991). Transmission of measles in medical settings—United States, 1985–1989. *American Journal of Medicine, 91*(3B), 320S–324S.

Baker, E. L., & Matte, T. P. (1992). Surveillance of occupational illness and injury. In W. Halperin & E. L. Baker (Eds.), *Public Health Surveillance* (pp. 178–194). New York: Van Nostrand Reinhold.

Ballinger, J. (1995). Just do it—Or Else. *Multinational Monitor, 16*(6), 7–8.

Banco, L., Lapidus, G., & Braddock, M. (1992). Work-related injury among Connecticut minors. *Pediatrics, 89*(5), 957–960.

Beale, C. L. (1990). A taste of the country: A collection of Calvin Beale's writings. P.A. Morrison (Ed.). University Park, PA: The Pennsylvania State University Press.

Behling, D,. & Guy, J. (1993). Industry profile: Healthcare: Hazards of the health care professional. *Occupational Health and Safety, 62*(2), 54–57.

Belville, R., Pollack, S., Godbold, J., & Landrigan, P. (1993). Occupational injuries among working adolescents in New York State. *Journal of the American Health Association, 269*(21), 2754–2759.

Benenson, A. S. (Ed.), (1995). *Control of Communicable Diseases Manual* (16th Ed.). Washington, DC: American Public Health Association.

Biefang, S., & Potthoff, P. (1994). Screening process to discover insured persons in need of rehabilitation. *International Journal of Rehabilitation Research, 17*(3), 215–229.

Blair, A., & Zahn, S. H. (1991). Cancer among farmers. In D. H. Cordes & D. F. Rea (Eds.), *Occupational Medicine: Health Hazards of Farming. State of the Art Reviews, 6*(3) 335–354. Philadelphia: Hanley & Belfus, Inc.

Brimsek, T. A., & Bender, D. R. (1995). Making room for the virtual office. *Association Management, 47*(12), 71–86.

Brooks, D., & Davis, L. (1996). Work-related injuries to Massachusetts teens, 1987–1990. *American Journal of Industrial Medicine, 29*, 153–160.

Brooks, D., Davis, L., & Gallagher, S. (1993). Work-related injuries among Massachusetts children: A study based on emergency department data. *American Journal of Industrial Medicine, 24*, 313–324.

Broste, S. K., Hanson, D. A., Strand, R. L., & Stueland, D. T. (1989). Hearing loss among high school farm students. *American Journal of Public Health, 79*, 619–622.

Brown, W. D. (1991). Heat and cold in farm workers. In D. H. Cordes & D. F. Rea (Eds.), *Occupational Medicine: Health Hazards of Farming. State of the Art Reviews, 6*(3) 371–390. Philadelphia: Hanley & Belfus, Inc.

Bryce, R. (1995). *New York Times,* August 6, 1995.

Burke, R. J. (1995). Commuting to work. *Perpetual and Motor Skills, 80*(1), 49–50.

Burke, T. P., & Jain, R.S. (1995). Employee benefits survey: A BLS Reader. USDL Bulletin No. 2459, 90–96.

Cabral, R. (1996). Violence in the workplace: Policies for developing workplace violence prevention strategies. R. Harrison (Guest Ed.) In *Occupational Medicine: Violence in the Workplace:State of the Art Reviews, 1* (2), 303–314. Philadelphia: Hanley & Belfus, Inc.

Cahill, V. (1995). Labor and management in the '90s: A love affair or love-lost? *Foundry Management & Technology, 123*(3), 30.

Capell, P. (1995, November). The stress of relocating. *American Demographics, 17,* 15–16.

Carskadon, M. (1990a). Patterns of sleep and sleepiness in adolescents. *Pediatrician, 17,* 5–12.

Carskadon, M. (1990b). Adolescent sleepiness: Increased risk in a high risk population. *Alcohol, Drugs and Driving, 5*(4), *6*(1), 317–327.

Carson, R. (1993). Proper health management can reduce cumulative trauma disorder incidence. *Occupational Health and Safety, 62*(12), 41–4.

Castillo, D., & Jenkins, E. (1994). Industries and occupations at high risk for work-related homicide. *Journal of Occupational Medicine, 36*(2), 125–132.

Castillo, D., Landen, D., & Layne, L. (1994). Occupational injury deaths of 16- and 17-year-olds in the United States. *American Journal of Public Health, 84*(4), 646–649.

Castro, J. (1993, March 29). Disposable workers. *Time, 141*(13), 43–47.

Caudron, S. (1994, July). Contingent work force spurs HR planning. *Personnel Journal,* 52–60.

Centers for Disease Control and Prevention. (1988). Update: Universal precautions for prevention of transmission of human immunodeficiency virus, hepatitis B virus, and other blood-borne pathogens in health care settings. *Morbidity and Mortality Weekly Report, 37,* 377–388.

Centers for Disease Control and Prevention. (1990). Protection against viral hepatitis: Recommendations of the Immunization Practices Advisory Committee (ACIP). *Morbidity And Mortality Weekly Report, 39*(RR-2), 1–26.

Centers for Disease Control and Prevention. (1991). Recommendations for preventing transmission of human immunodeficiency virus and hepatitis B virus to clients during exposure-prone invasive procedures. *Morbidity And Mortality Weekly Report, 40*(RR-8), 1–9.

Centers for Disease Control and Prevention. (1994). Guidelines for preventing the transmission of mycobacterium tuberculosis in health care facilities. *Federal Register, 59*(208), 54242–54303.

Coats, S. (1995). Organizing and repression. *Multinational Monitor, 16*(6), 17–19

Connon, C.L., Freund, E., & Ehlers, J.K. (1993). The occupational health nurse in agricultural communities program: Identifying and preventing agriculturally related illnesses and injuries. *AAOHN Journal, 41,* 422–428.

Cordes, D. H., & Rea, D.F. (1991a). Farming: A hazardous occupation. In D. H. Cordes & D. F. Rea (Eds.), *Occupational Medicine: Health Hazards of Farming. State of the Art Reviews, 6*(3) 327–334. Philadelphia: Hanley & Belfus, Inc.

Cordes, D. H., & Rea, D. F. (1991b). Preventive measures in agricultural settings. In D. H. Cordes & D. F. Rea (Eds.), *Occupational Medicine: Health Hazards of Farming. State of the Art Reviews, 6*(3) 541–550. Philadelphia: Hanley & Belfus, Inc.

Crime: Death on the job. (1994). *The Economist, 333,* 39.

Daley, C. L., Small, P. M., Schecter, G. F., Schoolnik, G. K., McAdam, R. A., Jacobs, W. R., et al. (1992). An outbreak of tuberculosis with accelerated progression among persons infected with the human immunodeficiency virus: An analysis using restriction-fragment-length polymorphisms. *New England Journal of Medicine, 326,* 231–235.

Dear, J. A. (1995, November 1). Work stress and health '95: Creating healthier workplaces. *Vital Speeches of the Day, 62,* 39–42.

Dedobbeleer, N., Champaign, R., & German, P. (1990). Safety performance among union and nonunion workers in the construction industry. *Journal of Occupational Medicine, 32,* 1099–1103.

Dennis, A. (1995). A firm without walls. *Journal of Accountancy, 180*(6), 62–63.

DiBenedetto, D. V. (1995). Occupational hazards of the health care industry: Protecting health care workers. *AAOHN Journal 43* (3), 131–137.

DiBenedetto, D. V. (1995). OEM Occupational health and safety manual (2nd Ed.) Boston, MA: OEM Press.

Di Fabio, R. P., Mackey, G., & Holte, J. B. (1995). Disability and functional status in clients with low back pain receiving workers' compensation: A descriptive study with implications for the efficacy of physical therapy. *Physical Therapy, 75*(3), 180–93.

Ditlea, S. (1995). Home is where the office is. *Nation's Business, 83*(11), 41–44.

Doeglas, D., Suurmeijer, T., Krol, B., Sanderman, R., van Leeuwen, M., & van Rijswijk, M. (1995). *Annals of the Rheumatic Diseases, 54*(6), 455–460.

Dumas, K. (1991). House panels vote measures on worker health, safety. *Congressional Quarterly Weekly Report, 49*, 2081.

Dunbar, M. (1992, November/December). Women & minorities in construction. *Michigan Construction Users Council Newsletter, 12.*

Equal Employment Opportunity Commission. (1992). *A technical assistance manual on the employment provisions (Title I) of the Americans with Disabilities Act.* Washington DC: U. S. Government Printing Office.

Engleberg, A. L. (1994). Disability and workers' compensation. *Primary Care: Clinics in Office Practice, 21*(2), 275–289.

Felton, J. S. (1990). *Occupational Health Management.* Boston: Little, Brown.

Felton, J. S. (1993). Occupational violence: An intensified work concomitant. *OEM Report, 7*(12), 101–103.

Franks, J. R. (1988a). Noise in the construction industry and its effect on hearing. *Hearing Instruments, 41*(10), 18, 21.

Franks, J. R. (1988b). Number of workers exposed to occupational noise. *Seminars in Hearing, 9*(4) (Reprinted in *NIOSH Publications on Noise and Hearing,* USDHSS, 1991, 287–298.).

Fuhrer, M. J. (1995). Conference report: An agenda for health rehabilitation outcomes research. *Journal of Allied Health, 24*(1), 79–87.

Fyock, C. D. (1990). *America's work force is coming of age.* Lexington, MA: Lexington Books.

Genasci, L. (1995, September 14). Firms pump $100 million into day care. *The Ann Arbor News: Business Section,* B6.

Glazner, L. K. (1991). Shiftwork: Its effect on workers. *AAOHN Journal, 39*(9), 416–421.

Gliniecki, C. M., & Burgel, B. J. (1995). Temporary work restrictions: Guidelines for the primary care provider. *Nurse Practitioner Forum, 6*(2), 79–89.

Government Accounting Office (GAO). (1990). *Child Labor: Increases in detected child labor violations throughout the United States.* GAO publication HRD-90-116, Washington, DC.

Government Accounting Office (GAO). (1991). *Child Labor: Characteristics of working children.* GAO publication HRD-91-83BR, Washington, DC.

Greenberger, E., & Steinberg, L. (1986). *When teenagers work: The psychological and social costs of adolescent employment.* New York: Basic Books, Inc.

Groeneveld, B. (1995). Unions rally to boost waning rolls. *Minneapolis–St. Paul City Business, 48,* 18.

Harber, P., & Fedoruk, M. J. (1993). Personal risk assessment under the Americans with Disabilities Act: A decision analysis approach. *Journal of Occupational Medicine, 35*(10), 1000–1010.

Harber, P., & Fedoruk, M. J. (1994). Work placement and worker fitness: Implications of the Americans with Disabilities Act for pulmonary medicine. *Chest, 105*(5), 1564–1571.

Hardy, I. R., & Gershon, A. A. (1990). Prospects for use of a varicella vaccine in adults. *Infectious Disease Clinics of North America, 4*(1), 159–173.

Harvey, M. G., & Cosier, R. A. (1995, March–April). Homicides in the workplace: Crisis or false alarm? *Business Horizons, 38,* 11–20.

Hayden, M. J. (1992). Disability awareness workshop: Helping businesses comply with the Americans with Disabilities Act of 1990. *American Journal of Occupational Therapy, 46*(5), 461–465.

Hellman, S. L., & Gram, M. C. (1993). The resurgence of tuberculosis: Risk in health care settings. *AAOHN Journal, 40*(2), 66–71.

Herz, D. E., (1995, April). Work after early retirement: An increasing trend among men. *Monthly Labor Review,* 13–20.

Heyer, N., Franklin, G., Rivara, F., Parker, P., & Haug, J. (1992). Occupational injuries among minors doing farm work in Washington. *American Journal of Public Health, 82*(4), 557–560.

Himmelstein, J. S., & Pransky, G. S. (1994). Ability to work and disability evaluation. In B. S. Levy & D. H. Wegman (Eds.), *Occupational Health: Recognizing and Preventing Work-Related Disease* (3rd ed.) (pp. 221–239). Boston: Little, Brown and Company.

Hughson, W. G. (1994). Work-related disabilities. *Proceedings, Annual Meeting of the Health Section of the American Council of Life Insurance, 53–65.*

Jarratt, J., Coates, J. F., Mahaffie, J. B., & Hines, A. (1994). *Managing your future as an association: Thinking about trends and working with their consequences 1994–2020.* American Society of Association Executives.

Jenkins, E., Kisner, S., Fosbroke, D., Layne, L., Stout, N., Castillo, D., Cutlip, P., Cianfrocco, R., et al. (1993). *Fatal injuries to workers in the United States, 1980–1989: A decade of surveillance. National profile,* (DHHS publication NIOSH 93-108). Washington DC: U. S. Government Printing Office.

Johnson, C. (1995). Changing face of labor reflects new horizons for organizing. *AFL-CIO News* 40(19), 12.

Johnston, W. B., & Packer, A. E. (1987). *Workforce 2000: Work and workers for the twenty-first century.* Indianapolis, IN: Hudson Institute.

Johanning, E., Goldberg, M., & Kim, R. (1994). Asbestos hazard evaluation in South Korean textile production. *International Journal of Health Services, 24*(1), 131–144.

Jones, T. W. (1995, November). A warning on the future of U. S. pensions. *The Participant,* 3.

Karlovich, R. S., Wiley, T. L., Tweed, T., & Jensen, D. V. (1988). Hearing sensitivity in farmers. *Public Health Reports, 103*(1), 61–71.

Kaufman, L., Cohn, B., & Rhodes, S. (1995, May 22). Union solidarity forever? Sorry, not this year. *Newsweek,* 64.

Kiene, K., Hsu, B., Rowe, D., & Carruthers, A. (1994). Hepatitis, HIV, and the dermatologist: A risk review. *Journal of the American Academy of Dermatology, 30*(1), 108–115.

Kligman, E. W., Peate, W. F., & Cordes, D. H. (1991). Occupational infections in farm workers. In D. H. Cordes & D. F. Rea (Eds.), *Occupational Medicine: Health Hazards of Farming. State of the Art Reviews, 6*(3), 429–446. Philadelphia: Hanley & Belfus, Inc.

Kraus, J. F., & McArthur, D. L. (1996) Violence in the workplace: Epidemiology of violent injury in the workplace. R. Harrison (Guest Ed.) In *Occupational Medicine: State of the Art Reviews, 11*(2), 201–218. Philadelphia: Hanley & Belfus, Inc

Kraus, L. E., & Stoddard, S. (1991). *Chartbook on work disability in the United States.* An InfoUse report. Washington DC: U. S. National Institute on Disability and Rehabilitation Research.

LaDou, J. (1992). The exposure of hazardous industries to newly industrialized countries (editorial). *Polish Journal of Occupational Medicine and Environmental Health, 5*(3), 223–226.

Lambert, V. (1995). Give your company a checkup. *Personnel Journal, 74,* 143–149.

Lange, J. E., & Mills, D. Q. (1979). *The Construction Industry: Balance wheel of the economy.* Lexington, MA: Lexington Books.

Laube-Morgan, J. (1992). The professional's psychological response in disaster: Implications for practice. *Journal of Psychosocial Nursing and Mental Health Services, 30*(2), 17–22.

Layne, L., Castillo, D., Stout, N., & Cutlip, P. (1994). Adolescent occupational injuries requiring hospital emergency department treatment: A nationally representative sample. *American Journal of Public Health, 84*(4), 657–660.

Lechner, D. E., Jackson, J. R., Roth, D. L., & Straaton, K. V. (1994). Reliability and validity of a newly developed test of physical work performance. *Journal of Occupational Medicine, 36*(9), 997–1004.

Leigh, J. P., & Fries, J. F. (1992). Disability in occupations in a national sample. *American Journal of Public Health, 82*(11), 1517–1524.

Lenz, E. A. (1994). Employer liability issues in staffing services arrangements. *Co-employment* (2nd ed.). Virginia: National Association of Temporary Services.

Levy, B. S. (1995). Health and social effects of worldwide economic transformation: Focus on occupational and environmental health. *Social Justice, 22,* 77–84.

Levy, B. S. (1996). The context of hazards in the international setting, with a focus on developing countries, In L. Fleming, J. Herzstein, & W. Bunn (Eds.). *International Occupational and Environmental Health*. Beverly, MA: OEM Publishing.

Levy, B. S., & Rest, K. M. (1996). Policies to protect and promote workers' health are necessary for sustainable human development. In G. Shahi, B. S. Levy, A. Binger, T. Kjellstrom, & R. Lawrence (Eds.), *International Perspectives in Environment, Health and Development: Toward a Sustainable World*. New York: Springer.

Levy, B. S., & Wegman, D. H. (1995). *Occupational Health: Recognizing and Preventing Work-Related Disease*, (3rd ed.). Boston: Little, Brown and Company.

Lewin, T. (1995, October 29). Workers of both sexes make trade-offs for family, study shows. *The New York Times: National*, 25.

Lippman, H. (1995, November). The new variety in managed care. *Business & Health*, 46–53.

Lipscomb, J. A. (1992). Violence toward health care workers: An emerging occupational hazard. *AAOHN Journal, 40*(5), 219–228.

Longbottom, H. M., Cox, K., & Sokas, R. K. (1993). Body fluid exposure in an urban tertiary care health center. *American Journal of Industrial Medicine, 23*(5), 703–710.

Lund, J. (1993). Varicella zoster virus in the health care setting: Risk and management. *AAOHN Journal, 41*(8), 369–373.

Lund, S., Jackson, J., Leggett, J., Hales, L., Dworkin, R., & Gilbert, D. (1994). Reality of glove use and handwashing in a community hospital. *American Journal of Infection Control, 22*(6), 352–357.

Lusk, S. L. (1995). Linking practice & research: Health promotion by mail. *AAOHN Journal, 43*(6), 346–348.

Lusk, S. L. (1993). Preventing noise induced hearing loss in construction workers. Grant proposal funded by National Institute for Occupational Safety & Health. Grant No. R01 OH03136–03.

Lusk, S. L., Ronis, D. L., & Hogan, M. M. (In press). Test of the Health Promotion Model as a causal model of construction workers' use of heavy protection. *Research in Nursing and Health*.

Lusk, S. L., Ronis, D. L., & Kerr, M. J. (1995). Predictors of hearing protection use among workers: Implications for training programs. *Human Factors, 37*(3), 635–640.

Markowitz, S. B. (1994). Epidemiology of tuberculosis among health care workers. *Occupational Medicine, 9*(4), 589–608.

Marquardt, M. J., & Engel, D. W. (1993). *Global human resource development*. Englewood Cliffs, NJ: Prentice-Hall.

Martin, K. J. (1995). Workers' compensation: Case management strategies. *AAOHN Journal, 43*(5), 245–250.

Mathiason, G. G., & Schuyler, M. (1996). Violence in the workplace: The law of workplace violence. In R. Harrison (Guest Ed.) *Occupational Medicine: State of the Art Reviews, 11*(2), 315–334. Philadelphia: Hanley & Belfus, Inc.

Mayall, D. (1995). Temporary work and labor market detachment: New mechanisms and new opportunities. In D. B. Bills, *The New Modern Times: Factors Reshaping the World of Work* (pp. 163–192). Albany, NY: State University of New York Press.

McGaughey, M. J., Kiernan, W. E., McNally, L. C., & Gilmore, D. S. (1995). A peaceful coexistence? State MR/DD agency trends in integrated employment and facility-based services. *Mental Retardation, 33*(3), 170–180.

McNaught, W., Barth, M. C., & Henderson, P. H. (1989). The human resource potential of Americans over 50. *Human Resource Management, 28*, 455–473.

McNerney, D. J. (1995). Telecommuting: An idea whose time has come. *HR Focus, 72*(11), 1, 4–5.

Menzies, D., Fanning, A., Yuan, L., & Fitzgerald, M. (1995). Tuberculosis among health care workers. *New England Journal of Medicine, 332*(2), 92–98.

Merchant, J. A. (1991). Agricultural injuries. In D. H. Cordes & D. F. Rea (Eds.), *Occupational Medicine: Health Hazards of Farming. State of the Art Reviews, 6*(3) 529–539. Philadelphia: Hanley & Belfus, Inc.

Mergenhagen, P. (1994, June). Rethinking retirement. *American Demographics*, 28–34.

Miller, M. (1995, March). *Occupational injuries among adolescents in Washington State, 1988–1991: A review of workers' compensation data* (Technical Report Number 35-1-1995). Safety and Health Assessment and Research for Prevention. Olympia, WA: Washington State Department of Labor and Industries.

Morris, J. (1995). Factors influencing the injury experience of temporary workers in a manufacturing setting. Unpublished Master's Dissertation, University of Michigan School of Nursing, Ann Arbor, MI.

Morris, R., & Bass, S. A. (1988). *Retirement reconsidered: Economic and social roles for older people.* New York: Springer Publishing Company.

Morrow, L. (1993, March 29). The temping of America. *Time, 40–47.*

Morehouse, R. L. (1995). Shiftwork: The special challenges for women. *AAOHN Journal, 43*(10), 532–535.

National Center for Health Statistics, (1990). Prevention profile. Health, United States, 1989. DHHS Pub No. (PHS)90-1232. Hyattsville, MD: U. S. Department of Health and Human Services, 1990.

National Center for Health Statistics. J. G. Collins & O. T. Thombery. (1989). Health characteristics of workers by occupation and sex: United States 1983–95. Advance Data from Vital and Health Statistics, No. 168, DHHS Pub no. (PHS)89-1250. Hyattsville, MD: U.S. Public Health Service.

National Institute for Occupational Safety and Health. (1996). *National Occupational Research Agenda.* Atlanta: U.S. Department of Health and Human Services.

National Institute for Occupational Safety and Health (NIOSH) (1995, May). *NIOSH Alert: Request for assistance in preventing deaths and injuries of adolescent workers,* (DHHS [NIOSH] Publication No. 95-125). Cincinnati, OH: U. S. Department of Health and Human Services.

National Safe Worksite Institute. (1992). *Sacrificing America's youth: The problem of child labor and the response of government.* Chicago, IL: Author.

National Safety Council. (1993). *Accident Facts, 1993 Edition.* Chicago, IL: Author.

National Safety Council. (1995). *Accident Facts, 1995 Edition.* Itasca, IL: Author.

Nitze, W. A. (1993, Summer). The economic case for sustainable development. *Issues in Science and Technology, 29–32.*

Office of Disease Prevention and Health Promotion, National Institute for Occupational Safety and Health, & Institute for Alternative Futures. (1987). The future of work and health: Implications for health strategies. Alexandria, VA: Institute for Alternative Futures.

Olmsted, B., & Smith, S. (1994). *Creating a flexible workplace: How to select & manage alternative work options.* New York: American Management Association, (2nd ed.)

Palchak, R. B., & Schmidt, R. T. (1996, February). Protecting the health of employees abroad. *Occupational Health & Safety, 65*(2), 53–56.

Parker, D., Carl, W., French, L., & Martin, F. (1994a). Nature and incidence of self-reported adolescent work injury in Minnesota. *American Journal of Industrial Medicine, 26,* 529–541.

Parker, D., Carl, W., French, L., & Martin, F. (1994b). Characteristics of adolescent work injuries reported to the Minnesota Department of Labor and Industry. *American Journal of Public Health, 84*(4), 606–611.

Parker, D., Clay, R., Mandel, J., Gunderson, P., & Salkowicz, L. (1991). Adolescent occupational injuries in Minnesota: A descriptive study. *Minnesota Medicine, 74,* 25–28.

Pollack, S., & Landrigan, P. (1990). Child labor in 1990: Prevalence and health hazards. *Annual Review of Public Health, 11,* 359–375.

Pruitt, R. H. (1995). Preplacement evaluation: Thriving within the ADA guidelines. *AAOHN Journal, 43*(3), 124–130.

Randolph, S. A., & Migliozzi, A. A. (1993). The role of the agricultural health nurse: Bringing together community and occupational health. *AAOHN Journal, 41,* 429–433.

Rekus, J. F. (1994, May). Chronic risks in construction. *Occupational Health & Safety, 103–104, 106–108, 129.*

Richter, E., & Jacobs, J. (1991). Work injuries and exposures in children and young adults: Review and recommendation for action. *American Journal of Industrial Medicine, 19,* 747–769.

Richman, L. S. (1995, September 4). Why baby-boomers won't be able to retire. *Fortune,* 48.

Ringen, K., Englund, A., & Seegal, J. (1995). Safety and health in the construction industry. *Annual Review of Public Health, 16,* 165–188.

Ringen, K., Englund, A., Welch, L., Weeks, J. L., & Seegal, J. L. (1995). Perspectives of the future. Ringen, et al. (Eds.), *Occupational Medicine: Construction Safety and Health. State of the Art Reviews, 10*(2), 445–451. Philadelphia, Hanley & Belfus, Inc.

Ringen, K., Pollak, E., Finklea, J. F., Melius, J., & Engllund, J. (1995). Health insurance and workers' compensation: The delivery of medical and rehabilitation services for construction workers. Ringen, et al. (Guest Eds.). In *Occupational Medicine: Construction Safety and Health: State of the Art Reviews, 10*(2), 435–444. Philadelphia: Hanley & Belfus, Inc.

Rivara, F. P. (1985). Fatal and nonfatal farm injuries to children and adolescents in the United States. *Pediatrics, 76,* 567–573.

Robinson, J. P., & Godbey, G. (1995, September/October). Are average Americans really overworked? *The American Enterprise, 6,* 43.

Rogers, B. (1994). *Occupational Health Nursing: Concepts and Practice.* Philadelphia: W. B. Saunders.

Russi, M. (1993). Environmental health issues for travelers. In F. J. Bia (Ed.) *Travel Medicine Advisor* (TCI. 1–TCI. 8). Atlanta, GA: American Health Consultants, Inc.

Rust, C. S. (1990). Health status of migrant farmworkers: A literature review and commentary. *American Journal of Public Health, 80,* 1213–1217.

Schober, S., Jandke, J., Halperin, W., Moll, M., & Thun, M. (1988). Work-related injuries in minors. *American Journal of Industrial Medicine, 14,* 585–595.

Scott, M. B. (1995). Focus on work & family: Work/family programs: Their role in the new workplace. *Employee Benefit Plan Review, 50,* 32–33.

Segal, L. M., & Sullivan, D. G. (1995, March–April). The temporary labor force. *Ergonomic Perspectives,* 2–19.

Sepkowitz, K. A., & Raffalli, J. (1994). Tuberculosis at the end of the twentieth century. *European Journal of Clinical Microbiology and Infectious Diseases,* 13(11), 902–907.

Service, M. (1995, March 20–28). Why health costs got smaller in 1994. *Business & Health, 13,* 20–22, 26, 28.

Simkiss, P., & Floyd, M. (1995). Developing a computerized information system for visually disabled people to assist with job placement. *International Journal of Rehabilitation Research, 18*(2), 133–141.

Smith, K. G. (1986). The hazards of migrant farm work: An overview for rural public health nurses. *Public Health Nursing, 3*(1), 48–56.

Smith, W. A., & White, M. C. (1993). Home health care: Occupational health issues. *AAOHN Journal, 41*(4), 180–185.

Solomon, C. M. (1994). Global operations demand that HR rethink diversity. *Personnel Journal, 73*(7), 40–50.

Staff. (1994, July/August). Post-NAFTA labor abuses. *Multinational Monitor, 15*(7), 4–5.

Steinberg, L., & Dornbusch, S. (1991). Negative correlates of part-time employment during adolescence: Replication and elaboration. *Developmental Psychology, 27,* 304–313.

Stone, R. A. (1995 March–April). Workplace homicide: A time for action. *Business Horizons, 38,* 3–10.

Sussman, G. L., & Beezhold, D. H. (1995). Allergy to latex rubber. *Annals of Internal Medicine, 122*(1), 43–46.

Tanzillo, K. (1995). Georgia Power workers use remote centers for telecommuting. *Successful Telecommuting, 32*(12), 14.

Tate, D. G. (1992). Workers' disability and return to work. *American Journal of Physical Medicine and Rehabilitation, 71*(2), 92–96.

Thelin, J. W., Joseph, D. J., Davis, W. E., Baker, D. E., & Hosokawa, M. C. (1983). High-frequency hearing loss in male farmers of Missouri. *Public Health Reports, 98*(3), 268–272.

Thomas, D. L., Factor, S. H., Kelen, G. D., Washington, A. S., Taylor, E., Jr., & Quinn, T. C. (1993). Viral hepatitis in health care personnel at The Johns Hopkins Hospital: The seroprevalence of and risk factors for hepatitis B virus and hepatitis C virus infection. *Archives of Internal Medicine, 153*(14), 1705–1712.

Toscano, G. (1994). Compensation and working conditions. *U. S. Department of Labor Bureau of Labor Statistics.* Washington, DC: U. S. Government Printing Office.

U. S. Bureau of the Census. (1995). *Statistical abstract of the United States 1995: The national data book* (115th edition). Washington, DC., 1995. (pp. 386, 440).

U. S. Bureau of the Census. (1992). *Statistical abstract of the United States* (112th ed.). Washington, DC: U. S. Government Printing Office.

U. S. Bureau of the Census. (1989). Current population reports, Series P-23, No. 160. *Labor Force status and other characteristics of persons with a work disability: 1982.* Special Studies, Washington, DC: U. S. Department of Commerce.

U. S. Department of Agriculture. (1989). Rural and rural farm population: 1988. In *Current Population Reports,* Series P-20, No. 439. Washington, DC: U. S. Government Printing Office.

U. S. Department of Health and Human Services. U. S. Public Health Service. (1991). *Healthy people 2000: National health promotion and disease prevention objectives: Full report with commentary.* (National Institutes of Health Publication No. 91–50212). Washington, DC: U. S. Government Printing Office.

U. S. Department of Labor, Occupational Safety and Health Administration. (1996). *Guidelines for preventing workplace violence for health care and social service workers* (OSHA 348). Washington, DC: U.S. Government Printing Office.

U. S. Department of Labor, Bureau of Labor Statistics. (1995a). BLS Releases New 1994–2005 Employment Projections, (Bulletin 95-485, December 1995). Washington, DC: U. S. Government Printing Office.

U. S. Department of Labor, Bureau of Labor Statistics. (1995b). Employee benefits survey: A BLS reader, (Bulletin 2459, February 1995). Washington, DC: U. S. Government Printing Office, 97–109.

U.S. Department of Labor, Bureau of Labor Statistics. (1994). The American Workforce: 1992–2005, (Bulletin 2452, April 1994). Washington, DC: U. S. Government Printing Office.

U. S. Department of Labor, Women's Bureau. (1994). *1993 Handbook on Women Workers: Trends & Issues.* Washington, DC: U. S. Government Printing Office.

Verbrugge, L. M. & Wingard, D. L. (1987). Sex differentials in health and mortality. *Women & Health Review.* Washington, DC: Author.

Wakefield, M. K. (1990). Health care in rural America: A view from the nation's capital. *Nursing Economics, 8,* 83–89.

Waller, J. A., Payne, S. R., & Skelly, J. M. (1989) Injuries to carpenters. *Journal of Occupational Medicine, 31*(8), 687–692.

Weeks, J. L., & McVittie, D. J. (1995). Controlling injury hazards in construction. In K. Ringen, et al. (Eds.). In *Occupational Medicine: Construction Safety and Health. State of the Art Reviews, 6*(2), 395–406. Philadelphia: Hanley & Belfus, Inc.

Wenzel, R. P., & Pfaller, M. A. (1991). Handwashing: efficacy versus acceptance. A brief essay. *Journal of Hospital Infection,* June, *18,* Supplement B., 65–68.

West, M. D. (1995). Aspects of the worksite and return to work for persons with brain injury in supported employment. *Brain Injury, 9*(3), 301–313.

Wilkinson, W. E., Salazar, M. K., Uhl, J. E., Koepsell, T. D., DeRoos, R. L., & Long, R. J. (1992). Occupational injuries: A study of health care workers at a Northwestern health science center and teaching hospital. *AAOHN Journal, 40*(6), 287–293.

Windau, J., & Toscano, G. (1994). Workplace homicides in 1992. *U.S. Department of Labor, Bureau of Labor Statistics.* Washington, DC: U.S. Government Printing Office.

Wright, K. A. (1993). Management of agricultural injuries and illness. *Nursing Clinics of North America, 28,* 253–266.

Yassi, A., Murdzak, C., Cheang, M., Tran, N., & Aoki, F. Y. (1994). Influenza immunization: Knowledge, attitude and behaviour of health care workers. *Canadian Journal of Infection Control, 9*(4), 103–108.

Zieger, R. H. (1994). *American workers, American unions.* Baltimore: John Hopkins University Press (pp. 193–205).

Zimakoff, J., Stormark, M., & Larsen, S. O. (1993). Use of gloves and handwashing behaviour among health care workers in intensive care units. *Journal of Hospital Infection, 24*(1), 63–67

CHAPTER

4

Legal and Ethical Issues

MAJOR TOPICS

- *Sources of law*
- *Federal acts and agencies*
- *Documentation and recordkeeping*
- *Workers' compensation*
- *Ethical principles*
- *Ethical conflicts*

Legal and ethical issues frequently arise in the occupational setting. It is essential that occupational health nurses be familiar with state and federal regulations that affect employees in their work settings and that nurses clearly understand their professional responsibility with regard to those regulations. Furthermore, they must be prepared to respond effectively to the various ethical concerns that may arise in a competitive environment, which often breeds conflicting opinions and moral dilemmas. The information in this chapter provides a broad overview of government regulations and ethical principles that can serve as a guide to occupational health nursing practice.

Legal Issues

I

Sources of Law

A. *Common law* is law that is made by courts in deciding individual disputes; this law creates legal precedents that must be relied upon in similar future cases.
1. Deference is accorded decisions made by higher courts; i.e., state courts have precedence over local courts, and federal over state.
2. Courts follow past precedents to promote the uniform and predictable application of common law rules based on changing societal values, norms, and cultures; however, courts can reinterpret prior decisions or the application of law to a subject matter in current, future, and/or past cases.

B. *Statutes* are legal rules created by federal legislatures.
1. Statutes may modify existing law or regulate new subject matter.
2. The legislature may delegate the responsibility for promulgating rules and regulations about a particular matter to an administrative agency.

3. Statutes may preempt rules and regulations of administrative agencies.
4. Statutes reflect societal norms and social order; thus, laws are enacted or codified as a result of societal changes.

C. *Federal law* is based on the United States Constitution and is the supreme rule of the land; that is, state statutes must be consistent with federal law.

D. *State law* regulates activities within the state's jurisdiction.
1. *Civil law* addresses the rights and duties of persons; an example is the Nurse Practice Act.
2. *Criminal law* is enacted to preserve public order.
3. *Administrative law* is regulated by administrative agencies within the states; for example, State Boards of Nursing are administrative agencies that oversee, monitor, and enforce the Nurse Practice Act.

II

Basic Legal Concepts

A. *Tort* refers to a private legal wrong against the person or property of another; examples include assault, battery, and defamation; this wrong is compensated with money damages.

B. *Negligence* is the failure to perform one's duties according to acceptable standards.
1. *Standard of care* refers to what the average, reasonable, and prudent occupational health nurse would do in the same or similar circumstances; it is also known as "reasonable and customary care."
2. *Exceptional circumstances,* such as emergencies, are taken into consideration when determining negligence.
3. *Duties* include coming to the aid of others and preventing forseeable harm.
   a. In the occupational setting, this includes harm that occurs in the course of employment.
   b. This duty applies if there is no unreasonable risk of harm to the occupational health nurse.
4. *Breach* occurs when one fails to maintain the customary standard of care.

C. Examples of negligence include:
1. Failure to take action
2. Failure to communicate danger
3. Delay in obtaining assistance
4. Medication errors
5. Failure to obtain informed consent

D. *Informed consent* implies that a decision is made with a clear understanding of a treatment or action, including material risks, benefits, and alternative treatments.
1. Content of the informed consent includes:
   a. Nature and purpose of proposed treatment
   b. Diagnosis
   c. Material risks of proposed treatment
   d. Alternative treatments
   e. Consequences of lack of treatment
2. Purposes of informed consent
   a. Provides worker with opportunity to make autonomous decision
   b. Protects the worker from harm
   c. Ensures accountability among health professionals

   3. Characteristics of informed consent
      a. Must be given freely and without coercion
      b. Must be given with full understanding
   4. The person giving informed consent must be mentally, physically, and legally competent

E. *Malpractice* is a type of negligence that involves professional misconduct or unreasonable lack of skill.
   1. The civil action for misconduct by the occupational health nurse will be determined by the applicable state statutes.
   2. Malpractice applies to a higher standard of care than the negligence does; malpractice requires expert testimony to help the jury understand the standard of care owed to a client by the reasonably prudent occupational health nurse.

F. *Statute of limitation* is the period of time after a tort occurs within which a lawsuit must be filed.
   1. Typically, the statute of limitation for negligence is two years.
   2. The statute of limitation for malpractice is typically one year.

III

Legal Responsibilities of the Occupational Health Nurse

A. Occupational health nurses are responsible for maintaining a current knowledge of the laws affecting occupational health practice in the jurisdiction where they practice; these laws include:
   1. Proposed bills and state legislation
   2. Proposed and implemented administrative laws, such as the nurse practice, pharmacy, and medical acts
   3. Proposed bills and federal legislation
   4. Proposed and implemented federal administrative rules and regulations

B. Because of the dynamic and evolving nature of occupational health nursing practice, inconsistencies between actual practice and legal parameters of practice may exist.
   1. Laws, rules, and regulations that are enacted are dynamic; thus, they may be challenged as professional practice evolves.
   2. The interpretation of laws, rules, and regulations may change as new cases are decided (common law) and precedents are established.
   3. Laws, rules, and regulations must be changed by following established procedures and protocols.

The Federal Act and Agencies Relevant to Occupational Health and Safety
IV

Occupational Safety and Health Act (OSH Act)

   The purpose of the OSH Act—Public Law 91-596, signed on December 29, 1970, is to "assure so far as possible every working man and woman in the Nation safe and healthful working conditions and to preserve our human resources."

A. Overview of the Act
1. The OSH Act applies to employers and employees within the United States as well as any territory under United States' jurisdiction.
2. The OSH Act does not apply to:
    a. Self-employed persons
    b. Family farms
    c. Industries regulated by other federal agencies, such as mining, nuclear, or air transportation
    d. State and local governments

B. Occupational Safety and Health Administration (OSHA)
1. OSHA is a federal agency within the Department of Labor that has responsibility for enacting, administering, and enforcing standards to provide for workplace health and safety.
2. A state may administer its own occupational health and safety program, provided that:
    a. OSHA approves the state program;
    b. The state's program includes state and local employees.
    c. (See Table 4-1 for list of states with Occupational Safety and Health Administrations.)
3. Promulgation of OSHA occupational health and safety standards
    a. Occupational health and safety standards must be reasonably necessary or appropriate to provide safe or healthful employment and places of employment.
    b. Standards are developed to eliminate or reduce risks; compliance must occur to the technological and economic extent possible.
    c. OSHA standards are developed by a public rule-making process that includes:
        1) Public notice
        2) Public hearings
        3) Public comment
    d. OSHA can implement emergency standards as proposed permanent standards effective for six months.

TABLE 4-1

States and Territories with Occupational Safety and Health Administrations

Alaska	Arizona	California
Hawaii	Indiana	Iowa
Kentucky	Maryland	Michigan
Minnesota	Nevada	New Mexico
North Carolina	Oregon	Puerto Rico
South Carolina	Tennessee	Utah
Vermont	Virginia	Virgin Islands
Washington	Wyoming	

Connecticut and New York have plans that cover state and local government employees only.

Note: Employers should contact their state agency to determine the most current status of a state regulated OSHA

Source: Levy & Wegman (1995).

4. Examples of OSHA standards include the Bloodborne Pathogens Standard, Asbestos Standard, Lead Standard, and Hazard Communication Standard.
5. General Duty Clause of OSH Act: Employers are required to furnish all employees "employment and a place of employment which are free from recognized hazards that are causing or are likely to cause death or serious physical harm."
   a. The General Duty Clause can be invoked for hazards not covered by an OSHA standard.
   b. The general duty obligation is an important means of protecting workers since setting standards is often a slow process.
6. OSHA is authorized to enforce established standards by performing inspections, with or without advance notice to the employer.
   a. Inspections may include record review, walk-through, and/or employee interview.
   b. OSHA has established a system of inspection priorities that occur in the following order (USDL, 1995):
      • Imminent danger situations, that is, when there is reasonable certainty that danger exists that can be expected to cause death or serious physical harm immediately, or before the danger can be eliminated through normal enforcement procedures
      • Fatalities and catastrophes resulting in hospitalization of three or more employees; these situations must be reported to OSHA by the employer within eight hours of the incident
      • Employee complaints of alleged violation of standards or of unsafe or unhealthful working conditions
      • Planned inspections aimed at specific high hazard industries, occupations, or substances
      • Random inspections of low hazard and nonmanufacturing worksites
      • Follow-up inspections to determine if previously cited violations have been corrected
   c. Employees or authorized employee representatives may request OSHA to perform an inspection.
      • If an inspection occurs, the employer has a right to see a copy of the complaint.
      • The employee's name will be withheld from the complaint if the employee requests.
   d. Inspections can occur without advance notice; however, employers have a right to refuse entry without a court order.
   e. OSHA may issue citations identifying violations and specifying the penalty associated with each violation.
7. OSHA also provides consultative services: employers can request an OSHA consultation to:
   a. Identify and correct hazards
   b. Provide technical assistance related to worksite hazards
   c. Provide education and training to health and safety personnel
8. In 1988, the first occupational health nurse was hired by OSHA.
   a. Purpose: to have nursing input into policy making
   b. An Occupational Health Nurse Intern Program was introduced in 1989; it is available to nurses in graduate school who are specializing in occupational health.
   c. In 1993, the Office of Occupational Health Nursing was formally recognized and established (see Appendix E for address).

C. Occupational Safety and Health Review Commission (OSHRC)
  1. OSHRC is an "independent" regulatory commission, authorized by the OSH Act, whose members are appointed by the President with Senate approval.
  2. OSHRC is responsible for handling the appeals filed by employers who have received OSHA citations.
     a. Employers must file a Notice of Contest within 15 days of receiving an OSHA citation.
     b. OSHRC assigns the appeal to an administrative appeal judge.
     c. Appeal of an OSHRC decision is made to a U.S. Court of Appeals.
D. National Institute for Occupational Safety and Health (NIOSH)
  1. NIOSH is an institute within the Centers for Disease Control and Prevention, U.S. Department of Health and Human Services.
  2. NIOSH conducts or funds occupational health and safety research in order to:
     a. Establish safe levels of toxic materials
     b. Form the basis for OSHA standards
  3. NIOSH also provides training and education to occupational health and safety professionals.

V

Equal Employment Opportunity Commission (EEOC)

A. EEOC is a federal administrative agency responsible for implementing and enforcing federal legislation relating to discrimination issues, such as affirmative action, disabilities, and drug use in the workplace.

B. Affirmative action issues are generally limited to age, sex, race, religion.

VI

Americans with Disabilities Act of 1990 (ADA)

A. The ADA was intended to counter the effects of discrimination for disabled individuals; its employment provision prohibits discrimination of an otherwise qualified individual on account of a disability. (See Chapter 3 for ADA definitions.)
  1. A person is qualified if he or she can perform the essential functions of the job with or without "reasonable accommodations."
  2. Title I of the ADA applies to the following employment activities: application procedures, hiring, firing, transfers, promotion, training, and employment-related health care activities (AAOHN, 1994b).
  3. Employment-related health care activities include: health data collection, drug screening, determination of job suitability, and confidentiality of health records (AAOHN, 1994b).
  4. The Equal Employment Opportunity Commission (EEOC) has enforcement responsibility for Title I.
B. According to the ADA, a disabled individual is a person who:
  1. Has a physical or mental impairment that substantially limits one or more major life activities,
  2. Has a record of such an impairment, or
  3. Being regarded as having such an impairment.
C. As of July 26, 1994, the ADA applies to a "covered entity" with more than 15 employees; "covered entity" includes private and public employers, labor unions, and joint labor-management committees.

D. ADA requirements for preplacement health assessments
  1. Must be performed after an applicant has been offered a position
  2. Can only evaluate the applicant's ability to perform the identified critical functions of the job being offered
E. Approach to Reasonable Accommodation (AAOHN, 1994b)
  1. Decisions regarding reasonable accommodation should be made by a multidisciplinary team that includes health and safety professionals, human resources, and management.
  2. The affected employee should be consulted regarding accommodations.
  3. Community resources and national agencies can provide information that can assist with the process of accommodation.
  4. The "reasonableness" of accommodation is based on cost and impact on the business.

VII

Drug-Free Workplace Act of 1988

This act applies to all federal grantees and contractors who receive contracts worth more than $25,000.

A. The act mandates that federal contractors and grant recipients:
  1. Notify employees that the unlawful manufacture, distribution, dispensing, possession, or use of a controlled substance is prohibited in the workplace
  2. Specify actions to be taken against employees for violating this prohibition
  3. Establish a drug awareness program
  4. Provide employees with a copy of the policy statement
B. The employee's responsibilities are as follows:
  1. Abide by the terms of the policy statement
  2. Notify the employer within five days of any criminal conviction for a drug statute violation occurring in the workplace
C. The act does not require drug testing as part of the employer's drug-free workplace program.

VIII

Department of Transportation Drug and Alcohol Testing

A. Omnibus Transportation Employee Testing Act of 1991 requires alcohol and drug testing of safety-sensitive employees in the aviation, motor carrier, railroad, and mass transit industries (see Table 4-2).
B. The DOT published rules (49 CFR Part 40) mandating antidrug and alcohol misuse prevention programs in February and August 1994.
C. The DOT rules include a drug and alcohol testing procedure rule, which establishes procedures for drug testing and breath alcohol testing (see Chapter 12: Drug and Alcohol Testing Program).
D. All drug and alcohol testing results and records are maintained under strict confidentiality by the employer, the drug testing laboratory, and the medical review officer.

TABLE 4-2

Safety-Sensitive Employees Covered by the Department of Transportation (DOT) Omnibus Transportation Employee Testing Act of 1991

DOT/Industry	Covered Safety-Sensitive Employees
Federal Highway Administration (FHWA)/Commercial	Holders of commercial drivers' licenses Commercial Vehicle Drivers
Federal Aviation Administration (FAA)/Aviation	Flight crews, attendants, instructors, air traffic controllers, aircraft dispatchers, maintenance personnel, screening, ground security
Federal Railroad Administration (FRA)/Railroads	Hours of Service Act employees, engine train and signal services, dispatchers, operators
Federal Transit Administration (FTA)/Mass Transit workers	Vehicle operators, controllers, maintenance workers
Research and Special Programs Administration (RSPA)/Pipelines	Operations, maintenance, emergency response personnel
United States Coast Guard (USCG)/Maritime*	Crew members, operating commercial vessels

*USCG has limited, existing rules that require drug testing and post-accident testing
Source: USDOT, FHWA Transportation Facts, Office of Public Affairs, February 3, 1994

IX

Family and Medical Leave Act (FMLA) of 1993 (29CFR825.118)

A. FMLA requires employers with 50 or more employees to provide up to 12 weeks of unpaid leave in any 12-month period in the following situations (AAOHN, 1995):
   1. The birth of the employee's child
   2. Adoption or foster placement of a child with the employee
   3. The employee is needed to care for a parent, spouse, or child with a serious health condition.
   4. The employee is unable to perform job functions because of a serious health condition.

B. Eligibility requires that the employees complete at least 12 months of employment and a total of 1,250 hours during the 12 months immediately prior to the leave.

C. Rights and responsibilities under FMLA (AAOHN, 1995)
   1. The employee will have the right to return to the same or equivalent position with equivalent benefits, compensation, and conditions of employment.
   2. The employee has a responsibility to provide employer with reasonable notice of the leave of at least 30 days when foreseeable.
   3. The employer has the right to require medical certification to support the employee's claim for leave related to health conditions of self or a family member.
   4. The employer has a responsibility to keep and maintain records regarding compliance with the act; they must also conspicuously post notice containing information about the FMLA.

D. Limitations of FMLA (AAOHN, 1995)
   1. Many employees are not aware of this law or its application to them.

    2. About half the workforce work in establishments with less than 50 employees; thus, they are not eligible for its benefits.

    3. Many employees cannot afford to take advantage of this unpaid leave.

X

Agency for Toxic Substances and Disease Registry (ATSDR)

A. The ATSDR is responsible for carrying out health-related respponsibilities of four federal statutes (Van Nostrand Reinhold, 1990)

    1. The Comprehensive Environmental Response, Compensations, and Liability Act of 1980 (CERCLA or "Superfund") which was amended as the Superfund Amendments and Reauthorization Act (SARA) of 1986 (see XI, C.)

    2. The Resource Conservation and Recovery Act of 1976 (RCRA), which was amended in 1984

    3. The Solid Waste Disposal Act, as amended by the Medical Waste Tracking Act (MWTA) of 1988

B. The functions of ATSDR include the provision of specialized services as follows (Van Nostrand Reinhold, 1990):

    1. Health assessment that consists of the evaluation of data and information on the release of hazardous substances into the environment

        a. Health assessments are used to assess any current or future effect of hazardous substances on public health.

        b. Health assessments provide information that is used in health advisories or other health recommendations.

        c. Health assessments help to identify studies or actions that are needed to evaluate and mitigate the human health effects of hazardous substances.

    2. Health consultations that are responses from ATSDR to specific questions or requests for information pertaining to hazardous substances or a hazardous facility

    3. Other functions and services including the development of toxicologic profiles of hazardous substances, health effects research, exposure and disease registries, emergency responses, health education, and case studies

XI

Environmental Protection Agency (EPA)

A. The EPA is an independent federal agency established in 1970 to protect the nation's environment from air and water pollution.

    1. The EPA establishes and enforces environmental protection standards such as the Toxic Substances Control Act (TSCA) and the Superfund Amendments and Reauthorization Act (SARA).

    2. The EPA conducts research on the effects of pollution.

B. Toxic Substances Control Act (TSCA) (40 CFR 717)

    1. Became effective in 1976

    2. Purpose: reduce the risk of injury to health or to the environment associated with the manufacture, processing, distributing, use, and disposal of chemical substances

    3. Requires manufacturers to provide information on any significant risks of chemicals they market

    4. Requires EPA approval of the manufacture and importing of "new" chemical substances (Travers & McDougall, 1995)

C. Superfund Amendments and Reauthorization Act (SARA)
1. Also known as SARA of 1986, Title III: amended the original Superfund Act, the Comprehensive Environmental Response, Compensation, and Liability Act of 1980.
2. Purpose: to provide for emergency planning in the community and training of workers who are either exposed to hazardous wastes or who must respond to emergencies related to hazardous wastes
3. Requires employers of facilities that manufacture or use hazardous substances to develop an emergency preparedness plan
4. Provides information on specific chemical emergency health treatment, even if this information is a trade secret.

Documentation and Recordkeeping in the Occupational Setting
XII

Documentation

Documentation is the written communication of information that is the basis of the legal occupational health record.

A. Purposes of documentation
1. Provides information to assist in planning care, for example, what measures have been implemented and the results of those measures
2. Provides a means to audit the quality of care and adherence to established policies and procedures
3. Establishes a frame of reference to gauge improvement or worsening of the client's condition
4. May be used as the basis for retrospective, current, or prospective research
5. Provides information which can be used for educational purposes

B. Characteristics of documentation
1. Documentation must be complete; if it wasn't written, it wasn't done.
2. Health documentation should be presented in a concise, descriptive, technical writing style, using accepted health abbreviations and terminology.
3. Health documentation must be legible.
   a. Black ink should be used for all entries in the health records since other colors may not produce legible photocopies.
   b. Errors should be corrected by striking through the notation with a single line and writing "error" above the notation; white-out or other correction techniques should never be utilized.
4. Stereotypes, generalizations, and judgmental statements should be avoided. For example, rather than "seems uncomfortable" ask the client to identify how much pain they are experiencing using a pain scale from 1 to 10.
5. Health documentation should be contemporaneous with the assessment performed or done as soon afterwards as possible.
   a. Information that was inadvertently omitted should be documented as soon as possible.
   b. Late entries should be preceded by the notation: "late entry."
   c. Late entries should identify the date of each entry and the date of the data being documented.

XIII

Types of Records

A. Occupational Safety and Health Administration Records

  1. The OSH Act requires most private sector employers with 11 or more employees at any time in a calendar year to prepare and maintain records of work-related injuries and illnesses. (See Table 4-3 for Standard Industrial Classification Codes for selected industries.)
  2. Recordable occupational injuries and illnesses resulting from a work accident or exposure include:
     a. Cases that result in a death
     b. Cases that result in an illness
     c. Cases that result in injury that involve:
        • Medical treatment other than first aid (Box 4-1)
        • Loss of consciousness
        • Restriction of work or body motion
        • Transfer to another job
        • Complication requiring medical treatment

TABLE 4-3

Standard Industrial Classification (SIC) Codes for Selected Industries

Industry	SIC Codes
Agriculture, forestry, and fishing	01–02 and 07–09
Oil and gas extraction	13 and 1477
Construction	15–17
Manufacturing	20–39
Transportation and public utilities	41–42 and 44–49
Wholesale trade	50–51
Building materials and garden supplies	52
General merchandise and food stores	53 and 54
Hotels and other lodging places	70
Repair services	75 and 76
Health services	80

BOX 4-1

Comparison of Medical Treatment and First Aid

Medical Treatment is any treatment, other than first aid (which is defined here), administered to injured employees. Medical treatment involves the provision of medical or surgical care for injuries that are not minor, through the specific application of procedures or systematic therapeutic measures.

First Aid is any one-time treatment and may include a follow-up visit for the purpose of observation of minor scratches, cuts, burns, splinters, and so forth, which do not ordinarily require medical care.

3. Employers and individuals not required to maintain OSHA injury and illness records include the following:
   a. Private employers, such as self-employed individuals, partners with no employees, and employers of domestics in the employers' private residences
   b. Employers engaged in the conduct of religious services or rites
   c. State and local government agencies are usually exempt; however, in certain states, agencies of the state and local governments are required to keep injury and illness records in accordance with state regulations.
4. Occupational health nurses are often responsible for ensuring that proper records are kept, and thus they must have current and up-to-date knowledge of record-keeping rules and regulations of OSHA (federal and state) and other regulatory agencies.

B. Employee exposure records include the following:
   1. Records of environmental (workplace) monitoring or measuring of a toxic substance or harmful physical agent
   2. Records reporting the results of biological monitoring
   3. Material Safety Data Sheets
   4. Chemical inventory or any other record that reveals the identity (e.g., chemical, common, or trade name) of a toxic substance or harmful physical agent as well as where and when the substance is (or was) used

C. The employee health (medical) record concerns the health status of an employee and is established and maintained by a physician, nurse, or other health care personnel.
   1. Content of employee health record may include (Table 4-4):
      a. Data include work injury/illness and follow-up care, physical assessments, diagnostic procedures, medications administered, consent forms, progress notes, and recommendations.
      b. The employee's health record does not include records concerning health insurance claims, records created solely in preparation for litigation, or voluntary employee assistance programs (EAP).
   2. Source of information includes (AAOHN, 1996):
      a. Routine health evaluations, such as preplacement, surveillance, and fitness for duty

TABLE 4-4

Example of Occupational Health Documentation Content

Criteria	Description
Reason for Visit	Why client is seeing you
Subjective Assessment	Location, quality, quantity, timing, setting, aggravating and alleviating factors, associated manifestations
Objective Assessment	Inspection, percussion, palpation, auscultation
Diagnosis	Medical versus nursing
Treatment/Plan	Diagnostic studies to be performed, medications prescribed, oral and/or written instructions, teaching, counseling, referral, follow-up

Source: Bates, (1995).

   b. Treatment of injuries and illnesses (whether related to work or not)
   c. Health promotion and disease prevention activities, such as cholesterol or
      blood pressure screening
3. A written policy for the management, access, and retention of individual
   health records should be in place; the policy should address (AAOHN, 1996):
   a. Where and how records are stored and secured
   b. Managing records when an employee resigns, transfers, or is terminated
   c. Mechanism for employee access and consent for disclosure
4. Employees' health records should be maintained in a secure place (i.e.,
   locked files) in the exclusive custody and control of company occupational
   health professionals (AAOHN, 1996).

XIV

Preservation of Employee Health (Medical) and Exposure Records

A. OSHA requires that certain health records must be retained for at least 30 years
plus the employee's term of employment.
   1. Records of injuries that involve health treatment, loss of consciousness, re-
      striction of work or motion, or transfer to another job are retained.
   2. Records of first aid or one-time treatment and subsequent observation of
      minor scratches, cuts, burns, splinters, and the like do not have to be retained.
   3. The health record of an employee who has worked for less than one year
      need not be retained beyond the term of employment if they are provided to
      the employee upon the termination of employment.

B. An employee's exposure records and analyses using the health and exposure
records are to be kept for at least 30 years beyond the worker's term of employment (AAOHN, 1996).

C. Biological monitoring records must be kept as specified by OSHA standards.

D. Records may be preserved in any manner (including microfilm) as long as the
information contained in the record is preserved and retrievable. Note: Chest X-
ray films shall be preserved in their original state.

XV

Access to Employee Medical and Exposure Records

A. OSHA Access to Employee Exposure and Medical Records Standard (29CFR-
1910.20) requires that employee or representative have access to records:

(NOTE: While this standard uses the term "Medical" Records, these records
may also contain health information which is non-medical in nature; thus, in
this publication, these records are called "health" records except when reference
is made to published documents that use the term "Medical" record.)

   1. In a reasonable manner and place
   2. Free of charge within 15 working days of the initial request
   3. Employer must make provisions for copying of records.

B. The employee should sign a written consent prior to release of health information (see Figure 4-1 for sample of authorization letter); the authorization must
include the following information:

1. What records are to be released, including dates of services
2. Purpose of release
3. To whom the records are to be released
4. Period of time for which authorization is valid
5. Date of authorization
6. Authority by which a person is requesting records
7. Identifying data of employee, including date of birth and social security number
8. Signature of person requesting records
9. Signatures of witnesses present

FIGURE 4-1   *Authorization Letter for the Release of Employee Medical Record Information to a Designated Representative*

I, _____ (name of worker/patient), hereby authorize _____

(individual or organization holding the medical records) to release the following medical information from my personal medical records (describe generally the information desired to be released):

_____

_____

_____

I give permission for this medical information to be used for the following purposes:

_____

_____

(Note: Several extra lines are provided below so that you can place additional restriction on this authorization letter if you want to. You may, however, leave these lines blank. On the other hand, you may want to (1) specify a particular expiration date for this letter (if less than one year); (2) describe the medical information to be created in the future that you intend to be covered by this authorization letter; or (3) describe the portions of the medical information in your records which you do not intend to be released as a result of this letter.)

_____

_____

_____

_____

_____

Full name of Employee or Legal Representative

_____

Signature of Employee or Legal Representative

Date of Signature _____

Source: OSHA 29 CFR 1910.20

C. Request for health records with a subpoena signed by an attorney is not a substitute for an authorization for release of health records.

D. Under no circumstances should the original health record, reports, or X-rays be released to the employee or representative before consulting with corporate legal counsel.

E. If it is believed that access to information contained in the records regarding a specific diagnosis of a terminal illness or a psychiatric condition could be detrimental to the employee's health, the employer may:
  1. Inform the employee that access will only be provided to a designated representative of the employee having specific written consent, and
  2. Deny the employee's request for direct access to this information only.

F. The occupational health nurse should notify an employer representative, preferably in the risk management department, whenever there is a request for records.

G. An employer may withhold trade secret information but must provide information needed to protect employee health; when it's necessary to release a trade secret, the employer may require a written agreement as a condition of release.

H. Each employee must be notified when beginning employment and at least annually thereafter of:
  1. The existence, location, and availability of any records covered by the OSHA Access to Employee Exposure and Medical Record Standard (29 CFR 1910.20)
  2. The person responsible for maintaining and providing access to records
  3. Right of access of the employee or a designated representative to these individual health and exposure records

I. All health and exposure records subject to 29 CFR 1910.20 must be transferred to the successor employer, to reserve and maintain these same records.

Workers' Compensation
XVI
Background Information

A. The workers' compensation system is intended to replace monetary loss resulting from injuries that occur as a result of a work-related injury, including the following:
  1. Salary continuation for disabled workers during actual disability
  2. Support for dependents in the event of occupational-related death
  3. Hospital, medical, and funeral expenses

B. In exchange for providing this salary continuation, the employer is immune from further legal action; that is, there is no employer negligence or fault.

XVII
Federal and State Programs

A. Federal civilian employees are covered by federal laws.

B. Each state and the District of Columbia have workers' compensation programs that apply to employees within their respective jurisdictions.
  1. Each jurisdiction has a workers' compensation statute.
  2. Courts in each jurisdiction interpret the language of their workers' compensation statute.

C. Work-related injuries and illnesses arise in the course of and out of employment.
  1. Compensable injuries are defined by statute in each jurisdiction and must be work-related.
  2. Compensable diseases are defined by statute, which may specifically identify conditions recognized within that jurisdiction.
      a. Identifying occupational disease can be complex and very difficult due to any of the following:
          • Time elapsed between exposure and onset of illness
          • Insidious onset of the illness
          • Multifactorial nature of the illness
          • Obscurity of exposure due to the inability to detect low levels of toxic substances
      b. Compensation for occupational diseases may require compliance with specified schedules.

D. Work-related disability can result from either work-related injury or illnesses that are rated by duration and degree of resulting disability.
  1. Disability is a legal concept determined by the state statutes.
      a. Legal disability is determined by the court or workers' compensation agency in evaluating a case.
      b. Impairment is a medical determination that includes the objective loss of body function.
  2. The duration of disability can be either permanent or partial.
  3. The degree of disability is the extent of disability, either temporary or total.
  4. The administrative determination of disability may be facilitated by an independent medical evaluation (IME), where another physician evaluates the employee and provides an opinion regarding:
      a. The employee's health condition
      b. Whether the employee can return to work
      c. Recommendation of physical limitations
      d. The length of time that the employee will be off work
      e. Recommendation of current and future treatment
      f. The etiology of the health condition
  5. When the ill or injured employee seeks to return to work, the employer must take into consideration any potential Americans with Disability Act implications. (See ADA discussion in Section VI.)
  6. Strategies for returning the employee to work include:
      a. Return-to-work programs that plan for progressively re-incorporating the injured or ill employee into the work setting
      b. Work-conditioning or work-hardening programs which are defined by the Commission on Accreditation of Rehabilitation Facilities (CARF) as ". . . a highly structured, goal-oriented, individualized treatment program designed to maximize the person's ability to return to work. Work hardening programs are interdisciplinary in nature with a capability of addressing the functional, physical, behavioral and vocational needs of the person served."
      c. Transfer to a different job with the same employer
      d. Transfer to a different job with a different employer
      e. Complete (100%) recovery with no work restrictions

Ethics and the Occupational Health Nurse

XVIII

Professional Position on Ethics

A. AAOHN Standards of Occupational Health Nursing Practice, Standard V, Ethics: The Occupational Health Nurse uses an ethical framework as a guide for decision making in practice (AAOHN, 1994a).

1. Occupational health nurses are confronted with complex ethical dilemmas that require careful communication with both management and the recipients of care.
2. An ethical framework provides the parameters within which the nurse makes ethical judgments.
3. The occupational health nurse is an advocate for clients to receive accessible, equitable, and quality health services, including a safe and healthful work environment.

B. The AAOHN Code of Ethics (Appendix B) provides the ethical framework for conduct by the occupational health nurse.

XIX

Ethics: Definitions and Principles

A. Definitions
1. *Ethics:* the philosophical study of conduct and moral judgment
2. *Morals:* principles of right and wrong
3. *Morality:* Society's expectations as to what people should or should not do
4. *Value:* worth or goodness
5. *Moral justification:* the reason for conduct

B. Ethical principles
1. *Autonomy* means self-governance: the ability to make individual decisions and choices, to act, and to think; self-determination
2. *Nonmaleficence* is the principle of doing no harm to others.
3. *Beneficence* is the principle of acting to do good for others.
4. *Distributive justice* means that benefits should be equally distributed and equally shared; there are three types of equality:
   a. Equality of moral worth
   b. Equality of opportunity
   c. Equality of outcome

C. Other principles important to occupational health nursing practice:
1. *Confidentiality* is the implicit promise that information divulged to another will be respected and not released or repeated (see Section XX.A).
2. *Veracity* is the observance of truth.
3. *Honesty* means freedom from deceit.
4. *Promise-keeping* is the act of following through on a pledge.
5. *Integrity* refers to unimpaired moral principles.

D. The value of nursing ethics in occupational health nursing lies in:
1. Recognition of the nurse's own values
2. Recognition of clients' values
3. Assisting clients to articulate their own values
4. Facilitating client's exercise of informed consent based upon their own values

$\overline{\underline{XX}}$

Ethical Conflicts

A. Confidentiality

1. Employers are charged with the responsibility for maintaining the occupational health and safety records of their employees.
2. The occupational health nurse is an agent of the employer; the occupational health nurse is charged with providing occupational health services to employees and maintaining health records; the occupational health nurse has a duty to:
   a. Document care or services provided to a client
   b. Maintain the confidentiality of the client's health records
3. If asked to divulge information contained in an employee's health records or to provide health records, the occupational health nurse should consider the following issues:
   a. For what purpose is the information being sought?
   b. Is the requested information work-related or not?
   c. Who is requesting the information?
   d. Is the requested information aggregate data or individual data?
   e. Why was the information gathered?
   f. Is the information being sought pursuant to an authorization for release of health records signed by the employee?
4. Unauthorized release of health records could result in personal liability, suspension of license to practice nursing by the state agency responsible for regulating the practice of nursing, or termination of employment by the employer.

B. Conflicts of interest and other ethical dilemmas

1. The occupational health nurse has multiple roles in the workplace, including employee, health care provider, client advocate, and co-worker; these multiple roles may result in ethical dilemmas that require a choice between two or more compelling ethical or moral values.
2. The occupational health nurse may be asked to provide the employer with information about the health needs of employees for use in developing health benefit plans, planning health education programs, and identifying worksite health issues.
   a. The occupational health nurse may be involved in prioritizing program needs.
   b. The occupational health nurse may participate in the decision-making process regarding allocation of scarce economic and personnel resources among work-site health programs.
3. The occupational health nurse may provide non-work-related health care, such as periodic health assessments and screening programs.
   a. The occupational health nurse must document the results of these evaluations and retain such documentation as health records.
   b. The occupational health nurse has an ethical and legal duty to maintain the confidentiality of the employee's non-work-related health information.
   c. Release of non-work-related health records requires an authorization for release of health records signed by the client whose records are being released.

BIBLIOGRAPHY

American Association of Occupational Health Nurses (1994a). *AAOHN Standards of Occupational Health Nursing Practice.* Atlanta: AAOHN Publications.

American Association of Occupational Health Nurses. (1994b). *The Americans with Disabilities Act.* AAOHN Advisory. Atlanta, GA: AAOHN Publications.

American Association of Occupational Health Nurses. (1995). *The Family Medical Leave Act.* AAOHN Advisory. Atlanta, GA: AAOHN Publications.

American Association of Occupational Health Nurses. (1996). *Employee health records: Requirements, retention, and access.* AAOHN Advisory. Atlanta, GA: AAOHN Publications.

Americans with Disabilities Act. (1990). P.L. 101-356, 42 U.S.C. §12101 et seq.

Bates, B. (1995). *A Guide to Physical Examination and History Taking.* Philadelphia: Lippincott.

Commission on Accreditation of Rehabilitation Facilities. (1992). *Standards Manual for Organizations Serving People with Disabilities.* Tucson, AZ: CARF.

DiBenedetto, D. V. (1995). *OEM Occupational Health & Safety Manual* (2nd ed). Boston, MA: OEM Press.

Equal Employment Opportunity Commission. (1992). *A technical assistance manual on the employment provisions (Title I) of the Americans with Disabilities Act.* EEOC-M-1A. Washington, DC, 1192: US Government Printing Office.

Furrow, B. R., Johnson, S. H., Jost, T. S., & Schwartz, R. L. (1991). *Liability and Quality Issues in Health Care.* St. Paul, MN: West.

Haas, T. F. (1987). On Reintegrating Workers' Compensation and Employers' Liability, *Georgia Law Review, 21,* 843.

Isernhagen, S. J. (1995). *The Comprehensive Guide to Work Injury Management.* Gaithersburg, MD: Aspen.

Larson, A. (1991). *The Law of Workmen's Compensation.* New York: Bender.

Levy, B. S., & Wegman, D. H. (1995). *Occupational Health: Recognizing and Preventing Work-Related Disease* (3rd ed.). Boston: Little, Brown and Company.

Mappes, T. A., & DeGrazia, D. (1996). *Biomedical Ethics* (4th ed.), New York: McGraw-Hill.

Pryor, E. S. (1990). Flawed Promises: A critical evaluation of the American Medical Association's Guides to the Evaluation of Permanent Impairment. *Harvard Law Review, 103,* 964.

Rogers, B. (1994). *Occupational Health Nursing Concepts and Practice.* Philadelphia: Saunders.

Shrey, D. E., & Lacerte, M. (1995). *Principles and Practices of Disability Management in Industry.* Winter Park, FL: GR Press.

Tate, D. (1992, June). Workers' Disability and Return to Work. *American Journal of Physical Med. & Rehabilitation, 71,* 92–96.

Travers, P. H., & McDougall, C. (1995). *Guidelines for an Occupational Health and Safety Service.* Atlanta, GA: AAOHN Publications.

U.S. Chamber of Commerce. (1993). *Analysis of Workers' Compensation Laws.*

U.S. Department of Labor, Occupational Safety and Health Administration. (1993). OSHA safety and health standards 29 CFR 1910.000, et seq. Washington DC: US Government Printing Office.

USDOT. (1994, February 3). *FHWA Transportation Facts,* Office of Public Affairs.

Veatch, R. (1986). *The Foundations of Justice.* Oxford University Press.

Van Nostrand Reinhold (1990). *Health Hazards of the Workplace Report.* Vol. 1 (8).

CHAPTER

5

Economic, Political, and Business Forces

MAJOR TOPICS
- *Economic forces*
- *Political forces*
- *International trade*
- *Global marketplace*
- *Business trends*
- *Managed care*

Economic, political, and business forces (including that of managed care) shape the way business is conducted in both the national and the global marketplaces. It is essential that occupational health nurses understand the basics of the economics, political forces, and business trends that shape the business environment in which they practice. This chapter presents an overview of these trends and discusses how they can affect occupational health nursing practice.

Economic and Political Forces

Ī

Introduction to Economics

A. *Economics* is concerned with the way in which limited resources are allocated; specifically, it involves the following:
   1. Allocation and management of the income and expenditures of a household, business, community, or government:
      a. Production, distribution, and consumption of wealth
      b. Satisfaction of the material needs of people
   2. The study of the world economy that is essentially a macroeconomic survey
   3. Societal establishment of economic systems that serve as a means of achieving the society's economic goals

B. Key economic terms
   1. *Capitalism:* Allows private ownership of property; income from property or capital accrues to the individual or firms that accumulate it and own it; individual firms are relatively free to compete with others for their own economic gain; the profit motive is basic to economic life.

2. *Communism:* Production systems are government or state owned, and production decisions are made by official policy and not directed by market action.

3. *Consumer Price Index (CPI):* Measures price changes of goods consumed by an urban family of four on a moderate income; CPI is also known as the cost-of-living index.

4. *Disposable Income (DI):* The gross national product (GNP) minus depreciation, business and personal taxes, and transfer payments (such as social security, welfare payments, and so on); "the money in people's pockets" to spend as they want

5. *Federal Reserve Discount Rate:* The rate at which the Federal Reserve Bank lends funds to its member banks

6. *Gross National Product (GNP):* The total final value of domestic goods and services produced in a national economy over a particular period of time, usually for one year
   a. GNP is the primary indicator of the national economy.
   b. GNP measures production in the economy by aggregating all goods and services produced by their current prices, for example, bushels of fruits, numbers of automobiles sold.
   c. GNP measures only goods and services that have a market.
   d. International comparisons of GNP are difficult.
   e. GNP does not measure quality of life.

7. *Microeconomics:* Deals with the economic behavior of individual units such as consumers, firms, and resource owners

8. *Macroeconomics:* Concerned with the behaviors of economic aggregates, such as the gross national (domestic) product (national income), consumption, the level of employment, investment, money supply, inflation, and international trade and production relationships

9. *Net National Product:* The GNP less capital consumption allowance (allocated costs for depreciation of capital equipment)

10. *Political Economy:* A term used to describe macroeconomics due to the influence of political and social institutions on the aggregate economy

11. *Prime Rate:* The rate that banks charge their commercial customers (those with good credit ratings and lowest risk) for short-term loans

12. *Producer Price Index (PPI):* Measures wholesale price of goods

13. *Socialism:* An economic system in which government owns or controls many major industries, but may allow markets to set prices in many areas

C. Major economic systems include capitalism, socialism, and communism.

D. *Economic indicators* measure the relative standing of one economic system (country) versus that of another.
1. Economic indicators include the gross national (domestic) product (GNP), net national product, and disposable income (DI).
2. Price indicators that reflect a nation's economic standing include the consumer price index (CPI) and the producer price index (PPI).

E. *Labor force statistics* measure how many noninstitutionalized people are currently working at paid jobs or who are willing to work; it indicates the employable population of the economy.
1. Persons in the military, jails, hospitals/sanitariums (patients), and full-time students are excluded in calculations of the labor force.

2. Labor force statistics that include military personnel are also published.
3. Unemployment statistics indicate the number of people looking for paid work and indicates changes in the labor market.

F. *Interest rates* are a percentage of a sum of money charged for its use; two major types of interest rates are prime rate and federal reserve discount rate.

G. *Balance of trade* refers to a country's value of imports and exports of merchandise.
1. The balance of trade consists of transactions in merchandise (such as automobiles, computers, etc.).
2. When a country exports more than it imports, it has a surplus, or *favorable*, balance of trade.
3. When a country's imports predominate, the balance of trade is in deficit and is called *unfavorable*.

II

Economic State of the Nation

A. During the 1980s, America's economy grew or "expanded" due to the following:
1. Decreased taxation (tax cuts) on business and citizens
2. Deregulation of businesses such as telecommunications, air travel, banking, and many others
3. Increased consumer spending, investment, and construction
4. The beginning trend of privatizing government services toward the end of the 1980s

B. The government release of money to the private sector, along with deregulation of business, made the 1980s the longest period of peacetime growth (Bagby, 1995).

C. Government cuts in spending did not keep pace with the growth of the national economy.
1. Tax cuts had a negative impact on government revenue.
2. Planned spending and reform of national entitlement programs, such as Medicare/Medicaid and Social Security, were not politically supported.
3. Entitlement program cuts were not large enough to cover the reduction in tax revenue.
4. American government started to spend more than it took in; this gave rise to deficit spending by the government, resulting in high deficits.

D. The United States went from the largest creditor nation to the largest debtor nation in the global economy.

E. Negative effects on Americans living with high national budget deficits include (Bagby, 1995):
- Higher interest rates
- Less investment
- Lower economic growth rate
- Lost revenue to pay interest on debt
- Being a debtor to foreign countries
- Lower sales of exports
- Long-term decrease in the standard of living for citizens

F. By the end of the 1980s, the American economy was in a recession.

III

The Impact of Economics on the Individual

A. In unstable, poorly functioning economies:
1. People have difficulty finding jobs that match their abilities and education.
2. Continually rising prices render savings worthless, thus affecting the ability of people, especially retirees, to survive.
3. The manager of a firm in a poorly functioning economy may have difficulty obtaining a sufficient quantity or quality of materials for the company at a reasonable price.
4. A company may have difficulty distributing its products and finding buyers able to purchase them.
5. Investment opportunities may be hard to find in a depressed economy.
6. Expending accumulated personal assets may be very difficult, since available goods and services may be limited or of poor quality.

B. In a thriving economy, both individuals and society as a whole can benefit from the efficient production of goods and services.
1. People are working (society may be at the level of full employment, and unemployment levels are low).
2. Families are receiving income and are consumers of goods and services that they need and/or want.
3. Economic progress gives people access to technologically advanced products.
4. A strong market for technologically advanced products stimulates research and investment for further technological progress.
5. A well-functioning economy is attractive to foreigners for investment of capital or purchasing goods.
6. A stable, advancing economy aids social progress in the following ways:
   a. More students pursue higher levels of education.
   b. Although students are absent from the workforce while in school, they enter the workforce at a higher level of skill and knowledge.
   c. Well-educated workers function at a higher productivity level and thus benefit the economy.

C. A thriving economy allows managers to:
1. Plan production and personnel programs with reasonable confidence that they will reap the benefits of the economy and projections for sales, productivity costs, and profits
2. Evaluate company and individual performance factors that have an impact on their "bottom line" without being hindered by an unstable economy
3. Expand businesses or add personnel to payroll

D. A well-run economy facilitates the production and exchange of goods and services.

IV

Changes in the National Economy

The transition in the national economy is from protected markets to international competition.

A. Economic competitiveness depends on a nation's financial, industrial and demographic characteristics, such as its unemployment rate, GNP, per capita income, average hours and conditions of work, and distribution of wealth (Potter & Youngman, 1995).

B. The economic competitiveness of a nation depends on the ability of its individual businesses to sell their goods and services at a profit in both domestic (national) and foreign markets.

C. America's ability to prosper depends on the ability of U.S. companies to produce and market goods and services that can compete successfully in terms of price, quality, innovativeness, customization, and serviceability with those of other nations.

V

Factors Affecting National and Global Competitiveness
(Potter & Youngman, 1995)

A. After World War II, America became the leading economic power due to the destructive impact of the war on the economies of Japan and Europe.
 1. Post-war benefits, such as the GI Bill, provided housing and educational opportunities to returning veterans, thus creating a competitive labor force, boosting the construction industry, and encouraging local community development.
 2. National and global economies and industrialization surged from 1953 to 1975 increasing world industrial output an average of 6% a year.
 3. The post-war economic boom in the United States was facilitated by the deregulation of industry as well as industrial developments and manpower planning that occurred during the war.
 4. Business, no longer hampered by wartime government constraints, returned to "free markets" and focused on meeting consumers' (rather than the government's) needs.

B. During the immediate post-war decades, the world was divided into domestic and international marketplaces.
 1. U.S. companies produced primarily for domestic or regional markets with minimal competition from imports and few multinational companies.
 2. American companies led the industrialized markets with increasing technological advances, mass production, and higher workers' wages through the 1970s.
 3. Government regulation and collective bargaining added to costs of American businesses.
 4. Europe, Japan, and the Pacific Rim countries, fully rebuilt after World War II, became increasingly competitive with the United States in the world market.

C. Customers both at home and abroad have become "global shoppers," seeking the best product at the most affordable price without regard to the country in which it was produced.

D. Imports to the United States grew 260% between 1975 and 1993, the increase fueled by increased American purchasing power.

E. U.S. exports account for:
 1. One out of every six American jobs in manufacturing
 2. $115 billion annually in services
 3. One-sixth of all U.S. agricultural production
 4. Overall, foreign trade accounts for almost 25% of America's GDP—over $1 trillion per year.
    a. Declining economic competitiveness means potentially fewer jobs, increased unemployment, lower per capita income, and larger budget deficits.

b. The economy entered into recession, and business retrenched during the 1970s, affecting manufacturing by decreasing mass production, job creation, wages, and employment levels.

c. The national economy expanded during the 1980s, but American manufacturing lost its competitive edge to foreign competitors who could produce goods at a lower cost than American companies.

d. The United States is no longer a primarily industrialized nation, a producer of manufactured goods; its economy depends more and more on the production of services and technology.

VI

International Trade Status of the Nation

A. Presently, the United States has a trade deficit: it imports more than it exports.

B. U.S. consumers buy more foreign products than foreigners buy U.S. goods.

C. Reasons for this trade imbalance include the following:
1. Some foreign countries have high trade barriers, making it difficult for the United States to sell products there.
2. The U.S. dollar has been high compared to other currencies, making it expensive for foreigners to buy American and inexpensive for Americans to buy foreign.
3. U.S. products are less competitive than foreign products in terms of price and availability.
4. U.S. services (such as architectural, engineering, and consulting) account for billions of dollars in trade, but are not accounted for in calculating the U.S. trade deficit.

D. The United States continues to produce one-fourth of the world's gross national product.

VII

The Global Marketplace

A. The global economy is becoming an integrated marketplace and is influenced by a variety of economic and political forces, such as the following:
1. General Agreement for Trade and Tariffs (GATT)
   a. GATT, which was created after World War II, works to reduce trade barriers and promote free trade among its member nations in the Free World.
   b. In 1994, the member nations of GATT agreed to create the World Trade Organization (WTO)—a more comprehensive and powerful organization to govern global trade in goods and services.
2. Unification of Europe to form the European Economic Community (EEC)
3. End of the "Cold War" and subsequent decline of communism
4. North American Free Trade Act (NAFTA), established in 1994, which opened up the borders of Canada, the United States, and Mexico to almost limitless trade.
   a. NAFTA will decrease trade barriers between the United States, Canada, and Mexico.
   b. NAFTA's long-term goal is to remove barriers to trade extending all the way from the state of Alaska to Argentina.
5. Increased economic growth of the Pacific Rim countries.

B. The world is moving toward "free trade," that is, trade without taxes or tariffs.

C. Fewer products are being produced entirely within any single nation; the world is moving towards a single economy—one marketplace (Naisbitt & Aberdene, 1990).

D. Economic and political forces are shaping a new globalized world.

VIII

Implications for the Occupational Health Nurse

A. The occupational health nurse is a company's primary resource regarding health care issues and the delivery of occupational health services.

B. Occupational health nurses ensure that the workforce is fit, healthy, and medically capable of performing work assignments, thus adding to the company's and the nation's productivity as well as ultimately to the GNP.

C. The role of the occupational health nurse will expand or contract throughout the business cycle and during periods of economic uncertainty (i.e., business contraction or expansion).

D. Occupational health practice will shift from the manufacturing sector to the service/technological sectors and will expand to include international issues of health and safety.

E. As the workforce expands past national borders (i.e., transfers to the geographical international market) the occupational health nurse will be responsible for:
  1. Ensuring the health of expatriates and their dependents: occupational health nursing duties may include:
      a. Immunizations for international travel
      b. Access to quality health care abroad
      c. Health education
      d. Psychological support systems (for example, access to employee assistance programs)
  2. Assisting with identifying international health and safety needs of the global workforce.
  3. Identifying national and international regulatory compliance issues that will affect the workforce, such as family leave and occupational health laws. (See Chapter 12 for sample International Travel program.)

Business Forces

IX

Business Trends

A. Megatrends (large social, economic, and technological trends) that shaped the 1980s in business include (Naisbitt and Aberdene, 1990):
  1. Shift from an industrial society to an information society
  2. Forced technology to high tech/high touch, for example, interactive technology
  3. National economy to a world economy
  4. Short-term to long-term planning
  5. Centralization to decentralization of company/business lines/units
  6. Institutional help to self-help
  7. Representative democracy to participatory democracy
  8. Hierarchies to networking teams
  9. Movement of business from northern states to southern states to save on labor and operating costs
  10. Limited options of "either/or" to multiple options

B. During the economic expansion in the 1980s, businesses invested, acquired additional product lines, and increased their workforces.
1. Many businesses established operations in southern states, where operating costs were lower.
2. Companies established decentralized business operations where operating divisions became dedicated "strategic business units," accountable for their own profits and losses.
3. Businesses merged "horizontally," acquiring companies that enhanced existing product lines.
4. During the latter part of the 1980s, the economy contracted, and business responded by:
   a. Divesting noncore or nonessential business units and product lines
   b. Downsizing workforces through layoffs or reorganizations
   c. Initiating vertical mergers (businesses acquiring similar businesses)

$\overline{\text{X}}$

Trends Impacting Business

Those trends that will affect both business and consumers in the 1990s (Naisbitt and Aberdene, 1990) include:

A. An expanding global economy

B. A renaissance in the arts

C. The emergence of free-market socialism

D. Global lifestyles and cultural nationalism

E. The privatization of the welfare state

F. The rise of the Pacific Rim nations

G. Increasing role of women in leadership

H. Advances in biology and genetics

I. The religious revival

J. Empowerment of the individual

$\overline{\text{XI}}$

Major Business Issues

A. Increased Federalism or regulatory constraints on business include mandatory compliance with regulations set forth by the following:
1. Occupational Safety and Health Administration (OSHA)
2. Department of Transportation (DOT)
3. Environmental Protection Agency (EPA)
4. Employee Retirement Income Security Act (ERISA)
5. Consolidated Omnibus Budget Reconciliation Act (COBRA)
6. Family Medical Leave Act (FMLA)
7. Americans with Disabilities Act (ADA)
8. State workers' compensation statutes

B. Cost shifting of social insurance programs (Social Security, Medicare, Medicaid) from government to privately funded sources.

C. Increasing costs of employee health and welfare benefits, such as workers' compensation and nonoccupational health and disability

D. Employers' trends such as:
1. Shift towards managed care for health benefit plans
2. Increased cost sharing of health care expenses and benefits with employees through increased deductibles and coinsurance rates, increasing their out-of-pocket expenditures
3. Increased involvement of employees in health-care decisions
4. Aggressive negotiation with health providers and packaging of provider services
5. Aggressive management of health care costs through utilization review, second opinions, pre-admission certification, concurrent review, case management, and retrospective reviews
6. Increased communication with employees regarding health care costs
7. Encouragement of managed care enrollments
8. Establishment of wellness programs
9. Emphasis on balancing employee work/lifestyle issues
10. Movement towards a "24-hour" system of health care—that is, the integration of occupational and nonoccupational medical care
11. Shift towards integrated benefits and disability management arrangements

E. Issues related to Workers' Compensation (DiBenedetto, 1996)
1. Estimated annual costs to the nation and business are $60 billion per year.
2. Direct costs of workers' compensation include medical care costs and indemnity (wage replacement) payments.
3. Indirect costs include: lost productivity, required replacement employee overtime, training, accident investigation, and broken equipment.
4. Identification and correction of the root causes of workers' compensation claims will facilitate a safer workplace and decrease workers' compensation claims, thus increasing workforce productivity.

F. Methods being used by businesses to control the cost of workers' compensation include (DiBenedetto, Harris, & McCunney, 1996):
1. Preclaim strategies, such as:
   - Assignment of responsibilities
   - Communications
   - Occupational safety and health programs
   - Injury prevention programs
   - Development of job responsibilities (essential functions and physical requirements)
   - Return-to-work programs
   - Identification of modified or transitional work assignments
   - Third-party administration (TPA) performance standards
   - Medical and case management requirements
   - Negotiated discounts of fee schedules and managed medical care arrangements
2. At-claim strategies, such as:
   - Immediate reporting of accidents to management and the carrier (TPA)
   - Timely accident investigation
   - Claim setup and initiation of medical and case management
   - Use of disability duration guidelines
   - Use of treatment guidelines or protocols
   - Use of independent medical examinations
   - Fraud investigation
   - Establishment of appropriate claim reserves

3. Post-claim strategies, such as:
    • Third Party Administration (TPA) audits
    • Utilization review
    • Quality assurance reviews
4. Additional trends include the integration of workers' compensation and non-occupational disability management to manage costs and facilitate the injured employee's return to work.

G. Increasing occurrence of violence in the workplace (see Chapter 3)

H. Need for advanced information technology and information processing

XII

Implications for Occupational Health Nursing
(DiBenedetto et al., 1996)

A. The occupational health nurse plays a primary role in helping the workforce attain its maximum level of health and thus adds to workforce productivity.

B. The occupational health nurse performs health care and management functions that vary according to the work setting, the employer's needs and expectations, the company philosophy, and the occupational health nurse's knowledge of the regulatory requirements that govern occupational health care, safety, and workers' compensation in that particular industry.

C. The occupational health nurse may have the following specific responsibilities:
1. Establish and implement health-related policies and procedures
2. Develop and maintain the company's regulatory compliance programs related to OSHA, EPA, DOT, ADA, FMLA, and workers' compensation requirements
3. Prevent injury and illness through health promotion and health education activities
4. Provide workers' compensation and nonoccupational case management (also referred to as integrated disability management), coordinate independent health examinations, arrange for second-opinion examinations, and perform case management functions to facilitate early return to work of ill and injured workers
5. Identify real and potential hazards in the workplace by conducting facility assessments and report those conditions to appropriate members of management for correction

D. The role of the occupational health nurse and funding for occupational health and safety programs will expand or contract throughout the business cycle.

E. Many companies continue to outsource occupational health and safety services; many occupational health providers are now contract providers or vendors.

F. As the workforce contracts through downsizing/layoffs, employees are most likely to file for workers' compensation; claims for on-the-job injuries may be fraudulent.

G. Occupational health nurses are increasingly involved in employee benefits, from evaluating plan sponsors, benefit components, use of second opinions, employee education and health promotion, lifestyle/life-skill education, and integration of health promotion to include family needs and requirements.

Managed Care

XIII

Health Care Reform and Managed Health Care

A. The major arguments for health care reform are these:
   1. The delivery of care is bogged down in administration and insurance underwriting.
   2. Health care costs are escalating.
   3. At least 37 million Americans lack health insurance or are underinsured.

B. Health reform components that have broad support include:
   1. A standard minimum benefit package
   2. Insurance market reform
   3. Health plan "report cards"
   4. Consumer choice of plans
   5. Voluntary purchasing pools

C. Major components of health care reform proposals have included insurance market reforms, cost containment mechanisms, managed care, and subsidies for low-income persons.

D. In past proposals, financing of health care reform would have come from employer or individual premium mandates or from voluntary plans that were based upon the present health care system.

E. Federal efforts to mandate health care reform failed to pass Congress in 1994.

F. Currently, market-driven reforms have moved the delivery of health care for the consumer from "free choice" to managed care.

XIV

Overview of Managed Care

A. *Managed care* is a broad concept generally applied to "pre-payment arrangement, negotiated discounts, and agreements for prior authorization and audits of performance" (Madison & Konrad, 1988, cited in Wassel, 1995).

B. Managed care plans generally provide some restrictions on the traditional unlimited access to providers and payment of reasonable and customary charges for their health care services (Wassel, 1995).

C. Managed care plans place responsibilities on both consumers and providers in the form of a binding contract (Wassel, 1995).

D. A managed care plan is any form of health plan that initiates selective contracting between providers, employers, and/or insurers to channel employees/patients to a specified set of cost-effective providers (a provider network). These providers have procedures in place to assure that only medically necessary and appropriate use of health care services occurs.

E. Three basic types of health care deliverers under managed care arrangements are the health maintenance organization (HMO), preferred provider organization (PPO), and point of service (POS) plan (Wassel, 1995).
   1. A *health maintenance organization (HMO)* provides a specified scope of services or benefits to members for a fixed fee.
      a. There are four types of HMOs: Staff, group, network, and independent practice associations (IPAs).
      b. HMOs provide 10-40% savings over traditional health plans.

2. A *preferred provider organization (PPO)* provides greater consumer choice through use of a limited provider panel, negotiated fee schedules, a utilization review, and the physician as gatekeeper.
   a. In exchange for reduced rates, providers frequently receive expedited claim payments and/or reasonable market share
   b. Employees have financial incentives to use PPO providers
3. A *point of service plan (POS)* is a health benefit plan through which several different types of insurance coverage are available. The employee chooses the insurance plan and provider at the time health care services are sought.
   a. POS plans provide incentives for employees to choose cost-effective providers.
   b. If managed care providers are not utilized by the employee, the extra cost of service is borne by the employee.

F. The *"24-hour"* model of health care incorporates both occupational (workers' compensation) and nonoccupational (disability) health care into one health care delivery system to improve continuity of care, manage and reduce claim costs, minimize redundancies in coverage, simplify adjudication, and reduce administrative efforts and costs. Approaches to 24-hour care include (Abbott, 1994):
1. 24-hour medical coverage where health benefits for all accidents or injuries fall under an integrated health plan. Disability or lost-time benefits would be paid by workers' compensation.
2. 24-hour disability coverage where disability benefits for both occupational and nonoccupational concerns would be paid from an integrated plan, but health payments would still be divided.
3. Integrated 24-hour medical and disability coverage where both medical and indemnity payments would be integrated under one plan.
4. *Accident only* and *sickness only* medical programs may also exist as a subset to these three major categories.

G. Managed workers' compensation is characterized by negotiated fee schedules, capitated rates, and the use of PPOs as well as other provider arrangements.

H. *Integrated disability management* is a comprehensive approach to integrating all disability benefits, programs, and services to help control the employer's disability costs while returning the employee to work as soon as possible and maximizing the employee's functional capacity (Mercer, 1995).

XV

Quality Controls in Managed Care
(Employee Benefit Research Institute [EBRI], 1995)

A. Maintaining the quality of health care is Americans' primary concern in the changing health care system.

B. Concern over health care cost inflation has led private employers and public programs to adopt various strategies to manage health care costs.

C. The aim of all these strategies is to purchase the highest quality health care at the lowest cost.

D. Defining and measuring health care quality are controversial and costly endeavors.

E. Health care quality can be viewed narrowly as clinical effectiveness.

F. Health care quality can be viewed in a broader sense as all the attributes of medical care that clients value.

XVI

Measuring the Quality of Care

Donabedian (1988) classified attempts to measure quality of care as studies of structure, process, and outcome.

A. *Structure* refers to attributes of care, such as caregiver's qualifications and resources available at the site of care.

B. *Process* examines the caregiver's activities, decisions made at various points in an episode of illness, and appropriateness of care.

C. *Outcome* measures the effects of care on health status and patient satisfaction.

XVII

Judging Standards of Care

Private organizations independently review quality standards in hospitals and other institutions and provide accreditation of those organizations.

A. Joint Commission for Accreditation of Healthcare Organizations (JCAHO)

B. Health Care Financing Administration (HCFA)

C. National Committee for Quality Assurance (NCQA)

D. Accreditation Association for Ambulatory Health Care

XVIII

Defining Quality Outcomes

A. Managed care relies on monitoring physicians' treatment patterns (through utilization review, physician profiling, and case management) and changing providers' financial incentives.

B. Health Plan Employer Data and Information Set (HEDIS) was established by the private sector (several employers and managed care organizations in 1989) as a tool for large purchasers of health care to use in judging the comparative value of competing health care plans. HEDIS:
1. Is a core set of performance measures that can be adapted to serve the needs of other purchasers
2. Provides benchmarks for performance in specific areas such as health plan quality, access and patient satisfaction, membership and utilization, finance and management, and activities
3. Relies primarily on structural and process measures of quality; major outcome measures are patient satisfaction and readmission rates for major disorders

C. Many analysts believe that the future evolution of the health care delivery system will be driven by the development of measures of the quality of care.

XIX

Implications for Occupational Health Nursing
(DiBenedetto et al., 1996)

A. Occupational health nurses are providing case management services, return-to-work planning, and management of integrated disability and workers' compensation services.

B. As market driven health care reform continues, the role and scope of occupational health nursing will expand into the managed care arena as an integrated model that combines both workers' compensation and disability management.

C. Occupational health nurses may be involved in the assessment, evaluation, and implementation of managed health care arrangements and programs.

D. Occupational health nurses will provide value-added knowledge and services as managed care vendors expand services into the occupational health/managed workers' compensation market.

E. Occupational health nurses will increasingly become involved in managed health care benefits for:
1. Employers
2. Employee populations
3. Managed health care vendors/organizations

F. Occupational health nurses may become the liaison between employer benefit plans and managed care organizations, thus facilitating lines of communication, professional cooperation, benefit services, and health care deliveries.

BIBLIOGRAPHY

Abbott, R. K. (1994, Sept/Oct). 24 Hour Medical Care: A Primer. *Innovations in Human Resources,* 12–14.

Bagby, M. E. (1995). *The First Annual Report of the United States of America: An Account to American Citizens of Where We Stand Economically, Socially, and Internationally.* New York: Harper Business.

DiBenedetto, D. V., Harris, J. S, & McCunney, R. J. (1996). *Occupational Health & Safety Manual,* (2nd ed.). Massachusetts: OEM Press.

Donabadien, A. (1988, Spring). Quality assessment and assurance: Unity of purpose, diversity of means. *Inquiry, 25,* 173–192.

Drucker, P. F. (1993). *Managing for the Future: The 1990s and Beyond,* (Sections 1C, 9A). New York: Truman Talley Books/Plume.

Drucker, P. F. (1989). *The New Realities: In Government and Politics/In Economics and Business/In Society and World View.* New York: Harper and Row.

Employee Benefit Research Institute (EBRI). (1995, March). *Measuring the Quality of Health Care, EBRI Brief No. 159*: Washington, DC: Author.

Epping, R. C. (1995). *A Beginner's Guide to World Economy.* New York: Vintage Books.

Friedman, J. P. (1987). *Dictionary of Business Terms.* New York: Barron's.

Heilbroner R., & Thurow, L. (1994). *Economics Explained: Everything You Need to Know About How the Economy Works and Where It's Going.* New York: Touchstone.

Katzenbach, J. R., & Smith, D. K. (1994). *The Wisdom of Teams: Creating the High Performance Organization.* New York: Harper Business.

Madison, D. L., & Konrad, T.R. (1988). Large medical group-practice organizations and employee physicians: A relationship in transition. *Milbank Memorial Quarterly, 66*(2), 240–282.

Mansfield, E. (1988). *Micro-Economics: Theory and Applications* (Shorter 6th ed.). New York: W. W. Norton & Company.

McRae, H. (1994). *The World in 2020: Power, Culture and Prosperity.* Boston: Harvard Business School Press.

Mercer, W. (1995). *The Language of Managed Disability.* New York: Mercer/Met Disability.

Naisbitt, J., & Aburdene, P. (1990). *Megatrends 2000: Ten New Directions for the 1990s.* New York: William Morrow & Company.

Peters, T. (1992). *Liberation Management: Necessary Disorganization for the Nanosecond Nineties.* New York: Fawcett Columbine.

Potter, E. E., & Youngman, J. A. (1995). *Keeping America Competitive: Employment Policy for the Twenty-First Century.* Lakewood, CO: Glenbridge Publishing Ltd.

Thurow, L. (1993). *Head to Head: The Coming Economic Battle Among Japan, Europe and America.* New York: Warner Books.

Traska, M. R. (1995). *Managed Care Strategies 1996.* New York: Faulkner and Gray.

Wassel, M. L. (1995). Occupational Health Nursing and the Advent of Managed Care: Meeting the Challenges of the Current Health Care Environment, *AAOHN Journal,* 43(1), 23–28.

Webster's New World Dictionary of Business Terms. (1985). New York: Simon & Schuster.

6

Principles of Administration and Management

MAJOR TOPICS

- *Leadership*
- *Strategic planning*
- *Managing occupational health services*
- *Tools for the occupational health nurse manager*
- *Information management systems*
- *Time management*
- *Evaluating occupational health services*
- *Total quality management*

Occupational health nurses must have leadership, management, and administrative skills to give the direction, provide the services, manage the resources, and document the outcomes related to employee health in the organization. As business and industry in America seek new solutions to the high cost of health care, these abilities will enable occupational health nurse managers to promote, maintain, and restore the health of workers and positively affect corporate profits.

Leadership and Strategic Planning

I̲

Leadership

Leadership is the "process of influencing the activities of an individual or a group in efforts toward the achievement of goals" (Adams, 1991, p. 22).

A. Leadership tasks include (Kouzes & Posner, 1987):
   1. Challenging the process
   2. Inspiring others to share a vision and see its exciting possibilities
   3. Enabling others to act by building teams based on trust and respect
   4. Modeling the way for others
   5. Recognizing individual and team achievements

B. Leadership styles include:
   1. Authoritarian/autocratic style, or a "do as I say" approach:
      a. Most effective in emergency situations
      b. Used when followers have little experience or limited motivation

2. Democratic/participative style:
   a. Most effective in long-term situations when followers are motivated and possess interpersonal and organizational skills
   b. Empowers followers through collaborative teamwork; focuses on communication and constructive relationships
3. Bureaucratic style, or "the book says so" approach:
   a. Often used by managers who do not tolerate creative problem-solving but rather want order and consistency in the way situations are handled day to day
   b. Tends to be impersonal
4. Laissez-faire, or permissive, style, sometimes called "anything goes":
   a. Allows for a full utilization of talents; may work well with highly motivated employees
   b. Requires an awareness of the level of competence and personal integrity of employees; may fail due to lack of direction

II

Strategic Planning

Strategic, or *long-range, planning* sets the course for the organization.

A. The philosophy, mission statement, goals, and objectives of occupational health services should reflect those of the greater organization (Marriner-Tomey, 1992).
1. The philosophy in an occupational health unit should articulate:
   a. The inherent worth of individual workers to the company
   b. A commitment to quality care based on standards of nursing practice
   c. An expectation that nursing practice be research-based
   d. An emphasis on health-promotion and risk-reduction services
   e. An emphasis on continuing education and appropriate certifications
2. The mission aims to promote, protect, and restore the health of workers.
3. Goals and objectives clarify the essential actions necessary to achieving the philosophy and mission (Marriner-Tomey, 1992), such as services provided and resources utilized.
4. Philosophy, mission, goals, and objectives need to be developed by management and staff of the health unit, approved by upper management, and revised periodically to fit the ever-changing business environment.

B. Strategic planning process involves:
1. Assessment of the internal and external environments
2. Identification of strengths and weaknesses as well as threats and opportunities
3. Recommendations regarding future direction and goals of an organization

---

TABLE 6-1

Stages of Planned Change

- **Unfreezing:** when workers become aware of the need for change and realize that the change could be positive

- **Moving:** when the change is actually being implemented and problems related to the change are resolved

- **Refreezing:** when the change is accepted as part of the organization's culture and workers are no longer tempted to revert to "prechange" ways

---

Source: Lewin (1951).

BOX 6-1

Case Study Using Lewin's Stages of Planned Change

Unfreezing: The occupational health nurse manager of Company X was displeased with the quality of service provided by three contract physicians. They were often late for appointments with workers, tended to keep workers off the job for extended periods, and often missed critical details in assessing workers during preplacement and occupational injury examinations.

Moving: It was determined by occupational health unit staff, line management, safety staff, and human resource staff that the occupational health unit needed a full-time provider with prescriptive authority at a cost less than or equal to current costs. After much research and discussion, it was decided to hire an occupational health nurse practitioner and retain one physician as a consultant to the occupational health unit staff and a preceptor to the occupational health nurse practitioner.

Refreezing: The change was made, and within a few months, feedback from managers and workers was positive regarding the occupational health nurse practitioner's competence, availability, professionalism, and attitude. Within a year, the occupational health nurse practitioner left for personal reasons, but the company immediately hired another occupational health nurse practitioner to replace her.

C. The goals of strategic planning include:
1. Improved efficiency, targeted resources, clear communication, coordinated activities, adaptation to change, and goal achievement (Marriner-Tomey, 1992)
2. Elimination of underused or duplicate services/programs
3. The development of philosophy, mission, and goals

D. Planned change involves mutual goal-setting between workers and the change agent. (See Table 6-1 for Stages of Planned Change.)
1. The role of the occupational health nurse as an agent for change includes:
   a. Identifying problems
   b. Assessing the forces that will drive or restrain the change
   c. Determining costs and benefits of the change
   d. Establishing a helping relationship with management and workers
   e. Ensuring that the change will last until it is time to change again
2. Planned change may relate to programs/services, staffing, facilities, cost containment, or health outcomes of workers. (See Box 6-1 for a case study.)

Managing Occupational Health Services
III

The Management Process

The *management process* "consists of achieving organizational objectives through planning, organizing, directing, and controlling human and physical resources and technology" (Douglass, 1992, p. 7).

A. Management theories can be used to guide the occupational health nurse manager's activities (see Table 6-2).

B. Occupational health nurses, as managers, must develop power bases in order to implement decisions regarding the health and safety of workers (see Table 6-3).

IV

The Organization: Its Culture, Climate, and Structure

A. Organizational culture

1. *Organizational culture* is a set of assumptions about the organization, outside the awareness of but known by the workers, that guide the collective organization in dealing with internal and external situations and challenges (Moran & Volkwein, 1992).

2. An organization's culture is rooted in the founding, the history, and the leadership of that organization.

3. Paradigms explaining origin of organizational culture (Zamanou & Glaser, 1994, p. 476):

   a. Fundamentalist: "Organizations produce culture."

   b. Interpretive: "Organizations are culture" because they are the product of interaction among people.

TABLE 6-2

Overview of Management Theories

Classical Theory (Taylor, 1911) focuses on efficiency through design.
- Work is reduced to specific tasks, and workers are trained to do those tasks (division of labor).
- A hierarchy of supervisors and managers provide direction to workers (chain of command) and workers are expected to obey supervisors, be loyal to the organization, and be rewarded for production (Sullivan & Decker, 1992).

Neoclassical Theory
- Begins with the principles of classical theory
- Adds the human-relations approach, the desire for social relationships in the workplace, group pressure, and personal fulfillment (Sullivan & Decker, 1992)
- Assumes workers can create a rational structure through participation, cooperation, and motivation

Theory X and Y (McGregor)
- Theory X managers believe people intensely dislike working and must be "coerced, controlled, and directed" by management in doing the work required (Grohar-Murray & DiCroce, 1992, p. 118).
- Theory Y managers believe that people enjoy work and are "self-directed, responsible, and capable of solving their own problems" (Grohar-Murray & DiCroce, 1992, p. 118).

Theory Z (Ouchi)
- Derived from studies of Japanese organization
- Uses the concepts of "collective decision making, long-term employment, slower promotions, indirect supervision, and holistic concern for employees" as the centerpiece of the theory (Tappen, 1989, p. 45)

Contingency Theory (Fiedler)
- Situational theory
- Argues that workers, managers, and the environment are a unique blend, and the effectiveness of a particular management approach is *contingent* on the blend (Tappen, 1989)
- Argues that the most successful managers are those who adapt their approach to the situation

Other Theorists
- Herzberg focused on motivation.
- Argyris centered on organizational and individual goals.
- Likert developed a continuum of management systems from autocratic to participative.

TABLE 6-3

Sources of Power

- **Legitimate power** or authority arises from one's position within the organization.

- **Referent power** or charisma comes from one's personality and other personal characteristics; confidence, controlling emotions, and dress may all contribute to referent power.

- **Reward power** is based on one's ability to reward others, for example, with merit pay increases and employee recognitions that are controlled by the manager.

- **Expert power** allows the occupational health nurse manager to make health care decisions because others recognize a nurse's special knowledge, skills, and abilities.

- **Connection power** is created when individuals work together, as when health and safety professionals collaborate with human resources staff (Ellis & Hartley, 1991).

- **Information power** is held by those who control and possess information; they are often more powerful than those who need the information but are barred from access to it (Ellis & Hartley, 1991).

- **Coercive power** is often used by authoritarian managers to control the behavior of others through fear, threats, and punishment.

B. Organizational climate
  1. The *organizational climate* is a set of employee perceptions, environmental properties, or relatively enduring characteristics of an organization that describe how an organization operates, what is important to an organization, and what ultimately influences worker behavior (Butcher, 1994; Al-Shammari, 1992; Moran & Volkwein, 1992).
  2. Organizational climate both influences and is influenced by communication patterns within the organization and with the greater community.
  3. Organizational climates form as a result of (Moran & Volkwein, 1992):
     - Workers' perceptions of the organization's structure
     - Individual "descriptions of organization conditions" (p. 23)
     - Worker interaction
     - A shared culture
  4. Comparison of organizational culture and climate
     a. *Organizational culture* is an anthropologic concept, is highly enduring, emerges from a historical context, is often held in workers' unconscious, and influences the organization's climate (Moran & Volkwein, 1992).
     b. *Organizational climate* emerged from social psychology, is relatively enduring, is mediated by the organization's internal and external environments, is held in the awareness of workers, and is a manifestation of the organization's culture (Moran & Volkwein, 1992).

C. The *organizational structure* includes positions, job responsibilities, and the relationships among the positions (Ellis & Hartley, 1991; Marriner-Tomey, 1992).
  1. *Vertical structures* are associated with clear lines of authority; power is held by a few.
     a. Also called hierarchical, centralized, or bureaucratic
     b. Characterized by role clarity, specialization, delegation of authority
     c. Advantages include efficiency and clarity

d. Disadvantages include an inclination to autocratic leadership, lack of cooperation among workers, and a loss of worker creativity and commitment

2. *Horizontal structures* are associated with few layers of management.
   a. Also known as decentralized or organic culture
   b. Characterized by worker self-reliance, tolerance for ambiguity, open communication, acceptance of change, and risk-taking
   c. Advantages include speed in responding to challenges, job satisfaction, opportunities for staff development, and less need for higher-paid supervisory personnel
   d. Disadvantages include training costs, costs of poor decisions by inexperienced workers, time spent to reach consensus

3. Mixed structures:
   a. Use a more centralized approach for routine, day-to-day functions
   b. Use decentralized approach for managing change and innovation

V

Policies and Procedures

These measures provide uniform ways of responding to situations and meeting organizational challenges.

A. Policies and procedures must be developed through collaborative efforts; policies and procedures:
1. Require participation of all affected parties as well as the approval and support of management
2. Often are developed as a result of problems in the workplace or regulatory mandates
3. Must be reviewed and revised regularly
4. Need to be deleted once they have outlived their usefulness (after careful consideration)

B. *Policies* serve as guidelines for action (Aguilar, 1988; Travers & McDougall, 1995).

C. *Procedures* are the more specific chronological steps necessary to operationalize the policy (Marriner-Tomey, 1992).
1. Procedures include a definition, purpose, resources needed, steps in the process, expected results, precautions, legal implications, responsibilities, and documentation (Marriner-Tomey, 1992; Travers & McDougall, 1995).
2. Not all tasks performed in the occupational health unit require a procedure; if the task is a common one that staff members are all familiar with, then writing a procedure is not necessary.

D. Once the policy and procedures are developed and approved, the policy should be disseminated to affected workers through an employee handbook, newsletters, payroll stuffers, closed-circuit television, or in-house computer networks when available

VI

Fiscal Issues: Budgeting and Resource Management

A. *Budgeting* is the process of planning and managing financial resources for a given time period.
1. Budgets usually fall within two categories: operating and capital expenditure
   a. *Operating budgets* itemize the following:

- Expected revenues to be generated by the occupational health unit (i.e., cost avoidance or actual income from providing services to another organization)
- Expected expenses to be incurred, including personnel salaries, benefits, and contract payment; facility expenses (rent, utilities, maintenance, repairs, and depreciation); supplies; travel; staff development
  b. *Capital expenditure budgets* include major investments (equipment or facility renovation).
2. Methods of budgeting include:
  a. The *incremental budget method* begins with the previous year's budget and adds or subtracts from each line item to fund programs and services.
    - Advantages: the historical foundation requires little need to justify continuing services and programs.
    - Disadvantages: resources may be lost if not used in a given year; thus, there may be an incentive to overspend the budget to justify the need for increases the next year.
  b. The *zero-based budget method* requires annual justification for each program and service in terms of outcome and cost.
    - Advantages: it requires annual analyses of all occupational health programs and services to evaluate their productivity and cost.
    - Disadvantage: extra time is required to produce the analyses and provide prioritized alternatives for each program and service.
3. The budgeting process (Tappen, 1989)
  a. Planning is based on past service performance and predictions of next year's costs and revenues.
  b. Preparation involves translating objectives into costs and revenues, justifying all requests, and eliminating low-priority programs and services.
  c. Modification and approval
    - The proposed budget is presented to management along with an overview of programs and services and an explanation of fiscal requirements.
    - Management may discuss specifics of some programs and services in an attempt to refine the budget requests.
  d. Monitoring includes the analysis of projected versus actual expenses, with investigation of variances greater than 5%.
4. The occupational health provider has the primary responsibility for the control of the occupational health unit budget.
5. Demonstrating cost savings of services
  a. Use zero-based budgeting to determine which program and services are cost effective and which need to be modified or eliminated.
  b. Compare costs of providing services in-house with the price of outsourcing to community providers (see Table 6-4).

B. *Resource management* refers to the timely monitoring of fiscal resources. Managing resources involves:
  1. Determination of the costs of resources
  2. Identification of methods to reduce waste
  3. Maintenance of appropriate inventory (sufficient supplies without excess)

C. Quarterly and annual reports
  1. Regular reports can be used to document productivity, quality of services, and progress towards goal attainment.
  2. Quarterly or monthly reports should include (Marrelli, 1993; Travers & McDougall, 1995):

TABLE 6-4

Sample of Format for Demonstrating Cost Savings

Category	Number of Visits	Outsource Costs	In-house Costs	Net Costs or Savings
Clinical				
Preplacement Exams				
Clinical Follow-Up (Occupational)				
Clinical Follow-Up (Nonoccupational)				
Screening (vision, hearing)				
Health Risk Appraisals				
Health Surveillance				
Diagnostic				
Blood Pressure				
Blood Work, Urinalysis				
Pregnancy Test				
Strep Screen				
Electrocardiogram				
Drug/Alcohol Screen				
Treatment				
Immunization				
Physical Therapy Modalities				
Wound Care				
Health Education				
Counseling				
Miscellaneous & Administration				
Special Projects				
Health Promotion Programs				
Disability Management				
Case Management				
Professional Consultation				
Reports				

Source: Childre, F., personal communication, October 1995

a. Budget projections versus actual expenditures
b. Update on quality activities and measures
c. Human resource summary (i.e., hires, vacancies)
d. Staff-development activities
e. Outcomes such as participation in particular programs and services
f. Staff participation in interdepartmental and interdisciplinary activities
g. Trends related to injuries and illnesses
3. Annual reports provide an overview of accomplishments during the past year.

VII
Human Resource Issues

A. Assessment of job functions
1. Often a prerequisite to writing position descriptions (Zwanenberg & Wilkinson, 1993)
2. May serve as the basis for hiring and developing staff
3. Also serves as the foundation for performance appraisals, that is, the measurement of employees' job performance quality and productivity

B. Position descriptions
1. Position titles should be clearly described in terms of "knowledge and skills required, levels of complexity and responsibility, actual work effort, and work conditions" (Forsey, Cleland & Miller, 1993, p. 33).
2. Descriptions should include as a minimum a statement of line authority and responsibility, duties, and qualifications (Travers & McDougall, 1995; Forsey, Cleland & Miller, 1993).
3. Occupational health nurses can refer to the American Association of Occupational Health Nurses' (AAOHN) guidelines for job descriptions and other AAOHN resources for guidance in developing job descriptions.

C. The *screening* of applicants can take many forms, including background checks, psychological profiling, biofeedback, handwriting analysis, and interviews (Yarborough, 1994).
1. Screening techniques must be:
a. Linked to actual job requirements
b. Reliable and valid, meaning that the results would be the same if the screening were administered multiple times and the screening results are indeed predictive of worker success in a particular job
2. Interviews are a very common type of selection screening used in business and industry today (Yarborough, 1994).
a. Questions asked must be limited to job functions and performance requirements; acceptable questions relate to the applicant's ability to complete the job tasks with or without accommodation (Alfus, 1994; Lissy, 1995).
b. Interviewers often ask either how the applicant dealt with a situation in a prior position or provide hypothetical situations about how the applicant might respond in the future (Pulakos & Schmitt, 1995).
c. Managers want to assess the applicant's abilities to work within the organization but also are interested in what the applicant can bring to the organization that will further organizational goals (Alderman, 1995).

D. *Staff development activities* include mentoring and training (Wachs, 1992c).

1. *Mentoring* is a process whereby a seasoned, skilled, and influential worker (mentor) commits to a long-term relationship with a novice worker (mentee) for the purpose of enhancing the career of the mentee (Carey & Campbell, 1994; Hensler, 1994; Ondeck & Gingerich, 1994).

   a. The mentoring process can be either formal (managed by the organization) or informal (spontaneous relationship) (Bartlett, 1995; Burgess, 1995; Hernandez-Piloto Brito, 1992).

   b. Mentoring is directed at assuring professional competency.

   c. Mentoring is used to prepare occupational health nurses to effectively apply nursing and occupational health and safety principles in an occupational setting.

2. *Training* is a more structured process of preparing staff to meet the needs of the organization.

   a. Training begins with orientation to the department and the position.

   b. Training activities may include on-site, in-house presentations; on-site, vendor-generated seminars; off-site offerings; or independent study.

   c. Activities are based on individual needs of staff, annual performance appraisals, and organizational needs.

   d. Training priorities may result from legislative mandates, such as the Americans with Disabilities Act or the Drug Free Workplace Act.

   e. Staff development activities must be evaluated by workers and management in terms of:
      • The desired behavior change as a result of the training
      • The improvement in knowledge, skills, or attitudes
      • The usefulness to the organization of the knowledge, skills, or attitudes

3. The key to both mentoring and training is motivation.

   a. *Motivation* is an "intrinsic drive" resulting from an individual's instincts, needs, and actual or expected rewards that determines an individual's behavior (Tappen, 1989, p. 391; Sullivan & Decker, 1992).

   b. Motivation is stimulated by others, including managers, mentors, or a work team.

   c. Motivation is a key concept in both management and leadership theories.

   d. Motivating others requires effective communication skills, credibility, caring, praise, constructive criticism, and inclusion of others in the decision-making process (Ellis & Hartley, 1991).

4. Team building

   a. Team building is important when tasks are complex and work requires a collaborative effort.

   b. Team building results in mutual respect and appreciation of each member's contributions.

   c. Teams take a long time to develop into efficiently functioning entities, and thus the goals should be stability in team membership and frequent opportunities for team members to collaborate.

5. Interdisciplinary occupational health and safety teams

   a. The interdisciplinary team may include the occupational health nurse, occupational physician, industrial hygienist, safety manager, ergonomists, toxicologists, and others.

   b. The coordination of the interdisciplinary team is often the responsibility of the occupational health nurse manager.

   c. The mission and goal of each discipline's contribution to the interdisciplinary team must be clearly articulated.

E. *Performance appraisals* are based on position descriptions, particularly job responsibilities, and standards of performance.
1. The purpose of performance appraisals is to develop the individual employee as well as to strengthen the organization through improved productivity and quality outcomes (Webb & Cantone, 1993).
2. Methods of appraisal include verbal feedback, corrective demonstration, conferences, memos, and other forms of communication (AAOHN, 1994).
3. Standards of performance "specify for the employee the conditions that will exist when the job is done to the manager's satisfaction" (Webb & Cantone, 1993).
   a. Each job responsibility should have a companion performance standard.
   b. Example of performance standards are as follows:
     • Provides professional nursing care appropriate to worker needs
     • Identifies worker health needs accurately using health history and physical assessment skills for 95% of the workers who present in the occupational health unit
     • Following signed protocols, prescribes appropriate treatment to meet identified health needs for 100% of workers who present in the occupational health unit
4. Documentation of progress toward standards of performance is important; it serves to justify salary increases and promotions.

F. Other appraisals that can be used to evaluate occupational health services include surveys of workers who use health services, upper management, community resources and vendors, professional colleagues, and occupational health unit staff (Eckes, 1994; Weber, 1995).

Tools for the Occupational Health Nurse Manager
VIII
Communication

A. *Listening* is hearing plus the thought processes that allow an "accurate perception of what is being communicated" (Meiss, 1991, Tape 1; Wachs, 1995b).
1. Obstacles to effective listening include:
   a. Multiple demands on occupational health nurses
   b. Biases and beliefs of the occupational health nurse
   c. Misunderstanding the meaning of words
   d. The differences in the rates of speech and listening
   e. The need to solve the problem rather than listen to the person
2. Effective listening requires:
   a. Encouraging the speaker to continue through the use of verbal and non-verbal behaviors
   b. Attempting to "understand the message that is spoken as well as the feelings being communicated and the congruence between verbal and non-verbal messages" (Tappen, 1989)
3. The listening role is a powerful one, often making the difference in whether or not agreements can be reached and work can be accomplished.

B. Negotiation and conflict resolution
1. These skills are most effective when both parties listen and aim for a win-win solution (Badawy, 1994).

2. "The most common sources of conflict are personal differences, lack of information, role incompatibility, and environmental stress" (Lemieux-Charles, 1994, p. 1129).
3. Approaches to conflict resolution include:
   a. *Competition:* the manager "overpowers the opposition" to meet their needs or goals (Lemieux-Charles, 1994).
   b. *Accommodation:* the manager is more concerned with working relationships than with outcomes and thus will allow others to achieve their goals.
   c. *Avoidance:* the manager refuses to address the issue (Fowler, Bushardt & Jones, 1993; Jones, Fowler & Bushardt, 1992).
   d. *Compromise:* the manager attempts to find a "middle ground . . . a mutually acceptable solution that partially satisfies both parties" (Lemieux-Charles, 1994).
   e. *Collaboration:* all parties work together to find the most satisfying solution for everyone involved.
4. *Negotiation* is "working side by side with another party to achieve mutually satisfactory results" (Dolan, 1990).
   a. A distributive approach tends to be competitive; each party is attempting both to resolve the issue and to gain something.
   b. An integrative approach focuses on problem solving, a win-win situation for all (Lemieux-Charles, 1994).
5. Successful negotiation requires:
   a. *Preparation:* clarifying the goal of the negotiation, seeing the issue from the other party's viewpoint, and planning to concede (Susskind & McKearnan, 1995; Neale & Bazerman, 1992; Wachs & Wachs, 1992)
   b. *Agenda:* agreed to by all and subject to modification as the negotiations progress (Karrass, 1995; Wachs & Wachs, 1992)
   c. *Clear communication:* essential to win-win outcomes

C. *Networking* is a process of establishing connections through introductions, promoting and supporting others, and helping others connect (Wachs, 1991).
1. Methods of networking include:
   a. Identifying essential contacts in the organization and in the community
   b. Being involved in community activities, such as serving on health-related advisory boards or attending community events
   c. Serving as a mentor
2. Networking is beneficial not only for the occupational health nurse manager but also for the organization.
   a. It helps to recruit and retain employees.
   b. It increases visibility within the community and is excellent publicity for the organization.

D. Day-to-day communication is handled with meetings.
1. Meetings serve as a means of disseminating information, brainstorming, planning, problem solving, or motivating (Wachs, 1992b).
2. Keys to an effective meeting include:
   a. Drawing up an agenda that describes the who, what, when, where, and why of the meeting
   b. Reviewing the purpose of the meeting and establishing the ground rules
   c. Reserving sufficient time for the meeting
   d. Using audiovisuals as needed to assist in conveying information
   e. Distributing the minutes or a written summary of the meeting to all participants and other interested parties

E. Other methods of communication include:
1. Electronic or voice mail
2. Memos and briefs

IX

Occupational Health Information Management Systems

A. The purpose of information management is to provide a means to collect, access, and use large amounts of information from many sources in order to effectively manage all aspects of the occupational health unit.

B. Information management systems (IMS) are essential because of:
1. Rapidly evolving regulations and emerging health issues
2. The need to communicate with members of an interdisciplinary health team
3. The changing nature of the workforce

C. Traditional methods of information management in occupational health include:
1. Demographics collected and stored locally as single records, independent of groups
2. Paper-based, hard-copy records of interventions
3. Transfer of intervention records by manually inserting them into the health records of individual employees
4. Manual tabulation to generate reports
5. Reports, primarily text-based summaries using the information available
6. A written log of employees' appointments and scheduled meetings with the occupational health unit
7. Budget, expenditures, orders, and other financial transactions, tracked by generating and distributing paper copies to various departments

D. Automated methods of information management in occupational health include:
1. Demographics collected, entered, updated, and maintained in central databases in both individual and group formats
2. Electronic records maintained for each intervention or interface
3. Automatic, electronic transfer of information to users with a verified "need to know"
4. Mechanized categorization of information within and across employee files.
5. Reports presented logically and visually, using graphs and charts that highlight progress toward meeting objectives and trends
6. Generating notices, scheduling appointments, and tracking interim examinations and tests
7. Tracking expenses and revenue to observe and monitor financial status
8. Developing algorithms and workflow diagrams to ensure consistency and minimize practice errors

E. Occupational health and safety information stored on automated information systems serves multiple purposes.
1. Useful data for the occupational health and safety team (occupational health nurses, physicians, industrial hygienists, safety professionals, ergonomists, and toxicologists) include:
   a. Work-related injury notification
   b. Hazard-recognition reports
   c. Surveillance-testing results
   d. Risk-factor tracking/trending reports
   e. Information required by the Occupational Safety and Health Administration (OSHA) (days lost, health treatment and work restrictions)

2. Health-related data provided to the human resources department include:
   a. Preplacement assessment reports
   b. Fitness-for-duty recommendations
   c. Work-restriction or accommodation requirements
3. Data provided to vendors and community providers of products and services include:
   a. Electronic orders, detailed requests, or protocols for services
   b. Forms required for reporting examinations and test results
   c. Mechanized invoicing and bill payment
4. Health-related data shared with managers or supervisors include:
   a. Notice of work-related illness or injury
   b. Return-to-work notices
   c. Recommendations for modification of workplace, job tasks, or work schedule
   d. Notice of need for work restrictions or accommodations
   e. Results of fitness-for-duty evaluations
   f. Notice of procedures required by law or by the company for employees (e.g., Department of Transportation [DOT] examinations, blood lead tests, or audiograms)
   g. Results of hazard-recognition or surveillance procedures conducted in their departments
5. Communication with workers includes:
   a. Notice of appointments for work-related procedures
   b. Results of examinations or tests performed
   c. Notice of screenings or health promotion offerings

F. Occupational health unit activities that are stored on automated information systems include activity reports, program participation rates, and units of service.

G. Automated information systems facilitate the implementation and management of health surveillance programs through:
1. Identification of target populations by exposure, risk factor, or job specifications
2. Selection of appropriate intervention, test, or examination
3. Notification of occupational health team members, employees, and managers of an examination schedule
4. Documentation of individual surveillance results and statistical analysis of group data
5. Reports to be generated may include:
   a. Trend data, such as the collection and tracking of audiogram results to describe the effects of environmental noise on employees
   b. Predictive data, such as the identification of a target population at risk of a particular injury by using data from another group doing similar work

H. Automated information systems can guide applied research to:
1. Generate hypotheses using current and past data
2. Conduct a literature search
3. Identify the target population by demographics, risk factors, exposures, and test results
4. Analyze results, using mechanized statistical packages
5. Generate the study report using narrative as well as charts, graphs, and other graphics to display data

6. Use the results to justify necessary changes or modifications that contribute to health and safety of workers

I. Information management systems can be used to evaluate services in terms of process, cost effectiveness, quality outcomes, and future direction by:
1. Tracking outcomes of activities (How many program participants quit smoking?)
2. Evaluating the level of resources required to produce the desired outcomes
3. Demonstrating the cost-benefit and cost-effectiveness of providing the service (Was the cost of mammography screening justified by the cost savings when two cases of breast cancer were detected in earlier, more treatable stages?)

J. Information systems can be used to ensure the effectiveness of processes and programs by:
1. Establishing and maintaining appropriate staffing patterns, ratios, and assignments
2. Maintaining an inventory of supplies and equipment, including data regarding cost, suppliers, expiration dates, calibration dates, and lease information
3. Conducting staff development activities, including performance appraisal and review formats and documentation; training and experience documentation; and setting staff goals, objectives, and timeframes for progress reviews
4. Generating required reports to management, the corporation, headquarters, and regulatory bodies
5. Conducting and managing results of annual audits
6. Tracking lost time, work-related injuries, and OSHA-recordable or workers' compensation cases

K. The use of automated information systems has several legal, ethical, and professional implications.
1. To safeguard the security and integrity of electronic health records:
   a. Develop policies and procedures for computer use.
   b. Require that all employees with access to health records sign a "statement of protection of confidentiality."
   c. Provide guidelines for disclosure to all users.
   d. Establish and impose penalties for system/information misuse.
   e. Establish and maintain audit trails or records of who and when a record was accessed and for what purpose.
   f. Back up information frequently and store it separately from other files.
2. To safeguard the confidentiality of employee health records:
   a. Establish and maintain lists of approved users, signatures, titles, and "need-to-know" status, including:
      • Who may access a record
      • Who may write on a particular record
      • Who may read only a particular record
      • Who may retrieve or transmit a record
   b. Block specific information, restricting access to those with a "need-to-know" status and those on user approval lists.
   c. Establish and use client identifiers, such as employee numbers for use during transmission of data.
   d. Encode sensitive information.

EXAMPLE OF APPLICATION OF DATA TO PREPLACEMENT PROCESS

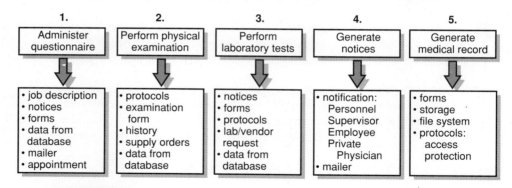

FIGURE 6-1

e. Require multilevel clearance for accessing coded information to:
   • The occupational health, safety, or benefits departments
   • Registered nurses or physicians
   • The assigned case manager
f. Change passwords frequently on an unscheduled basis.
g. Never leave an employee file open on a screen when not in use.
h. Never fax records to an unsecured or unattended receiver.
i. Never print copies of a record or part of a record unless the copy is required for a validated reason, such as subpoena, client access, OSHA request, or established protocol.
j. Never modify or change a previous entry but rather use the same process as for a paper record: identify the entry to be modified, state the reason for the change, make the change, and date and sign the entry.

L. Procedures for selecting and implementing an occupational health information management system:
   1. Identify and define the information needs of the unit:
      a. List all services and organizational functions provided.
      b. Develop work flow for each process.
      c. Identify the data needs for each step (see Figure 6-1).
         • Identify all forms, questionnaires, notices required for that step in the process.
         • Specify all interfaces and information exchanges required.
         • Specify the method of communication desired or required, (automated notices, electronic mail, reports or newsletters).
      d. Define report requirements.
      e. Identify security measures necessary.
   2. To investigate and assess information systems that are available commercially:
      a. Attend trade shows or exhibits at conferences.
      b. Network with other occupational health nurses who are users of automated systems.
      c. Use lists of systems available from the American Association of Occupational Health Nurses (AAOHN), the American College of Occupational

and Environmental Medicine (ACOEM), and the *Computers in Nursing* journal to identify appropriate products.

  d. Access and review literature on specific products from journals and newsletters of professional organizations.

  e. Request a demonstration of products from the supplier, the developer, or the vendor.

3. Considerations when selecting an automated information system include:

  a. Can the system be tailored to meet specific needs not embedded or included at the time of purchase?

  b. How much time and cost (over and above the purchase price) will be involved in making modifications?

  c. Is the vendor able and willing to provide training?

  d. Will the vendor provide ongoing support for both users and the system?

  e. How flexible is the system to accommodate future changes in the occupational health unit organizational structure and range of services?

  f. What are the costs and benefits of buying a commercially available product over building a system internally?

  g. What is the connectivity and compatibility of the system to existing systems with which it will have to interface in order to transmit and share information?

  h. What built-in security mechanisms does the system have?

4. Once the selection of a system has been made, an implementation plan must be developed:

  a. Assign an implementation team.

  b. Select a pilot site to test the system.
     • Begin with simple maneuvers involving minimal interfaces, such as documentation of visits in an employee record.
     • Progress to more complex multidisciplinary functions, such as electronic transmission of environmental sampling results to members of the team at diverse locations.

  c. Make modifications based on pilot feedback as appropriate.

  d. Work with the vendor or supplier to resolve issues before full implementation.

  e. Establish a time line for implementation.

  f. Assure integration of the system with other systems in the corporate network as appropriate.

  g. Evaluate the effectiveness of the system in terms of time saved, improved legibility, costs savings, accuracy, and staff needs.

  h. Measure satisfaction of users over time.

  i. Identify and implement modifications necessary to make the system more efficient and acceptable by users.

  j. Assign responsibility for continuous improvement by monitoring effectiveness, applicability, usability, and quality of outputs.

5. The transition to an automated system requires technical, functional, and philosophical changes for the occupational health unit staff, which can be facilitated by:

  a. Involving as many staff members as practical in all stages of decision making

  b. Providing sufficient training

  c. Recognizing that individuals learn and adapt at different rates

  d. Supporting members as they become comfortable with the new technology

M. Nursing informatics is a new and growing specialty.
1. *Informatics nurse specialists* (INS) are nurses who develop and evaluate information applications, tools, processes, and structures intended to assist nurses to manage the data that support the practice of nursing.
2. The "practice" of nursing informatics has the following characteristics:
   a. The content of the information is related to nursing.
   b. The technology is designed to facilitate handling, communication, and transformation of nursing information.
   c. The focus of activity is information handling, communication, or transformation rather than patient care, education, research, or administration (American Nurses Association, 1994).

$\overline{X}$

Time Management

A. The principal benefits of managing time are:
1. Feelings of accomplishment and control over work, resulting in job satisfaction
2. Long-term commitment to the profession and the organization (Wachs, 1993).

B. To manage time:
1. Set realistic, prioritized goals for the occupational health unit and allow staff adequate time to devote to achieve them.
2. Limit additional programs and services the occupational health unit may be called upon to provide (Wachs, 1993).
3. Develop a "to do" list, avoid time wasters and paper shuffling, use technologies such as computers, create a supportive work environment, and reward oneself for a job well done (Wachs, 1993).

C. Delegating responsibility and commensurate authority to occupational health unit staff is not only effective time management but also effective nursing management (Pollock, 1994; Klock, 1995).

$\overline{XI}$

Critical Thinking

Critical thinking is the "process of examining underlying assumptions about current evidence and interpreting and evaluating arguments for the purpose of reaching a conclusion from a new perspective" (Sullivan & Decker, 1992, p. 226).

A. *Problem solving* is a "process used when a gap is perceived between an existing state and a desired state" (Sullivan & Decker, 1992, p. 228); the steps of the problem-solving process include assessment, data analysis, solution definition, implementation, and evaluation.

B. *Decision making* is the "process of establishing the criteria by which alternative courses of action are developed and selected" (Sullivan & Decker, 1992, p. 233).
1. Decisions can be made under conditions of certainty, uncertainty, or risk.
2. The decision-making process includes (Sullivan & Decker, 1992):
   a. Identifying the gap between what is and what should be
   b. Establishing parameters for solutions, such as deciding which factors are acceptable and which are not
   c. Seeking and testing alternative solutions
   d. Exploring what could go wrong
   e. Evaluating the action

C. *Creativity* is the "ability to develop and implement new and better solutions" (Sullivan & Decker, 1992, p. 243).

1. Challenge staff to think creatively by generating many ideas (brainstorming) or by generating one unique idea (synectics) (Sullivan & Decker, 1992).
2. Foster creative problem solving:
   a. Establish a safe environment to try innovative practices without fear of failure.
   b. Promote interaction between occupational health unit staff and others both within and outside the organization.
   c. Reward staff for unique approaches to occupational health unit problems.

XII

The Image of the Occupational Health Nurse

The occupational health nurse should be seen as a competent business person who has particular expertise in health and safety.

A. *Image* is created through the display of personal characteristics and interpersonal skills.

1. Personal appearance plays a major role in the occupational health nurse's image.
2. Professionalism displayed through interactions with workers, management, and the greater community attests to the positive image of nurses.
   a. Caring and competence are frequently evaluated by workers and management.
   b. Dealings with community providers, vendors, and other business people will color the community's perception of not only an individual occupational health nurse but of nurses in general.
3. The occupational health nurse can also positively affect the image of nurses by:
   a. Publishing articles in the organization's newsletter and the community newspaper
   b. Belonging to professional organizations, such as the American Association of Occupational Health Nurses
   c. Recognizing and publicizing excellence among staff members (Brown, 1989)

B. The image of the occupational health nurse relates directly to the nurse's influence and ability to promote health and safety in the organization.

Evaluating the Quality of Occupational Health Services

XIII

Total Quality Management (TQM)

A. *Total quality management* (TQM) and *continuous quality improvement* (CQI) are processes used to put customer needs and quality products first.

1. TQM is a business strategy that focuses on work processes and outcomes.
2. In health care, a similar strategy is known as continuous quality improvement (CQI).

3. Quality improvement is defined as conformance to customer requirements and specifications, fitness for use, buyer satisfaction, and value at an affordable price (Harrington, 1987).
4. The quality improvement process is a disciplined, ongoing process for producing outputs and preventing errors in products and services.

B. Approaches to total quality management
1. W. Edwards Deming's TQM program, called the Deming Cycle, includes the following steps (Deming, 1986):
   a. Plan a work process.
   b. Do or implement a work process.
   c. Check or measure a work process.
   d. Act on results to continuously improve the process.
2. Joseph Juran's program focuses on quality planning, quality control, and quality improvement of processes (Juran, 1988).
3. Philip B. Crosby's program is based on organizational development, with the following absolutes for quality management (Crosby, 1979):
   a. Conformance to requirements
   b. Prevention
   c. Zero defects
   d. Cost of quality

C. According to the conceptual framework of TQM or CQI (Figure 6-2), interpersonal behaviors are at the center of total quality management or continuous quality improvement.

D. Task behaviors that get work done include:
1. Proposing a new idea or suggestion
2. Building on another's idea or suggestion
3. Seeking information by soliciting facts, data, experiences, or clarifications from others
4. Giving information by offering facts, data, experiences, or clarifications to others
5. Seeking opinion by soliciting values, beliefs, or sentiments from others
6. Giving opinion by offering values, beliefs, or sentiments to others
7. Disagreeing by opposing or raising doubts about an issue, not a person
8. Summarizing by restating the content of previously shared dialogue in condensed form
9. Testing comprehension by asking questions for one's own understanding of previous communication
10. Checking to find out if consensus has been reached or if more discussion is needed.

E. Group maintenance and facilitation behaviors are important elements of TQM.
1. Encourage others by supporting or recognizing their contributions.
2. Resolve disagreements and conflict by searching for alternatives and/or agreements.
3. Checking performance by temporarily suspending task operations in order to facilitate the internal group process.
4. Set standards to improve the quality of the group's process.
5. Relieve tension by and increase enjoyment by suggesting breaks or proposing fun approaches to work.

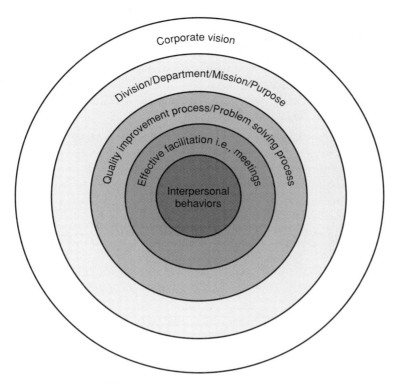

FIGURE 6-2 *Conceptual Framework for Total Quality Management*

Adapted from Honeywell Total Quality Management User's Guide, 1995; Reprinted with permission of Xerox Quality Services.

XIV

Benchmarking in TQM

A. *Benchmarking* is the "continuous process of measuring a company's products, services and practices against industry leading competitors" (Collins, 1995, p. 50) and "against industry's best practice" (Landwehr, 1995, p. 120).

B. The purposes of benchmarking include (Beasley & Cook, 1995):
1. Modifying organizational culture or climate
2. Fostering competition
3. Creating an awareness of the quality standard within the industry
4. Measuring productivity and performance quality
5. Setting performance standards
6. Managing the organization to achieve the best results

C. The benchmarking process includes the following steps (Brown, 1995; Collins, 1995; Murray & Murray, 1992; Landwehr, 1995; Bergman, 1994):
1. Planning: deciding which processes will be benchmarked, the activities to assess, the development of measurement tools, and an assessment of internal functioning
2. Data collection: identifying best practice companies and sharing information

3. Data analysis: identifying performance gaps between the study company and the benchmark companies

4. Change: using the data to unfreeze workers to accept the need for modification in the work process under review and then implementing the change based on the benchmark criteria

5. Monitoring: not only overseeing the change process but also recalibrating benchmarks at regular intervals

D. Benchmarking has some potential problems, such as (McWilliams, 1995):
1. Choosing the wrong benchmark organizations for comparison
2. Failure to appreciate that while organizations may be comparable, they will also be unique in ways that may affect the legitimacy of the comparison
3. The need for common definitions of processes and criteria
4. The need to be the best no matter what the cost
5. Reluctance to use other quality interventions other than benchmarking

E. The occupational health nurse must understand the concepts in TQM and benchmarking sufficiently to communicate with others in the organization about the opportunities and challenges of quality management.

XV

Summary

A. To be an effective manager, the occupational health nurse must possess leadership and management skills, including the ability to budget and manage people and resources.

B. In addition, the occupational health nurse as a manager must have knowledge of both the organization and the occupational health unit.

C. Finally, the occupational health nurse manager must use various forms of communication, including meetings, memos, presentations, networking, delegating, and negotiating, in order to meet the health and safety needs of the workers and the organization.

D. Evaluation of occupational health unit programs and services should provide evidence of the quality of and need for services related to health and safety in the organization.

BIBLIOGRAPHY

Adams, C. (1991). An analysis of school nurse leadership styles. *School Nurse, 7*(2), 22–25.

Aguilar, F. E. (1988). *General managers in action.* New York: Oxford University Press.

Alderman, L. (1995). What you need to ace today's rough-and-tough job interviews. *Money, 24*(4), 35.

Alfus, P. (1994). Know new interview guidelines—or risk legal trouble. *Hotel and Motel Management, 209*(19), 16–17.

Al-Shammari, M. M. (1992). Organizational climate. *Leadership & Organization Development, 13*(6), 30–32.

Amann, M. (1994). Informatics: The application to occupational health nursing. *AAOHN Journal, 42*(8), 391–398.

American Association of Occupational Health Nurses. (1994). *AAOHN standards of occupational health nursing.* Atlanta: AAOHN Publications.

American Nurses Association. (1992). *Next generation nursing information systems: Essential characteristics for professional practice.* Publication #NSS-30. Washington, DC: Author.

American Nurses Association. (1994). *Scope of practice for nursing informatics.* Publication #NP90. Washington, DC: Author.

Axline, L. L. (1994). Ethical considerations of performance appraisals. *Management Review, 83*(3), 62.

Badawy, M. K. (1994). Listening is an art in negotiation. *Electronic Business Buyer, 20*(12), 19.

Bartlett, R. C. (1995). The mentoring message. *Chief Executive, 101,* 48–49.

Beasley, G., & Cook, J. (1995). The "what," "why," and "how" of benchmarking. *Agency Sales, 25*(6), 52–56.

Bergman, R. (1994). Hitting the mark. *Hospitals and Health Networks, 68*(8), 48–51.

Brown, S. (1995). Measures of perfection. *Sales & Marketing Management, 147*(5), 104–105.

Butcher, A. H. (1994). Supervisors matter more than you think: components of a mission-centered organizational climate. *Hospital & Health Services Administration, 39*(4), 505–521.

Burgess, L. (1995). Mentoring with the blindfold. *Employment Relations Today, 21*(4), 439–444.

Calano, J., & Salzman, J. (1988). *CareerTracking: 26 success shortcuts to the top.* New York: Simon & Schuster.

Carey, S. J., & Campbell, S. T. (1994). Preceptor, mentor and sponsor roles: Creative strategies for nurse retention. *Journal of Nursing Administration, 24*(12), 39–48.

Collins, M. J. (1995). Benchmarking with simulation: How it can help your production operations. *Production, 107*(7), 51–52.

Crosby, P. B. (1979). *Quality is free.* New York: New American Library.

Deming, W. E. (1986). *Out of the crisis.* Cambridge, MA: MIT-CAES.

Dolan, J. P. (1990). *Negotiate like the pros* (audiotape). Boulder, CO: CareerTrack.

Douglass, L. M. (1992). *The effective nurse: Leader and manager.* St. Louis: C.V. Mosby.

Eckes, G. (1994). Practical alternatives to performance appraisals. *Quality Progress, 27*(11), 57–60.

Ellis, J. R., & Hartley, C. L. (1991). *Managing and coordinating nursing care.* Philadelphia: J.B. Lippincott Company.

Finley, C. (1994). What is sexual harassment? *PT, 2*(12), 17–18.

Friley, E. (1994). Tools of the trade. *Supervision, 55*(4), 11–13.

Forsey, L. M., Cleland, V. S., & Miller, B. (1993). Job descriptions for differentiated nursing practice and differentiated pay. *Journal of Nursing Administration, 23*(5), 33–40.

Fowler, A. R., Bushardt, S. C., & Jones, M. A. (1993). Retaining nurses through conflict resolution. *Health Progress, 74*(5), 25–29.

Gabbard, G .O., Atkinson, S. D., & Jorgenson, L. M. (1995). Can patients sexually harass their physicians? *Archives of Family Medicine, 4*(3), 261–265.

Grohar-Murray, M. E., & DiCroce, H. R. (1992). *Leadership and management in nursing.* Norwalk, CT: Appleton & Lange.

Hagenow, N. R., & McCrea, M.A. (1994). A mentoring relationship: Two viewpoints. *Nursing Management, 25*(12), 42–43.

Haggard, T. R., & Alexander, M. G. (1994). Tips on drafting and enforcing a policy against sexual harassment. *Industrial Management, 36*(1), 2–5.

Harrington, H. J. (1987). *The improvement process: How America's leading companies improve quality.* New York: McGraw-Hill.

Heller, B. (1995). The power memo. *Executive Female, 18*(2), 42–46.

Helmer, D. C., Dunn, L. M., Eaton, K., Macedonio, C., & Lubritz, L. (1995). Implementing corporate wellness programs: A business approach to program planning. *AAOHN Journal, 43*(11), 558–563.

Hensler, D. J. (1994). Mentoring at the management level. *Industrial Management, 36*(6), 20–21.

Hernandez-Piloto Brito, H. (1992). Nurses in action: An innovative approach to mentoring. *Journal of Nursing Administration, 22*(5), 23–28.

Herrick, K., Hansten, R., O'Neil, L., Hayes, P., & Washburn, M. (1994). My license is not on the line: The art of delegation. *Nursing Management, 25*(2), 48–50.

Honeywell Solid State Electronics Center. (1990). *Quality improvement tools.* Minneapolis, MN: Author.

Houston, S., & Luquire, R. (1991). Measuring success: CNS performance appraisal. *Clinical Nurse Specialist, 5*(4), 204–209.

Jones, M. A., Fowler, A. R., & Bushardt, S. C. (1992). Job conflict resolution styles of nurses. *Journal of Nursing Administration, 22*(11), 63.

Juran, J. M. (Ed.). (1988). *Juran's quality control handbook* (4th ed). New York: Random House.

Kane, I., & Fickley, B. J. (1992). Correlating nursing care, nursing practice and nursing performance standards. *Perspectives in Psychiatric Care, 28*(3), 27–31.

Karrass, C. (1995). Take charge of the agenda. *Traffic Management, 34*(1), 45.

Kaye, J., Donald, C. G., & Merker, S. (1994). Sexual harassment of critical care nurses: A costly workplace issue. *American Journal of Critical Care, 3*(6), 409–415.

Klarman, K. L., & Mateo, M. A. (1994). An approach to presentation skill development of nurses. *Journal of Nursing Staff Development, 10*(6), 307–311.

Klock, J. P. (1995). Learn to be a master delegator! *Real Estate Today, 28*(3), 50–53.

Koba, H. (1995). U of T medical school uses multistep strategy to prevent sexual harassment. *Canadian Medical Association Journal, 152*(3), 414–415.

Koss, J. P. (1995). The benchmarking buzz. *Beverage World, 114*(1593), 114.

Kouzes, J. M., & Posner, B. Z. (1987). *Leadership challenge.* Palo Alto, CA: TPG/Learning Systems.

Laird, M. J. (1993). Sexual harassment: A look to the future. *Management Decision, 31*(5), 51–54.

Lam, E. (1994). Benchmarking best practice. *Nursing Times, 90*(46), 48–51.

Landwehr, W. R. (1995). Focus on benchmarking: Achieving world-class maintenance and superior competitive performance. *Plant Engineering, 49*(7), 120–121.

Lemieux-Charles, L. (1994). Physicians in health care management: Managing conflict through negotiation. *Canadian Medical Association Journal, 151*(8), 1129–1132.

Lewin, K. (1951). *Field theory in social sciences.* New York: Harper & Row.

Libbus, M. K., & Bowman, K. G. (1994). Sexual harassment of female registered nurses in hospitals. *Journal of Nursing Administration, 24*(6), 26–31.

Lissy, W. E. (1995). Interviewing job applicants under the ADA. *Supervision, 56*(3), 17.

Lukes, E. N. (1993). Performance appraisal: A motivational tool. *AAOHN Journal, 41*(12), 599–600.

Marrelli, T. M. (1993). *The nurse manager's survival guide.* St. Louis: C.V. Mosby.

Marriner-Tomey, A. (1992). *Guide to nursing management.* St. Louis: Mosby YearBook.

McBey, K. (1994). Perfecting performance appraisals. *Security Management, 38*(11), 23–25.

McWilliams, B. (1995). What's wrong with benchmarking? *CFO, 11*(5), 105–106.

Meiss, R. (1991). *Effective listening* (audiotape). Boulder, CO: CareerTrack Publications.

Moran, E. T., & Volkwein, J. F. (1992). The cultural approach to the formation of organizational climate. *Human Relations, 45*(1), 19–47.

Morgan, R. L. (1995). Guidelines for delegating effectively. *Supervision, 56*(4), 20–21.

Morzinski, J. A., Simpson, D. E., Bower, D. J., & Diehr, S. (1994). Faculty development through formal mentoring. *Academic Medicine, 69*(4), 267–269.

Murray, J. A., & Murray, M. H. (1992). Benchmarking: A tool for excellence in palliative care. *Journal of Palliative Care, 8*(4), 41–45.

Neale, M. A., & Bazerman, M. H. (1992). Negotiating rationally: The power and impact of the negotiator's frame. *Academy of Management Executive, 6*(3), 42–51.

Neuhs, H. P. (1994). Sexual harassment. A concern for nursing administrators. *Journal of Nursing Administration, 24*(5), 47–52.

Ninemeier, J. D. (1995). 10 tips for delegating tasks. *Hotels, 29*(6), 20.

Ondeck, D. A., & Gingerich, B. S. (1994). The mentoring relationship. *Journal of Home Health Care Practice, 6*(4), 1–7.

Outwater, L. C. (1994). Sexual harassment issues in home care: What employers should do about it. *Caring, 13*(5), 54–60.

Pollock, T. (1994). Secrets of successful delegation. *Production, 106*(12), 10–11.

Poor, E. (1992). The memo as project manager. *The Executive Female, 15*(3), 63–65.

Pulakos, E. D., & Schmitt, N. (1995). Experience-based and situational interview questions: Studies of validity. *Personnel Psychology, 48*(2), 289.

Rice, H. W. (1995). Teaching the art of the memo: Politics and precision. *Business Communication Quarterly, 59*(1), 31–34.

Rogers, B. (1994). *Occupational health nursing: Concepts and practice.* Philadelphia: W.B. Saunders Company.

Rogers, J. L., & Maurizio, S. J. (1993). Prevalence of sexual harassment among rural community care workers. *Home Healthcare Nurse, 11*(4), 37–40.

Schein, E. H. (1988). *Process consultation: Its role in organizational development.* Reading, MA: Addison-Wesley Publishing Company.

Seitel, F. P. (1993). Meaningful memos. *United States Banker, 103*(11), 77.

Sherer, J. L. (1994). Resolving conflict (the right way). *Hospitals & Health Networks, 68*(8), 52–55.

Sullivan, E. J., & Decker, P. J. (1992). *Effective management in nursing.* Redwood City, CA: Addison-Wesley Nursing.

Susskind, L., & McKearnan, S. (1995). Enlightened conflict resolution. *Technology Review, 98*(3), 70–72.

Tappen, R. M. (1989). *Nursing leadership and management: Concepts and practice.* Philadelphia: F.A. Davis.

Taylor, F. W. (1911). *The principles of scientific management.* New York: Harper & Brothers.

Travers, P. H., & McDougall, C. (1995). *Guidelines for an occupational health and safety service.* Atlanta: AAOHN.

Wachs, J. E. (1991). Strategies to develop "interconnectedness." Part I: Connections within the organization. *AAOHN Journal, 39*(12), 578–579.

Wachs, J. E. (1992a). Strategies to develop "interconnectedness." Part II: Connections within the community. *AAOHN Journal, 40*(3), 144–146.

Wachs, J. E. (1992b). Facilitating an effective meeting. *AAOHN Journal, 40*(6), 294–296.

Wachs, J. E. (1992c). Developing health service staff. *AAOHN Journal, 40*(9), 448–450.

Wachs, J. E. (1993). Managing time. *AAOHN Journal, 41*(6), 300–302.

Wachs, J. E. (1994a). Professional presentations: Transmitting information with polish and flair. Part I—Preparing the presentation. *AAOHN Journal, 42*(3), 141–143.

Wachs, J. E. (1994b). Professional presentations: Transmitting information with polish and flair. Part II—Delivering the presentation. *AAOHN Journal, 42*(6), 305–308.

Wachs, J. E. (1995a). Serving the community. *AAOHN Journal, 43*(2), 109–110.

Wachs, J. E. (1995b). Listening. *AAOHN Journal, 43*(11), 590–592.

Wachs, J. E., & Price, M. (1995). Asking questions: A management tool. *AAOHN Journal, 43*(5), 285–287.

Wachs, P. M., & Wachs, J. E. (1992). Negotiation without confrontation. *AAOHN Journal, 40*(12), 599–601.

Webb, P. R., & Cantone, J. M. (1993). Performance evaluation: Triumph or torture? *Journal of Home Health Care Practice, 5*(2), 14–19.

Weber, A. J. (1995). Making performance appraisals consistent with a quality environment. *Quality Progress, 28*(6), 65–69.

Williams, K. G. (1994). Responding to false charges of sexual harassment. *American Journal of Hospital Pharmacy, 51*(16), 2004–2005.

Wywialowski, E. (1993). *Managing client care.* St. Louis: C. V. Mosby.

Yarborough, M. H. (1994). New variations on recruitment prescreening. *HR Focus, 71*(10), 1–5.

Zamanou, S., & Glaser, S. R. (1994). Moving toward participation and involvement. *Group & Organization Management, 19*(4), 475–502.

Zwanenberg, N. V., & Wilkinson, L. J. (1993). The person specification—A problem masquerading as a solution? *Personnel Review, 22*(7), 54–65.

CHAPTER

7

Scientific Foundations of Occupational Health Nursing Practice

MAJOR TOPICS

- *Nursing science*
- *Environmental health*
- *Epidemiology*
- *Toxicology*
- *Industrial hygiene*
- *Ergonomics*
- *Injury prevention*
- *Social and behavioral sciences*

The science and practice of occupational health nursing is based on a synthesis of knowledge gained from multiple disciplines. It is essential that occupational health nurses understand the principles of the basic sciences that provide the theoretical, conceptual, and factual framework of the profession. In addition to the nursing and occupational health sciences (i.e., toxicology, industrial hygiene, and ergonomics), effective occupational health nursing practice requires knowledge and understanding of the public health (i.e., environmental health and epidemiology) and the social/behavioral sciences. This chapter provides an introduction and overview of these foundational disciplines.

Nursing Science
I

History of Nursing Science

A. Florence Nightingale established public health as an important focus for nursing.
1. She emphasized the need for nurses to improve environmental conditions in order to protect the health of clients, thus laying the foundation for occupational health nursing.
2. She provided the initial spark for development of nursing theory and research, although her major influence was on nursing education.

B. Development of nursing research and theory (Gortner & Nahm, 1977; Stevenson, 1992)

1. From 1950 to 1975, theories focused on nursing practice.
   a. *Nursing Research,* the first journal for nursing science, was established in 1953.
   b. Most grand theories for nursing practice developed during this time period (see Section III).
   c. Most early theories of practice require modification before they can be applied to care delivered in the occupational setting.
2. From 1975 to 1990, middle range theories began to be developed to guide research.
   a. Middle range theories, in contrast to grand theories, are more amenable to testing through research techniques, and they lend themselves better to testing the interventions used in occupational health nursing practice.
   b. As the commitment of nursing to be a research-based discipline grew, the implementation of research results into nursing practice became a major goal.
3. From 1990 to the present, clinical outcomes research, and particularly the study of nurse-sensitive outcomes, became the major focus for nurse researchers; examples of clinical outcomes of occupational health nursing intervention include:
   a. Prevention of work-related illness and injury
   b. The timely return-to-work of the ill or injured worker
   c. Decrease of the costs of health care and disability compensation
   d. Modification of the personal impact of illness and injury on the worker and the family

II

Research–Theory–Practice Linkages

A. Relationships between research and practice (Meleis, 1991)

1. Practice provides a unique context for nursing research.
   a. Problems regularly confronted in occupational health nursing practice should stimulate nursing research studies.
   b. Examples include the prevention of work-related hearing loss, organizational factors affecting the wearing of personal protective equipment, and the use of modified duty positions.
2. As a professional discipline, nursing practice should be research-based, and changes in practice should be driven by research findings.
3. Specialized research is required to develop effective ways to disseminate nursing research findings to appropriate audiences and implement them to improve practice.
4. Methods of informing occupational health nurses about research affecting their practice need to be further developed.

B. Relationships between research and theory (Meleis, 1991)

1. Qualitative research techniques (i.e,. ethnography and grounded theory)
   a. These techniques often lead to the development or refinement of theories about important concepts in nursing practice.
   b. Such research techniques might be used to develop theories about the management of work-related symptoms, workers' self-care, or organizational culture.

2. Quantitative research techniques
   a. These techniques may lead to the development or testing of theories.
   b. Epidemiological techniques, for example, might be used to test nursing theories about risk and risk reduction.

III

Early Nursing Theory: Grand Theories

Grand Theories are more useful as overall frameworks for making decisions in practice than for identifying specific research questions; three categories of grand theories are (Meleis, 1991; Reihl & Roy, 1988):

A. Needs-based theories
   1. These theories are based on the idea that nursing care is required to help clients meet specific functional needs (e.g., theories of Virginia Henderson, Dorothea Orem).
   2. Example: Orem's theory might be adapted to promote self-care related to the prevention of work-related symptoms or to modify the work setting for the disabled worker.

B. Interaction-based theories
   1. These are based on the idea that nursing care proceeds through a process of interaction between the nurse and the client (e.g., those of Hildegarde Peplau, Ida Jean Orlando, J. Travelbee, Imogene King, J. Paterson, and L. Zderad).
   2. These theories could be adapted to clarify the relationship between the occupational health nurse and the worker.

C. Outcome-based theories
   1. These are based on the idea that nursing focuses on outcomes of care related to energy conservation, balance, or harmony (e.g., theories of Dorothy Johnson, Myra Levine, Martha Rogers, Sister Callista Roy).
   2. Example: Johnson's theory might be adapted to examine physiological and behavioral outcomes of occupational health nursing interventions.

IV

The Domain of Nursing

Nursing is differentiated from other scientific disciplines by the way it defines the client, or recipient of care; the environment or context of care; the health and/or illness problems under consideration; and the therapeutic interventions applied. These domains emerged from the grand theories of nursing (Ellis, 1982; Flaskerud & Halloran, 1980; and Meleis, 1991).

A. Patient/client/recipient of care
   1. Under what conditions do human beings become recipients of nursing care?
   2. Risks to health, function, equilibrium, and/or self-care ability tend to define a person or group's need for nursing care.
   3. Occupational health nurses are concerned primarily with working-age adults and their families.

B. Environment of care
   1. What are the properties, components, and dimensions of the environment that influence the recipient's health status?
   2. For nursing, the environment includes physical, sociocultural, organizational, economic, political, and interpersonal dimensions.
   3. These dimensions of the environment are all essential considerations for occupational health nurses, indicating that this is a particularly important domain for occupational health nursing practice.

C. Health/illness problems
   1. What are the health or illness conditions that are influenced by nursing care?
   2. In nursing, health is considered to be more than absence of disease and includes dimensions of self-actualization as well as illness.
   3. Occupational health nurses focus primarily on work-related illnesses and injuries or potentially disabling conditions that might limit someone's ability to work or that might be worsened by work.
D. Nursing therapeutics
   1. What are the content and goals of nursing interventions?
   2. Nursing interventions are those nursing activities and actions deliberately designed for recipients of nursing care.
   3. Occupational health nurses, for example, perform interventions that are unique to the occupational setting or workers.

V

Modern Nursing Theory: Middle Range Theories

A. Characteristics of middle range theories
   1. Evolve from the daily practice considerations of nurses and focus on more specific practice problems than grand theories.
   2. Are often more amenable than grand theories to testing using research techniques.
   3. By contrast, narrow range theories focus on problems that are unique to individual settings or small groups of clients and are less useful for nursing as a whole.
B. Examples of middle range theories with applicability to occupational health nursing research include the following:
   1. Pender's theory of health promotion and health (protection) behaviors:
      a. Focuses on individual perceptions and the likelihood that an individual will perform a recommended preventive health action
      b. Such a theory has immediate implications for occupational health nursing research and might be applied to worker perceptions about work-related risks of illness and injury and safe work activities.
      c. A researcher might attempt to identify the factors that influence workers' use of hearing protection.
   2. Social support
      a. Multiple theories of social support describe the beneficial effects of support from others, including supervisors and co-workers.
      b. Social support within and among teams of supervisors and co-workers might be studied by occupational health nurses as a predictor of safer work activities and fewer injuries.
   3. Mischel's model of uncertainty
      a. This theory describes the concept of uncertainty and its effects on an individual's choices related to health care seeking and recovery from illness or injury (Mischel, 1988).
      b. An occupational health nurse researcher might adapt the theory to study recovery from an occupational injury or illness; uncertainty and fear of reinjury, for example, might be a factor in delaying the return to work of clients whose symptoms persist after carpal tunnel syndrome surgery.

VI

Occupational health nursing practice influences and is influenced by nursing science.

A. Occupational health nurses need to actively participate in national activities to ensure that the working population is considered when research priorities are set.

B. Occupational health nurses need to participate in determining which outcomes are important for the nursing care of working-age adults and their families and which outcomes are affected by occupational health nursing interventions.

C. Occupational health nursing participation in the development of taxonomies is critical to ensure the inclusion of data related to occupations, occupational health nursing and worksite interventions, prevention programs, worker participation, and work-related injuries and illnesses.

Environmental Health

VII

The Effects of the Environment on Health

Environmental health is the "freedom from illness or injury related to exposure to toxic agents and other environmental conditions that are potentially detrimental to health" (Institute of Medicine, 1995, p. 15).

A. An Institute of Medicine study (1995) identified three themes related to nursing and the environment (p. vi):

1. The environment is a primary determinant of health, and environmental health hazards affect all aspects of life and all areas of nursing practice.
2. Nurses are well positioned to address environmental health concerns of individuals and communities.
3. There is a need to enhance the awareness of and emphasis on environmental threats to the health of populations served by all nurses, regardless of their practice arena.

B. Some of the most significant environmental conditions that are capable of harming the health of humans are experienced at work.

C. Three factors are used to analyze the balance of health (Shortridge, 1992):

1. The *causative agent,* which is related to work processes or interactions
2. The *susceptible host,* the worker with the following characteristics
   a. Generally healthy enough to hold a job
   b. Of working age
   c. Often of childbearing age
3. The *environments,* or the work settings, which are highly variable

D. Workers are faced with multiple workplace hazards that place them at risk.

1. A *hazard* is defined as a substance capable of causing harm (see Chapter 2 for a description of categories of hazards).
2. *Risk* is the probability that harm will occur.

E. A systematic understanding of the agent-host-environment relationship as it exists in the work setting can provide the basis for the prevention of morbidity and mortality and for the promotion of health.

F. The chief disciplines that guide the occupational health nurse in an understanding of the agent-host-environment relationship are epidemiology, toxicology, and industrial hygiene; these are described in the following sections.

Epidemiology
VIII

Overview of Epidemiological Terms and Principles

Epidemiology is the public health science that is fundamental to describing and understanding relationships among agents, hosts, and their environments.

A. Definitions
1. The word *epidemiology* is of Greek derivation (from *epi,* meaning "upon"; *demos,* meaning "people"; and *logos,* meaning "science").
2. *Epidemiology* is the study of the distribution and determinants of health-related states or events in specified populations, and the application of this study to control of health problems (Last, 1988).
3. An *incidence rate* is an epidemiological term that describes the rate of disease development among persons at risk.
    a. The numerator includes only new cases of disease during a given time period; the denominator includes everyone at risk of developing the disease during that period.
    b. Incidence, therefore, measures the probability (or risk) of developing disease.
4. A *prevalence rate* is an epidemiological term that describes the proportion of the population that has the condition at a given point in time or during a given time period.
    a. The numerator includes new and existing cases; the denominator includes all who are at risk of developing the disease, including those who have it.
    b. Prevalence measures the current burden of disease and is useful for measuring and projecting health care needs.

B. Examples of epidemiological research include:
1. Control of infectious diseases, such as tuberculosis among migrant farm workers
2. Control of effects of chemical hazards, such as mesothelioma and lung cancers related to exposure to asbestos
3. Understanding genetic susceptibility to disease, such as coronary heart disease, which seems to result from a combination of hereditary and environmental factors
4. Understanding effects of nutritional status, such as the link between a high-fat diet and colorectal cancer
5. Linking pathogens to specific disease processes, such as the Human Immunodeficiency virus (HIV) to Acquired Immunodeficiency Disease Syndrome (AIDS)

C. Epidemiology has great relevance to occupational health nursing.
1. It serves as a tool for identifying and preventing hazardous worksite exposures.
2. Findings from epidemiological studies of worker populations are frequently reported in the occupational health literature.
3. Epidemiological studies of work-related problems will assist occupational health nurses to provide high-quality health services.

IX

Measures of Association

The study of association is key to epidemiology; criteria to evaluate causality of observed association include (Mausner & Kramer, 1985):

A. Strength of the association
   1. This refers to the magnitude (amount) of risk associated with an exposure.
   2. Magnitude of risk is often measured by the ratio of two rates.

B. Consistency of the association
   1. Similar findings result across several studies of the association.
   2. Conclusions are similar despite the use of different study designs.

C. Temporality of the association
   1. Studies demonstrate that the independent variable (cause) precedes the dependent variable (effect) chronologically.
   2. Temporality cannot be evaluated with a cross-sectional study.

D. Dose-response relationship
   1. As the degree of exposure increases, the risk for developing the outcome increases.
   2. Lack of a dose-response does not rule out a causal relationship.

E. Plausibility of the association
   1. The association is consistent with a plausible biologic explanation.
   2. Knowledge of the natural history of the disease and results of animal and other laboratory experiments need to be considered.

X

Existing Sources of Epidemiological Data

A. Health outcome data are available through a variety of public and private agencies.
   1. Census data (U.S. Census Bureau)
   2. Vital statistics (U.S. Census Bureau)
   3. National health surveys (National Center for Health Statistics)
   4. Disease registries (from state and federal agencies).

B. Exposure data are often more difficult to obtain, especially in environmental and occupational settings.
   1. Examples of exposure data are air monitoring data and biomarkers of exposure.
   2. Data may be obtained from exposure registries such as those maintained for heavy metal exposure, certain pharmaceuticals, and needlestick injuries.

XI

Comparisons of Rates

A. A *rate ratio* (also known as *relative risk*) is a measure of the relationship between two rates, that of the exposed and that of the unexposed population.

B. *"Odds ratio"* is a good estimate of the rate ratio, but is derived from case control or cross-sectional studies.

C. A *rate difference* is a measure of the difference between two rates, one for the exposed and one for the unexposed population. Because it describes the increased amount of risk attributed to the exposure, it is known as "attributable risk."

BOX 7-1

Using Crude, Specific, and Adjusted Rates to Describe a Health Problem

Crude Rates: The crude rates of lung cancer in a population will not reflect the fact that older individuals are at higher risk for lung cancer. To look at the association between smoking and lung cancer, it would not be fair to compare crude rates of lung cancer in groups of smokers and nonsmokers who differ in age distribution.

Specific Rates: Rates of lung cancer could be computed for age-specific groups, perhaps by decade of age, to examine differences in lung cancer rates by age.

Adjusted Rates: The age-adjusted rates of lung cancer in the smoking and nonsmoking groups could be compared to look meaningfully at the question of an association between smoking and cancer.

XII

Types of Rates
(See Box 7-1 for an example.)

A. *Crude rates* are based on the actual number of events for a given time period but do not reflect any important differences in risk among subgroups in the population.

B. *Characteristic-specific rates* allow one to compare rates for similar subgroups of two or more populations (e.g., age-specific or gender-specific rates).

C. *Adjusted* (or *standardized*) *rates* reflect population differences by taking into consideration important characteristics that may affect risk (e.g., age-adjusted rates).

XIII

Inferential Statistics
These are statistics from a sample of a population that are used to make inferences about the entire target population (Mausner & Kramer, 1985).

A. A *hypothesis* is a supposition, arrived at from observation or reflection.
  1. A hypothesis leads to predictions that can be tested.
  2. Hypothesis testing involves conducting a test of statistical significance and quantifying the degree to which sampling variability may account for the observed results.

B. Some well-known tests of statistical significance include the t-test and chi-square test.

C. A *p-value* is a quantitative statement of the probability that the observed difference (or association) in a particular study could have happened by chance alone.
  1. $p < 0.05$ means that the probability that the observed difference occurred by chance is less than 5%.
  2. $p < 0.05$ is the customary level of accepting an association as statistically significant.

D. A *confidence interval* provides an idea of the magnitude of the effect and the inherent variability in the estimate.
   1. A confidence interval is an alternative to a P-value.
   2. The calculation of the confidence level is based on the assumption that the distribution of observed rates can be approximated by the standard normal curve.
   3. A 95% confidence level means that there is a 95% probability that the true rate of an observation lies within the calculated interval.

E. The *power* of a study is its chance of detecting a real association; that power is affected by four variables:
   1. The magnitude of the effect (or association)
   2. The variability of the measures of interest
   3. The level of statistical significance that has been set (alpha)
   4. The size of the sample studied
      a. Larger sample sizes increase the stability of measurements made in an epidemiologic study.
      b. Power calculations based on the above variables suggest the appropriate sample size needed for an epidemiologic study.

XIV

Overview of Study Designs
(Also see Chapter 13: Methodology.)

A. *Experimental designs* are preferred for determining causality
   1. In an experimental study, the investigator assigns the exposure (or putative cause) to the study subjects.
   2. *Clinical trials* and *intervention studies* are both examples of experimental designs.
   3. Experiments are limited by ethical constraints.

B. *Nonexperimental designs* that attempt to simulate the results of an experiment, had one been possible, are primarily *descriptive studies* or *analytic* (ex post facto) *studies.*
   1. *Descriptive studies* are hypothesis generating and therefore are not intended to determine causality.
      a. A *cross-sectional study* examines the relationship between diseases (or other health-related characteristics) and other variables of interest as they exist in a defined population at one point in time.
      b. An *ecologic study* involves the group rather than the individual as the unit of analysis, usually because information is not available at the individual level.
   2. *Analytic studies:* the investigator systematically determines whether risk of disease is different for exposed and non-exposed individuals.
      a. A *cohort study* (also called a *prospective study* or *follow-up study*) is an analytic study in which persons who are initially free of the disease (or outcome) but vary in one or more factors (such as exposure), are followed over a period of time for the occurrence of the disease, or outcome.
      b. In a *case-control study,* a group of persons with a disease (cases) are compared to a group without the disease (controls) to study the characteristics (such as exposure factors) that might predict or cause the disease.
   3. Table 7-1 lists advantages and disadvantages of cohort, case-control, and cross-sectional study designs.

TABLE 7-1

Advantages and Disadvantages of Various Designs of Nonexperimental Epidemiologic Studies

Study Design	Advantages	Disadvantages
Cohort or Prospective	Good for study of rare exposures	Lengthy
	Allows classification of exposure before disease develops	Large sample size required
	Can determine incidence of disease	Generally expensive
	Can determine true relative risk	
	Can follow multiple outcomes	
Case-Control	Good for study of rare outcomes	Exposure histories may be difficult to construct
	Subject loss to follow-up a problem	Recall bias can be a problem
	Can estimate relative risk by odds ratio	Must select appropriate control group
	Takes less time	
	Less expensive	
	Requires smaller sample size	
	Can look at multiple risk factors	
Cross-Sectional	Generates hypotheses	Cannot determine causality
	Useful in study of exposures that do not change (e.g., blood type)	Current exposure does not always represent relevant past exposure

Source: Modified from Mausner & Kramer (1985).

XV

Bias and Confounding in Epidemiologic Studies

Detection of associations that are not real and have not occurred due to chance is the result of biased study methods or the presence of confounding variables (Mausner and Kramer, 1985).

A. *Bias* refers to systematic error in an epidemiologic study that results in an incorrect estimate of the association between exposure and risk of disease.
  1. Selection bias
      a. This type of bias occurs when the identification of subjects for inclusion into the study on the basis of either exposure (cohort study) or disease (case-control study) status depends in some way on the other axis of interest.
      b. Selection bias can result from differential surveillance, diagnosis, or referral of individuals into the study.

TABLE 7-2

Types of Bias in Epidemiologic Studies

Type of Bias	Description
Information	Exposure or outcome is ascertained differently from study groups.
Recall	Individuals with negative outcomes are more likely to remember and report exposure experience.
Interviewer	Interviewers' prior knowledge of outcome status affects ascertainment of exposure information in interview.
Lost to follow-up	Prospectively, those with negative outcomes may be lost to follow-up at greater rate than controls.
Misclassification	Ascertainment of either exposure or outcome status is incorrect for some subjects.
Selection	Entry into study or control group is affected by factors related to exposure (case-control) or outcome (cohort).
Self-selection	Individuals' participation is affected by their knowledge of disease or exposure status.

2. Information (or observation) bias
   a. This type of bias results from systematic differences in the way data on exposure or outcomes are obtained from various study groups.
   b. Examples of types of information bias include: recall bias, interviewer bias, loss of subjects to follow-up over time, and misclassification (see Table 7-2).
3. Study results may be biased either toward or away from the null hypothesis or in both directions.

B. *Confounding* results when the estimate of the effect of the exposure of interest is distorted because it is mixed with the effect of an extraneous factor; in occupational epidemiology studies, age and smoking status are usually important confounding variables.

C. Methods to avoid and/or manage study biases and confounding include:
   1. A strict study protocol with attention to how subjects are selected for study is a means of avoiding study bias in the design phase of the study.
   2. Systematic, standardized data collection techniques that are consistent for all study participants will help avoid bias in the data collection phase.
   3. Confounding can be avoided by making comparisons only among individuals with the same level of the confounding variable; this is also known as controlling for the effect of the confounding variable.
      a. Confounding is usually avoided by stratifying or adjusting during data analysis.
      b. Matching subjects is another way to control for confounding.
      c. In an experimental study, confounding is avoided by randomization of treatment between cases and controls.
      d. Subjects who are lost to follow-up should be evaluated to assess whether they differ in important characteristics from those who have remained in the study.

XVI

Screening

Screening is the application of a test to people who are as yet asymptomatic; its purpose is to classify them with respect to their likelihood of having a particular disease.

A. An implicit assumption of screening is that early detection will lead to prevention of death or disability; criteria for screening include:
  1. A recognizable presymptomatic stage of disease must exist.
  2. An effective treatment must be available.
  3. The screening test should have sufficient validity.

B. A highly valid screening test is one which is highly sensitive and specific.
  1. Sensitivity is the ability of a test to identify correctly those who have the disease; a sensitive test yields few false negatives.
  2. Specificity is the ability of a test to identify correctly those who do not have the disease; a specific test yields few false positives.
  3. Sensitivity and specificity do not change when the prevalence of the disease in the population changes.

C. The *predictive value* of screening tests is their ability to predict disease status from test results.
  1. *Positive predictive value* is the likelihood that an individual with a positive test truly has the disease.
  2. *Negative predictive value* is the likelihood that an individual with a negative test does not have the disease.
  3. Levels of predictive value do change when the prevalence of a disease in a population changes.
     a. As the prevalence of a disease in a population increases, the positive predictive value of the test will also increase.
     b. However, as the prevalence increases, the negative predictive value will decrease.

Toxicology

XVII

Overview of Toxicological Terms and Principles

Toxicology is the study of adverse effects of chemicals on biologic systems (Doull & Bruce, 1985).

A. A *target organ* is the organ that is selectively affected by a harmful agent.

B. A chemical is toxic—that is can cause harm—IF:
  1. Its properties make it capable of producing harm;
  2. It is present in sufficient amount;
  3. It is present for sufficient time;
  4. It is delivered by an exposure route that allows it to be absorbed; AND
  5. It reaches a susceptible body organ.

C. *Toxic agents* can be classified by their form of action on biologic systems.
  1. *Asphyxiants* deprive the body tissue of oxygen.
     a. Simple asphyxiants displace oxygen and cause suffocation; examples are carbon dioxide, nitrogen, and argon.

    b. Chemical asphyxiants prevent oxygen use by the cell, although enough oxygen may be present; examples are carbon monoxide and cyanide.

  2. *Corrosives* cause irreversible tissue death; ozone and acids are examples of corrosives.

  3. *Irritants* cause temporary, but sometimes severe, inflammation of the eyes, skin, or respiratory tract; an example is ammonia.

  4. *Sensitizers* cause allergic reactions after repeated exposure; examples are nickel and toluene diisocyanate.

  5. *Carcinogens* are capable of causing cancer; examples include asbestos, coal tar, and vinyl chloride monomer.

  6. *Mutagens* are toxins that cause changes to the genetic material of cells that can be passed on to future generations; known human mutagens include ethylene oxide and ionizing radiation.

  7. *Teratogens* cause malformations in an unborn child; some agents that are teratogenic are organic mercury compounds, ionizing radiation, and some pharmaceuticals.

  8. Toxins may have more than one form of action and may act at more than one site. For example, formaldehyde is irritating to the eyes and respiratory tract, can irritate and sensitize the skin, and is suspected of being a carcinogen.

D. Characteristics of exposure

  1. The *dose* of an agent is the amount that reaches the target organ.

    a. The dose is usually impossible to determine accurately.

    b. The dose is usually estimated by measuring the amount administered (as with drugs) or the amount to which a person has been exposed (as with work exposures).

    c. Vapors or gases are expressed as parts per million (ppm).

    d. Solids (dusts or fume) are expressed according to their weight per volume of air, usually as milligrams per cubic meter (mg/M^3).

    e. Higher concentrations of substances are generally absorbed in greater amounts.

    f. Longer or more frequent periods of exposure also lead to greater absorbed doses.

  2. Acute and chronic exposures

    a. *Acute exposure* occurs when exposure is short-term and absorption is fairly rapid.

    b. *Chronic exposure* refers to longer duration or repeated periods of contact.

    c. In general, acute toxic exposures tend to be at higher levels, and chronic exposures occur at lower concentrations.

  3. *Guidelines and standards* serve to evaluate the seriousness of an exposure.

    a. Examples of workplace guidelines are Threshold Limit Values (TLV); examples of workplace standards are Permissible Exposure Limits (PEL) (described in detail in the Industrial Hygiene section).

    b. Guidelines and standards indicate upper limits of exposure concentrations that are not felt to pose a danger to workers who are exposed over normal work hours.

    c. Published limits cannot be viewed as definitely "safe" levels.

    d. Guidelines and standards may be controversial due to lack of scientific data, lack of agreement over the levels associated with health effects, and the reality that levels that protect most individuals may yet affect susceptible subgroups.

XVIII

Major Exposure Routes

A. *Inhalation:* This is the most important route of exposure in the occupational environment because it is the most common route by which occupational exposures are absorbed.

1. Most absorption takes place in the alveoli, where blood flow is high and close to the inhaled air; to reach the alveoli, the substance must be a gas or a particulate ranging in size from approximately 1–10 microns in diameter.
2. Absorption by inhalation is highly influenced by the rate and depth of respirations; thus, workers performing heavy physical labor may absorb substances at a higher rate.
3. Although the lung may serve as the target organ of some inhaled toxins, other substances gain entry through the lungs but exert their effect elsewhere in the body; examples are solvents and carbon monoxide, which have systemic effects.

B. *Cutaneous:* The skin does provide a barrier to most substances, but its effectiveness as a barrier varies according to its condition, site, and the properties of the chemical agent.

1. Some substances cross the epidermal layer or enter through hair follicles.
2. Some substances may enter by the trauma of injection or impalement; this entry method is less common.
3. In general, gases penetrate most freely, liquids less freely, and solids that are insoluble in water or fats do not penetrate the skin.
4. Longer contact promotes higher levels of absorption.
5. Damage to the epidermal cells by a chemical may promote its further absorption.

C. *Ingestion:* In the occupational setting, ingestion is the least common route of entry.

1. Caustic or irritant chemicals, if ingested, may have a direct adverse effect on the gastrointestinal tract.
2. Some toxins act systemically following their absorption.
3. Smoking or eating at worksites can lead to consumption of toxins by way of contaminated hands, food, or smoking materials.

XIX

The Dose–Response Relationship

This is the relationship between levels of exposure and the resulting toxic effects in a susceptible population of humans or experimental animals (Klaassen, 1986b).

A. Higher doses are generally associated with effects in a greater proportion of individuals.

B. Identification of a dose-response relationship lends support to a theory that a substance causes a given effect.

C. Dose-response curves provide a basis for evaluating a chemical's relative toxicity; an agent is considered more toxic when a smaller dose is needed to produce effects comparable to those produced by a greater dose of a less toxic substance.

1. Terms that describe toxicity of a substance are *lethal dose, 50% (LD50)* and *lethal concentration, 50% (LC50)*.
2. These terms refer to the dose (LD50) or concentration (LC50) that produce death in 50% of a group of experimental animals.

3. These indices are smaller for more toxic agents. For example, the LD50 of acetone is 5,340 mg/kg, whereas hydrogen cyanide, a much more toxic compound, has a LD50 of 0.5 mg/kg (Dreisbach and Robertson, 1987, pp. 182, 252).

4. Animal studies are useful because they provide information about potential toxic effects or target organs in humans; however, they must be interpreted cautiously because of the many differences in response that exist among species.

XX

Nature of Effects

A. The effects of toxins with long latency periods may not be apparent until years after the exposure period.

B. Interactive effects may occur with two or more concurrent exposures (Klaassen, 1986b).

1. *Synergistic effects* are resultant effects that surpass the sum of the separate effects.

2. *Antagonism* results in an overall effect that is less than the sum of the separate effects.

3. *Potentiation* means that a chemical has no adverse effect on its own, but its presence increases the effect of another substance or makes that substance capable of exerting an effect.

XXI

The Fate of Toxins in the Body

Once absorbed, the fate of toxins in the body varies (Klaassen, 1986b).

A. Excretion

1. Some chemicals are excreted unchanged into expired air, urine, feces, bile, or perspiration.

2. Other avenues of excretion include milk, spinal fluid, saliva, and hair.

3. Most chemicals and their metabolic products are excreted through the kidney/urine pathway.

B. Transformation

1. Chemicals may be transformed into a substance that can be excreted by a process called *biotransformation.*

2. Products of biotransformation may be either less toxic or more toxic than their parent chemical.

3. This is an important concept when individuals differ in the rate at which they metabolize substances, for this rate can affect individual susceptibility to a toxin.

C. Factors affecting excretion

1. Many agents are not metabolized or excreted immediately but, instead, are deposited in body tissue and slowly released and excreted over time.

2. *Half-life* is the term that describes the time it takes for one-half of the total absorbed amount to be eliminated from the body.

3. The length of the half-life depends on both the agent and the tissue in which it is stored; for example, the half-life of lead is over 20 years in bone, compared to only about 25–30 days in blood.

XXII

Endogenous and Exogenous Host Factors
These factors can influence susceptibility and magnitude of the toxic response.

A. *Endogenous* factors are inherent to the individual and are beyond the control of that individual.
   1. *Gender* may influence susceptibility to some toxins, although the cause of this difference is not well understood in all cases.
      a. Some cancers and other diseases may be associated with gender.
      b. Women have a greater proportion of body fat and therefore may accumulate more lipid soluble toxins than men.
      c. Other differences in metabolism, anthropometry, and genetic types may account for varying susceptibility to toxins.
   2. *Genetic differences* may cause variation in metabolism, detoxification, excretion, and cellular response to toxins.
   3. *Aging* is related to rate and efficiency of metabolism, levels of organ function, and patterns of excretion.
      a. Age-related factors may increase toxic responses among older adults.
      b. Similarly, children may experience increased susceptibility because of their higher respiratory and metabolic rates, less mature nervous systems, and immature livers, which lack the detoxification mechanisms of adults.
      c. Children are also more susceptible than adults to some cancers because they are growing and their cells are dividing more rapidly.
      d. Pregnant mothers may be exposed to worksite agents that have the potential to cause perinatal malignancies.
   4. *Health conditions* can increase individual susceptibility to toxins; for example, heart disease can influence effects of exposure to asphyxiants that affect oxygen availability or utilization.

B. Individuals may be able to exert some control over *exogenous* factors, since those factors are related to behavior or environmental conditions.
   1. *Nutrition* factors can enhance or inhibit absorption or toxic responses.
   2. *Obesity* may promote more storage of lipid soluble substances.
   3. *Lifestyle* factors such as smoking or alcohol consumption increase overall chemical exposures that must be handled by the body.
   4. *Stress* may have an effect on the function of some organs, such as those in the cardiovascular, immune, and gastrointestinal systems.
   5. Some adverse health conditions are temporary and manageable but may affect an individual's vulnerability to toxins.

Note: Table 7-3 presents some major effects seen in various body systems and gives examples of worksite exposures that cause them.

Industrial Hygiene
XXIII

Overview of Industrial Hygiene
Industrial hygiene refers to the "science and art devoted to the anticipation, recognition, evaluation, and control of those environmental factors arising in or from the workplace that may result in injury, illness, impairment or affect the well-being of workers and members of the community" (American Industrial Hygiene Association, 1996)

TABLE 7-3

Potential Toxic Effects by System, with Examples of Toxins

System	Effects	Sources of Exposure
Respiratory	Irritation	hydrogen chloride, ammonia
	Sensitization	isocyanates
	Fibrosis	silica, asbestos, beryllium
	Carcinogens	asbestos, arsenic, chromium VI
Dermatologic	Irritation	acetone, carbon disulfide
	Corrosive burns	alkali, hydrogen fluoride
	Sensitization	chromate, nickel
	Carcinogenesis	ultraviolet light, arsenic
Nervous System	Depression/altered consciousness	carbon monoxide, solvents
	Behavior and mood disturbance	lead, mercury, manganese
	Cognitive disturbance	lead, solvent
	Cerebellar impairment	toluene, mercury
	Parkinson-like effects	carbon monoxide, manganese, pesticides
	Peripheral neuropathy	acrylamide, *n*-hexane, methyl *n*-butyl ketone
Hearing and Vision	Acid burns of eyes	hydrochloric and tannic acid
	Alkali burns of eyes	sodium hydroxide, calcium oxide
	Blindness	methanol
	Deafness	noise
Hematopoetic	Bone marrow suppression	ionizing radiation, benzene
	Red cell lysis	arsine, trinitrotoluene (TNT), naphthalene
Hepatic	Necrosis	carbon tetrachloride, chloroform, tetrachloroethane
	Cirrhosis	carbon tetrachloride
	Malignancy	vinyl chloride monomer
Renal and Bladder	Nephrotoxicity	heavy metals, carbon tetrachloride, chloroform
	Renal cancer	coke oven emissions
	Bladder cancer	benzidine, B-napthylamine
Reproductive	Decreased sperm production	ionizing radiation, heat
	Decreased female fertility	ionizing radiation, carbon disulfide
	Spontaneous abortions	ethylene oxide
	Congenital defects	rubella, varicella

A. The field of industrial hygiene draws upon knowledge from many occupations including engineering, physics, chemistry, and biology.

B. Industrial hygiene "involves evaluation of the extent of exposure and development of corrective measures to control health hazards by reducing or eliminating hazards" (Plog 1996, p. 3).

C. Professional organizations for industrial hygienists include the American Industrial Hygiene Association (AIHA) and the American Conference of Governmental Industrial Hygienists (ACGIH) (see Appendix E).

XXIV

Sources of Information for Hazard Recognition

A. *Qualitative assessment* of the worksite includes:
  1. Communication with key personnel, such as plant management representatives and supervisors, to learn about materials and processes
  2. Communication with other occupational health professionals to learn about health problems that may be related to exposure
  3. Conversations with workers to learn about their perceptions of exposure

B. *Observational assessments* are achieved through strategies such as walk-through surveys, focused inspections, and job hazard analyses. (A complete description of these and other strategies is detailed in Chapter 9.)

C. Material safety data sheets (MSDS)
  1. Information on MSDSs includes (Hathaway, 1994):
     a. Identification of the material and its manufacturer
     b. Hazardous ingredients and regulatory and/or advisory levels
     c. Physical and chemical properties
     d. Fire and explosion hazard data
     e. Reactivity data
     f. Health hazard data
     g. Precautions for safe handling and use
     h. Control measures
     i. Special precautions and comments
  2. Some caveats are in order when using information provided in the MSDS (Fowler, 1990).
     a. The quality of MSDSs is variable; the information is sometimes outdated, unclear, and inconsistent for the same materials across manufacturers.
     b. Recommended protective measures may be unnecessarily complex and need to be considered in the context of the specific material's actual use and control measures in effect.

XXV

Sampling Methods

Approaches for estimating the dose of an exposure received by workers include personal and environmental *sampling* as well as *biological* and *medical monitoring* (Plog, 1996). (For details on methods, see Chapter 9.)

A. Sampling techniques may measure exposure before absorption has occurred.
  1. Approaches to sampling depend on the type of agent and the route by which it is absorbed by workers (Smith, 1988).
     a. *Skin wipes* measure amounts of cutaneously absorbed materials that contact the skin.

   b. *Noise dosimeters,* worn near the worker's ear, record worksite noise levels.
   c. *Airborne contaminants* can be assessed by means of personal monitoring at the worker's breathing zone or environmental monitoring in the work area.
   2. Several important factors govern whether the sampling results will truly represent worker exposure (Gross and Morse, 1996).
      a. The location of the sampling device with regard to the worker and source of contaminant should be based on worker movements.
      b. The workers to be sampled usually are those who are most highly exposed.
      c. Timing of sampling should take into account seasonal changes, shifts, and other sources of variation.
      d. Length of sampling time generally represents a full shift.
      e. The number of samples depends on the type of instrumentation, concentration of contaminant, and purpose of sampling.

B. Biological and/or medical monitoring identify the presence of a chemical in the body following exposure.

C. Exposure records are extremely important and must be maintained for at least 30 years.

XXVI

Airborne Contaminants

   Levels of airborne contaminants can be compared to the following guidelines and standards.

A. Permissible Exposure Limit (PEL)
   1. PELs are promulgated by the Occupational Safety and Health Administration (OSHA) and are legally enforceable.
   2. These refer to 8-hour time-weighted averages of airborne exposure.

B. Threshold Limit Value (TLV)
   1. TLVs are guidelines developed by the American Conference of Governmental Industrial Hygienists (ACGIH) and are published annually by that organization (see Appendix E).
   2. These also refer to 8-hour time-weighted averages, with the following exceptions.
      a. *Ceiling levels,* or uppermost TLV levels, cannot be exceeded.
      b. *Short-term exposure levels* (STEL) are the maximum 15-minute time-weighted averages permitted over a work day, with at least 60 minutes between successive exposures.

C. Recommended Exposure Level (REL)
   1. RELs are developed by the National Institute for Occupational Safety and Health (NIOSH).
   2. These are the exposures that, in the judgment of NIOSH, will not cause adverse health effects in most workers.

XXVII

Control Strategies for Occupational Exposures

A. *Elimination* or *substitution* with less harmful materials—the preferred control strategy

B. *Engineering controls* to enclose or isolate operations, improve ventilation, or change the process

C. *Changes in work practices* of workers to minimize potential exposures to hazards

D. *Administrative controls* (such as worker rotation) to minimize exposure, the development of monitoring or surveillance programs, and worker training

E. *Personal protective equipment* (PPE) such as ear plugs and muffs, safety goggles, gloves, coveralls, and respirators—the least preferred control strategy

Ergonomics

XXVIII

Overview of Ergonomic Terms and Principles

The term *ergonomics* (also known as "human factors") refers to the study of the interaction between humans and their work.

A. The term literally means the laws (from the Greek word *nomos*) of work (*ergos*).

B. The field of ergonomics is concerned with the design of the worksite, equipment, physical environment, and organization of work.

C. The field is multidisciplinary, involving health professionals, engineers, behavioral scientists, physiologists, and others.

D. Its purpose is to prevent acute and chronic injuries, make worksites comfortable, enhance productivity, reduce fatigue and errors, and promote job satisfaction (Eastman Kodak Company, 1986).

E. Proper job design can make jobs appropriate for workers of both sexes and all ages; considerations are given to size, strength, visual capacity, hearing, capabilities, and limitations.

F. Ergonomics seeks to fit the job to the person rather than the person to the job.

XXIX

Musculoskeletal Disorders

Several *musculoskeletal health problems* can be caused or aggravated by worksite factors (NIOSH, 1988).

A. Affected tissue structures include muscles, tendons, ligaments, peripheral nerves, blood vessels, joints, cartilage, and bones.

B. Problems occur in the upper and sometimes lower extremities, cervical spine, and lower back; symptoms of musculoskeletal disorders include pain, swelling, erythema, numbness, and paresthesia.

C. Examples of work-related musculoskeletal disorders are: tendinitis, tenosynovitis, epicondylitis, DeQuervain's syndrome, synovitis, ganglion cysts, and rotator cuff tendinitis.

D. Nerve entrapment syndromes include carpal tunnel syndrome (median nerve entrapment at the wrist), tarsal tunnel syndrome (tibial nerve entrapment at the ankle), and ulnar nerve entrapment at the elbow or wrist.

E. Another form of peripheral nerve impairment has been termed hand-arm vibration syndrome; this is thought to be due to vibration such as that experienced with the use of power tools (NIOSH criteria document Occupational Exposure to Hand-Arm Vibration, 1989, #94-807).

XXX

Risk Factors for Musculoskeletal Problems

The major worksite risk factors that have been identified for musculoskeletal problems of the upper extremities are repetition, force, mechanical stresses, awkward postures, low temperatures, and vibration.

A. The goal in task and tool design is to avoid or minimize these risk factors.

B. *Repetition* refers to the performance of the same or similar tasks again and again; for example, if one work cycle (a series of motions that is then repeated) lasts less than 30 seconds, or if, in the case of cycles lasting several minutes, there are subcycles that comprise more than 50% of the overall cycle, the job is generally considered repetitive (NIOSH, 1988).

C. *Force* is exerted in tasks that require lifting weights, handling heavy tools, pinching with the fingers, or applying other grips while working.

D. Repetition seems to be a stronger risk factor than force for carpal tunnel syndrome (Silverstein, Fine & Armstrong, 1987).

E. *Mechanical stresses* refers to the forces that result from a worker's direct contact with work surfaces or tools.

F. The *compressive forces* that result from striking objects with hand-held tools or from leaning against hard surfaces or corners on work tables can lead to nerve compression disorders.

G. Work frequently requires workers to assume awkward positions for prolonged or repetitive periods; deviation from neutral posture has been identified as a risk factor in the following conditions:
1. Cervical spine—extreme neck flexion and twisting.
2. Back—twisting at the waist, lifting with legs straight, bending and reaching repetitively, maintaining awkward postures for long periods, carrying, pulling, pushing, or lifting heavy objects from below the knees or above the shoulders, or lifting weight beyond capabilities (Garg, 1995).
3. Shoulders—raising the arm or elbow above mid-torso without support, reaching behind one's body.
4. Forearm/elbow—repeated rotation (i.e., supination and pronation).
5. Wrist/hand—repeated wrist flexion and extension, holding the hand in ulnar deviation.

H. *Vibration* caused by power tools or other work equipment can adversely affect the upper extremities.

I. Whole-body vibration, such as that experienced by drivers of trucks and heavy equipment, can affect the back, lower extremities, and possibly shoulder and neck.

J. *Cold environmental conditions* have an effect on manual dexterity and muscle strength and may directly or indirectly cause hand disorders.

XXXI

High-Risk Jobs

Types of jobs that are considered particularly high risk in terms of ergonomic exposures include:

A. Office work
1. Work at video display terminals may require individuals to assume static and/or awkward positions for typing if workstations are not properly adjusted.

2. Other conditions in the office environment that may introduce hazards include poor lighting, obstructions in walkways, slippery floors, and heavy objects.

B. Manual materials handling—a part of many jobs, from loading trucks and moving heavy goods to working in grocery stores
   1. In addition to repeated bending, lifting, and twisting, this work sometimes involves exposures to vibration.
   2. The risks of back injury are high for these types of jobs.

C. Assembly work—often machine-paced, giving the worker little control over the speed at which he or she works
   1. Repetitive motions tend to be characteristic of this work.
   2. Sometimes work is performed in static or awkward postures or with poorly designed tools.

XXXII

Evaluating Risk Factors

Various methods can be used to evaluate worksites for ergonomic risk factors; each approach has its advantages and disadvantages.

A. *Interviews or questionnaires* that ask workers about their work
   1. Advantages: This method may reveal factors that might not otherwise be noted. Workers have the most complete view of their tasks throughout all work periods.
   2. Disadvantages: There may be high variability in the way workers report their perception of work performance; reports may be incomplete or biased.

B. *Observation and use of checklists*—observing workers while they work and noting any risk factors
   1. Advantages: Observers using the same methods will look at all workers in the same way and thus introduce less variability; this method is fairly efficient —that is, one observer can see many workers in their setting.
   2. Disadvantages: People may change the way they behave when they are under observation; the limited time period for observation may cause some things to be missed; and observers must be trained to be accurate and consistent.

C. *Videotaping and analysis*—taping the worker on the job and later conducting a detailed analysis of motions and other risk factors
   1. Advantages: Analysis is recorded and does not rely on one person's assessment; tape can be slowed or frozen to evaluate details of work tasks; measurement of time and motion can be highly accurate.
   2. Disadvantages: Videotaping requires expensive equipment and experienced personnel; behavior may change when being taped; only a small window of worker's time is recorded, and therefore it is not useful for evaluating highly variable tasks.

XXXIII

Ergonomic Improvements

Some considerations and guidelines for analyzing existing jobs or designing new jobs are as follows (Ross, 1994; U.S. Department of Labor, 1990):

A. General environment: Provide well-illuminated, comfortable levels of temperature and humidity; good visibility of labels and signs; clear, audible auditory signals.

B. Workstations and chairs: These should be adjustable to accommodate workers of different sizes.

C. Layout: Place tools, controls, and materials in front of the worker to prevent twisting, reaching, bending; keep work space free of obstacles.

D. Postures: Avoid static postures; locate and orient work to promote neutral positions.

E. Repetition: Engineer the product or process to reduce repetition; vary tasks; rotate workers to different jobs; provide mechanical devices; allow rest time.

F. Forces: Reduce the size and weight of objects held; employ power rather than pinch grips; balance tools; provide correctly fitting gloves, not tight or bulky; sharpen tools frequently.

G. Mechanical stresses: Ensure that handles on equipment fit the worker's hands; pad or eliminate sharp edges.

H. Vibration: Eliminate vibrating tools if possible; isolate sources of vibration; keep tools and equipment properly maintained; maintain even floor surfaces to reduce vibration from driving; reduce driving speeds.

I. Lifting: Reduce size and weight of tools and objects lifted frequently; use mechanical lifting devices; use gravity to move work; raise the work (or lower the operator); provide grips and handles; reduce friction where objects are slid; increase friction when objects are held; evaluate lifting tasks according to NIOSH lifting guidelines (Garg, 1995).

J. Work organization: Alternate physically demanding and mentally demanding tasks; vary the rate and nature of tasks as much as possible; provide breaks (frequent short breaks are generally better than long, less frequent breaks).

Injury Prevention and Control
XXXIV

Occupational Injury Epidemiology

The study of the natural history of injuries helps to define the host, agent, vector, and environmental (psychosocial and physical) factors that contribute to the injury occurrence.

A. Characteristics of occupational injury
   1. Occupational injuries are not random events.
   2. Injuries are predictable and preventable.
   3. Injuries result when energy is exchanged in a manner and dose sufficient to overcome the host's threshold of resistance in the presence or absence of certain environmental conditions (see Table 7-4 for an example).

TABLE 7-4

Example of Occupational Injury Occurrence: A Fracture

Host	Injury	Agent	Vector	Exposure Event	Physical Environment	Sociocultural Environment
Employee • Age • Sex • Health Status • Physical Condition	Fracture	Kinetic energy	Cement floor	Slip and fall	Oil, grease, dirt, and water on floor; painted cement floor; equipment and supplies on floor; lighting; integrity of floor	Attitude towards housekeeping; costs associated with injuries and lost time not accounted for under department budget

B. Examples of sources of injuries
1. *Mechanical or kinetic energy* sources: impact of an object, dashboard, floor, knife, noise, extreme air pressure (explosion)
2. *Thermal energy:* steam, flame, hot substances, and lasers
3. *Electric energy:* man-made sources, such as high-tension wires, and natural sources, such as lightning
4. *Radiation,* both ionizing and nonionizing, including radiotherapeutic devices, implants and pharmaceuticals, radioactive minerals, and sunlight
5. *Chemical energy:* effects of acids, bases, poisons/toxins, and irritants
6. Absence of energy-producing mechanisms necessary to sustain life, such as absence of respiration secondary to drowning

C. The energy-exchanging event causing an injury can be studied as a sequence of interactions viewed in pre-event, event, and post-event phases.

XXXV

Countermeasures

Strategies that are effective in preventing or reducing the extent of injuries were identified and categorized by William Haddon (1963, 1979) as control *countermeasures* (Table 7-5).

TABLE 7-5

Haddon Matrix *case example of control countermeasures = slips and falls on the same level in a maintenance area*

Phase	Human Factors	Environmental and Engineering Factors	Social, Legal, and Political Factors
Pre-event	• Shoes—non-skid soles • Safety training—increase awareness • Establish work practices, including housekeeping	• Non-skid floor (paint, strips) • Oil/grease absorbing material for spills • Good lighting • Proper storage of equipment and supplies	• OSHA inspections and regulation compliance • Safety audit • Risk Management—insurance losses and litigation
Event	• Padded clothing • Optimum physical condition of employees	• Energy absorbing floors (with non-skid surface) • Emergency notification system	• Injury investigation, reporting and tracking • Coordination of medical care
Post-event	• Effective first-aid response • Interface with ambulance and hospital emergency services	• Prompt access to work location • Access to first-aid equipment and supplies	• Emergency response system—triage, first aid, evacuation and definitive medical care

Source: Adapted from Haddon 1963, 1979 in Hayes (1990).

A. Pre-event countermeasures include:
  1. Preventing the creation of the workplace hazard
  2. Reducing the amount of the hazard
  3. Preventing the release of the hazard
  4. Modifying the rate of release of the hazard
  5. Separating the hazard from the employee

B. Event countermeasures include:
  1. Placing a physical barrier between the hazard and the person
  2. Modifying the basic qualities of the hazard
  3. Increasing the individual's resistance to injury

C. Post-event countermeasures include:
  1. Evaluating rapidly the injury that has occurred or is occurring and counter its continuation as well as extension of effects
  2. Following stabilization of the injured party, provision of definitive medical and surgical treatment and rehabilitative and reconstructive care, with a goal of restoration to an optimum level of functioning.

XXXVI

Implications for Occupational Health Nurses

A. An understanding of occupational injury epidemiology will enable occupational health nurses to analyze and characterize the potential for injury in their work setting.

B. The occupational health nurse can use injury prevention and control principles to study, prevent, and control the occurrence of injury-producing events and the extent of injury.

Social and Behavioral Sciences
XXXVII

Effects of Social Conditions and Behavior on Health

Social and behavioral sciences provide a means to examine the influences of workers' social milieus and lifestyles on their health.

A. Modern approaches to health services have been influenced by a variety of factors.
  1. Life expectancy has substantially increased.
  2. Patterns of disease have changed; the leading causes of death have shifted from infectious diseases to chronic diseases related to behaviors and environmental factors.
  3. Traditional approaches such as the medical paradigm are not responsive to many modern-day health problems.

B. Research in the behavioral sciences has provided a means to examine the relationship between human behavior and the occurrence of illness and injury.
  1. The behavior of individuals and groups is complex, and understanding behavior is a complicated process.
     a. People make certain choices, even those they know are not good for their health (e.g., not wearing hearing protection).
     b. The key to affecting behavioral change is understanding the human thought processes that affect behavior (e.g., ear plugs are not comfortable).

    c. Focusing on behavioral strategies may result in workers' making healthier behavioral choices (e.g., allowing worker participation in selection of hearing protection devices).

    d. Behavioral approaches to research may also facilitate a better understanding of the neurological and behavioral effects of certain exposures (to lead, for example).

2. A large set of theoretical approaches and models have been developed to understand behavior. (See Chapter 11 for examples of behavioral theories and models.)

    a. These theories and models explain why people behave as they do.

    b. They provide a rich source of ideas that can be used to further an understanding of behavior.

    c. They enable health care providers to develop more effective interventions.

C. Research in the social sciences has provided a means to examine the contribution of social environments to the occurrence of illness and injury.

1. There is increased recognition of the relationship of social phenomena to health and illness outcomes.

2. Examples of social indices that may affect occupational health include rates of violence, divorce, unemployment, and the number of dual-career families in a community.

3. The provision of appropriate health services depends on complete understanding and appreciation of the nature of work and the social context of the workplace.

D. Unique attributes of social and behavioral sciences

1. Qualitative techniques are more likely to be used as a data collection technique.

2. Quality of life is an important outcome for the social and behavioral sciences; quality of life considers emotional, social, intellectual, physical, and spiritual health.

XXXVIII

Health Promotion and Risk Reduction

    These are examples of areas that require an understanding of the psychosocial determinants of health.

A. There is a need to develop organizational "healthy policy" as a strategy to improve workers' health.

1. Healthy policy facilitates and supports healthy behaviors.

2. The health-promoting and/or the health-damaging policies of organizations are likely to receive increased scrutiny in the coming years (Pender, 1996).

3. Organizational change is a critical factor in achieving a healthy occupational environment.

B. A key area that would benefit from focus on social and behavioral sciences is health promotion that focuses on lifestyle and stress reduction.

C. Social and behavioral sciences can augment an understanding of factors that threaten the health of workers.

1. The psychosocial environment of the workplace plays a critical role in the occurrence of occupational injury and illness.

2. The organization of work is influenced by the ideologies, values, and beliefs of people both within the organization (managers and workers) and outside

of it (scientists and government); these ideologies affect the social dimensions of the workplace.

3. The organization of work has been identified as a research priority area by the National Institute for Occupational Safety and Health (NIOSH, 1996).

D. Implementing strategies based on findings from social and behavioral investigations is likely to result in cost savings to employers and a better quality of life for employees.

BIBLIOGRAPHY

American Industrial Hygiene Association (AIHA). (1996). Fairfax, Virginia: Author.

Cowan, M., Heinrich, J., Lucas, M., Sigmon H., & Hinshaw, A. (1993). Integration of biological and nursing sciences: A 10-year plan to enhance research and training. *Research in Nursing and Health, 16,* 3–9.

Doull, J., & Bruce, M. C. (1986). Origin and scope of toxicology. In C. D. Klaassen, M. O. Amdur, & J. Doull (Eds.), *Casarett and Doull's Toxicology: The Science of Poisons* (3rd ed.) pp. 3–10. New York: Macmillan Publishing Co.

Dreisbach, R. H., & Robertson, W. O. (1987). *Handbook of Poisoning: Prevention, Diagnosis, and Treatment* (12th ed.). Norwalk, Connecticut: Appleton & Lange.

Casarett and Doull's Toxicology: The Science of Poisons (3rd ed) (1986). (pp. 3–10). New York: Macmillan Publishing Co.

Eastman Kodak Company. (1983). *Ergonomic Design for People at Work* (Vol. 1). New York: Van Nostrand Reinhold.

Eastman Kodak Company. (1986). *Ergonomic Design for People at Work* (Vol. 2). New York: Van Nostrand Reinhold.

Ellis, R. (1982). Conceptual issues in nursing. *Nursing Outlook,* July/August, 406–410.

Ewart, C. K., & Fitzgerald, S. T. (1994). Changing behaviour and promoting well-being after heart attack: A social action theory approach. *Irish Journal of Psychology, 15,* 219–241.

Fitzgerald, S. (1991). Self-efficacy theory: Implications for the occupational health nurse. *AAOHN Journal, 39*(12), 552–557.

Fowler, D. P. (1990). Industrial Hygiene. In *Occupational Medicine.* J. LaDou (Ed.). (pp. 499–513). Norwalk, Connecticut: Appleton & Lange.

Flaskerud, J., & Halloran, E. (1980). Areas of agreement in nursing theory development. *Advances in Nursing Science, 3*(1), 1–7.

Garg, A. (1995). Revised NIOSH equation for manual lifting: A method for job evaluation. *AAOHN Journal, 43,* 211–216.

Gortner, S., & Nahm, H. (1977). An overview of nursing research in the United States. *Nursing Research, 26,* 10–33.

Gross, E. R., & Morse, E. P. (1996). Overview of industrial hygiene. In B. A. Plog, J. Niland, & P. J. Quinlan (Eds.), *Fundamentals of Industrial Hygiene* (4th ed.) (pp. 453–483). Itasca, Illinois: National Safety Council.

Hathaway, B. K. (1994). Understanding the material safety data sheet. *AAOHN Journal, 42,* 291–295.

Hayes, W. (1990). Nursing advances in occupational injury prevention and control. In J. M. Radford (Ed.) *Recent Advances in Nursing (26). Occupational Health Nursing,* Edinburgh, Churchill, Livingstone.

Henry, S. (1995). Informatics: Essential infrastructure for quality assessment and improvement in nursing. *Journal of the American Medical Informatics Association, 2,* 169–182.

Institute of Medicine. (1995). *Nursing, Health, and the Environment,* A. M. Pope, M. A. Snyder, & L.H. Mood (Eds.). Washington, DC: National Academy Press.

Klaassen, C. D. (1986a). Principles of toxicology. In C. D. Klaassen, M. O. Amdur & J. Doull (Eds), *Casarett and Doull's Toxicology: The Science of Poisons* (3rd ed.) (pp. 11–32). New York: Macmillan Publishing Co.

Klaassen, C. D. (1986b). Distribution, excretion, and absorption of toxicants. In C. D. Klaassen, M. O. Amdur & J. Doull (Eds), *Casarett and Doull's Toxicology: The Science of Poisons* (3rd ed.) (pp. 33–63). New York: Macmillan Publishing Co.

Landrigan, P. J. (1992). Commentary: Environmental disease—a preventable epidemic. *American Journal of Public Health, 82,* 941–943.

Last, J. M. (1988). *A Dictionary of Epidemiology* (2nd ed.). New York: Oxford University Press.

Mausner, J. S., & Kramer, S. (1985). *Mausner & Bahn Epidemiology—An Introductory Text* (2nd ed.). Philadelphia: W. B. Saunders Company.

Meleis, A. I. (1991). *Theoretical Nursing: Development and Progress.* (2nd ed.). St. Louis: Lippincott.

Mischel, M. H. (1988). Uncertainty in illness. Image–The Journal of Nursing Scholarship, 20, 225–232.

National Institute for Occupational Safety and Health (1988). *Cumulative Trauma Disorders: A Manual for Musculoskeletal Diseases of the Upper Limbs.* V. Putz-Anderson (Ed.). New York: Taylor & Frances.

National Institute for Occupational Safety and Health (1996). *National Occupational Research Agenda.* Atlanta: U.S. Department of Health and Human Services.

Pender, N. (1996). *Health Promotion in Nursing Practice.* (3rd ed.). Los Altos, CA: Appleton & Lange.

Plog, B. A. (1996). Overview of industrial hygiene. In *Fundamentals of Industrial Hygiene* (4th ed.) (pp. 3–32.). B. A. Plog, J. Niland and P. J. Quinlan (Eds.). Itasca, Illinois: National Safety Council.

Reihl, J. P., & Roy, Sister C. (1988). *Conceptual Models for Nursing Practice.* (3rd ed.). New York: Appleton-Century-Crofts.

Ross, P. (1994). Ergonomic hazards in the workplace: Assessment and prevention. *AAOHN Journal, 42*(4), 171–176.

Salazar, M. K. (1991). Comparison of four behavioral theories: A literature review. *AAOHN Journal, 39*(3), 128–135.

Shortridge, L., & Valanis, B. (1992). *The epidemiological model applied in community health nursing* (pp. 151–170). Baltimore: Mosby Year Book.

Silverstein, B. A., Fine, L. J., & Armstrong, T. J. (1987). Occupational factors and carpal tunnel syndrome. *American Journal of Industrial Medicine, 11,* 343–358.

Smith, T .J. (1988). Industrial hygiene. In B. S. Levy and D. H. Wegman (Eds.), *Occupational Health: Recognizing and Preventing Work-Related Disease,* (2nd ed.) (pp. 87–103). Boston: Little, Brown & Co.

Stevenson, J. (1992). Review of the first decade of the Annual Review of Nursing Research. *Annual Review of Nursing Research, 10,* 1–22.

U.S. Dept. of Labor, OSHA. (1990). *Ergonomics Program Management Guidelines for Meatpacking Plants.* OSHA publication No. 3123: Washington DC.

Weinstein, N. D. (1988). The precaution adoption process. *Health Psychology, 7*(4), 355–386.

Weinstein, N. D., and Sandman, P. M. (1992). A model of the precaution adoption process: Evidence from home radon testing. *Health Psychology, 11*(3), 170–180.

Section Two:
Strategies and Approaches to Occupational Health Nursing Practice

CHAPTER

8

Developing, Implementing, and Evaluating a Comprehensive Occupational Health and Safety Program

MAJOR TOPICS
- *Program development*
- *Assessment*
- *Program planning*
- *Program implementation*
- *Program evaluation*
- *Cost-benefit analyses*

The previous chapters have described the foundations of the occupational health and safety field. This information provides a framework for occupational health nursing practice. This chapter is intended to introduce the reader to the strategic processes that are essential to the development, implementation, and evaluation of comprehensive occupational health and safety programs. Chapters 9, 10, and 11 will discuss in detail specific components of these programs, and Chapter 12 will provide samples of programs that can be used as models in the occupational setting. Comprehensive health and safety programs are often designed to improve and protect both the work-related and non-work-related health of employees and their families. The purpose of these programs is to "assist employees in promoting health, preventing illness, detecting disease at its earliest stages, and rehabilitation" (Wachs & Parker-Conrad, 1990, p. 201).

Program Development: Assessment and Program Planning

Assessment

Assessment is a process used to gather important health and safety information.

A. Assessment data are used to:
1. Identify areas of need, value, or importance for health programs and topics
2. Target health and safety behaviors
3. Describe workers as well as the worksite environment

B. Worker-related assessment may involve:
   1. Description of work and home locations, and demographics of workers, dependents, and retirees
   2. Health status of worker population such as nutritional status, exercise habits, and personal behaviors and lifestyles related to risks (i.e., tobacco use)
   3. Health insurance coverage and utilization to determine the major costs and number of health problems affecting workers, their families, and retirees
   4. Disability information about type, severity, and cost, to assist in planning specific programs that will focus on early prevention or rehabilitation efforts
   5. Additional data, including premature death records, life insurance claims, and community arrest records, to determine problems stemming from alcohol and drug misuse/abuse that directly or indirectly affect company workers (Parker-Conrad, 1991)

C. Environmental assessment at the worksite identifies existing and potential health and safety hazards as well as organizational variables that may affect employees and thus call for special programs.
   1. Examples of work-related information to be collected include:
      a. Data concerning exposure to environmental hazards that may affect worker health and safety
      b. Worker injury and illness data
   3. Occupational health services activity reports should be reviewed to identify the nature of services provided, who utilizes the department, and whether nonoccupational problems/concerns are overshadowing time spent on work-related issues or on problems that can be prevented.

D. Other categories of information for workplace assessment include (Travers & McDougall, 1995):
   1. Description of the company
      a. Standard Industrial Classification (SIC) Code
      b. Number and type of facilities
      c. Company vision and mission
      d. Organization's culture and values
   2. Health service models already in place within the company
      a. Available health insurance options
      b. Description of on-site and/or vendored services
      c. Workers' compensation (self-insured, state funded, or other)
      d. Types of employee programs in place (i.e., employee assistance programs, wellness programs, light duty/alternative work programs)
      e. Safety committee
   3. Information included in health records (daily logs, surveillance and monitoring data, disability information, and other)

E. Workplace assessment should include input from multiple sources; for example:
   1. Data from and consultation with other corporate occupational health and safety professionals in the fields of nursing, medicine, safety, and industrial hygiene (IH)
   2. Data that can be obtained through an insurance company, an area university, or a private IH consultant
   3. External occupational medical consultation

F. Assessment Tools
   1. The following tools can be used to gather information for the assessment:
      • Questionnaires

- Health risk appraisals
- Workplace walk-throughs
- Employee health and safety records
- Interviews with employees and management
- Health insurance claims
- Workers' compensation forms
- OSHA records/logs
- Life insurance records
- Medical utilization data

2. The specific tool or tools one utilizes for the assessment is based upon the nature of the initial workplace diagnosis and the factors that led to the original need for the assessment, the financial backing available, the program goals, and the extensiveness of the study.
3. It is important to determine the specific focus of an assessment; assessments may focus on:
   a. Workplace hazard analysis
   b. Health evaluation
   c. Behavior analysis or social concern
   d. Legal/regulatory program compliance issue(s)
   e. Cost savings for the company
   f. Public relations/good will benefit(s)

II

Program Planning

Program planning is the recipe for implementing health services goals and objectives and is the blueprint or detailed guideline for directing activities and evaluating all programs and services conducted by or for the occupational health department. Program planning includes the following activities:

A. Analyze assessment data and target/prioritize areas where programs need to be developed to benefit the health of company employees.
   1. List strengths and limitations of the worker population and the organization.
   2. Review computerized materials and organize data in a manner that will assist in decision making.
   3. Select programs that will benefit most individuals and/or the organization's long-term goals (prioritize various data findings).
   4. Clarify the process and activities that will provide benefits and assist in reaching both short- and long-range goals.

B. Resource identification for program planning activities includes:
   1. *Personnel:* Determine the number and expertise of professionals and other employees needed to develop and implement specific programs. Are additional employees or consultants needed?
   2. *Financial resources:* Develop a budget that will include all expenditures for each program.
      a. Divide budget into sections similar to current workplace yearly categories.
      b. Determine direct and indirect costs that will add to existing or expected expenditures.
      c. Identify potential sources of funding for programs as well as ideal versus minimum costs required to complete each program.
   3. *Equipment:* List the equipment needed for the implementation and final evaluation of the program. Examples include:

   a. Audiovisual materials, such as a television, videotape player, camcorder, audio tape recorder/player, and portable overhead projector
   b. Medical equipment and related expenses, such as pulmonary function measurement devices, syringes, needles, and materials for blood analysis as well as blood pressure measurement
   c. Computers and software needed to produce health risk appraisals, questionnaires, reports, and program correspondence, and educational literature
   d. Other miscellaneous materials specific to the data collection, program implementation, or evaluation phase

4. *Supplies and other resources* needed to develop and implement a program can be costly.
   a. Paper, computer supplies, and mailing costs are expenses often forgotten in program planning.
   b. Public relations and marketing may require brochures, posters, television ads, and special incentives (T-shirts and caps, for example) that help to ensure program participation and completion.

5. *Facilities and space* are important.
   a. Determine if in-house facilities are available and adequate or if outside space will be needed.
   b. Estimate the cost of utilizing facilities, which may include heating, air conditioning, and lighting.

C. *Develop goals and objectives* that blend with the organizational philosophy and company culture.

1. Goals and objectives should be developed before presentation of a program plan to others for discussion and approval (see Box 8-1 for examples).
   a. Goals should be presented in broad, general terms that state the expected results of implementing a program.
   b. Objectives are much more specific and should be presented as measurable, limited to a given time period, and relevant to attaining the goal.

2. A program begins with broad, general goals for the health services department, such as: Provide quality clinical services for workers, both for work-related and non-occupational injuries and illnesses.

3. The success of a program will be linked to the original health behavior data, health insurance costs, or workers' compensation statistics to help determine program effectiveness (evaluation) for the entire company.

4. Methods that will be used to accomplish goals and objectives should be identified in the planning phase and may include educational activities, engineering controls, and administrative practices.

Program Implementation
III

Program Implementation
   Following the planning and approval phases, *program implementation* begins.

A. Processes involved in implementation

1. Activating the method of delivery
2. Monitoring the time frame, target populations, expected outcomes, and cost factors
3. Feeding information continuously back into the loop and using it for periodic program evaluation, redesign, and improvement.

BOX 8-1

Examples of Goals and Objectives

Work-Related Program

Goal: All employees will be in compliance with all OSHA health and safety requirements.

Objective 1) Given classes describing the appropriate health and safety rules for each area, 90% of the employees will not report work-related injuries in the following year. (Or company will experience a 10% decrease in reportable injuries in the next 6 months.)

Objective 2) Given monthly participation in health and safety orientation and inservice, all new employees will be able to pass written exams about OSHA requirements that relate to their specific worksite hazards.

Personal Health and Safety Program

Goal: Employees in the Health Promotion Awareness program will report a decrease in the overall incidence of premature deaths in the company.

Objective 1) Given classes on health awareness, 80% of the employees will participate in special health promotion programs in the next 6 months.

Objective 2) Given participation in health promotion programs, 70% of employees will report a decrease in significant changes or health findings to the occupational health nurse in the next 6 months.

(Other objectives could target specific nutrition education, exercise participation, smoking cessation.)

B. "The goal of the implementation phase is to make the transition from the program design or plan to the successfully operating program" (O'Donnell, 1987, p. 35).
   1. The program execution will involve progressive monitoring of activities, personnel, educational processes, and management support.
   2. Timetables and schedules should be evaluated periodically to assure operational success as the programs are developing and to identify who is responsible for their running according to schedule.
   3. Progress can be monitored by routinely comparing completed activities with predetermined standards and assignments.

C. Program implementation may be done either within the existing health services department or contracted to outside businesses in whole or part. Some of the positive and negative aspects of each are as follows:
   1. The "pros" of providing in-house programs include:
      a. They are convenient for the working population, since they eliminate costly commuting time.
      b. The current staff knows the workplace—the workers, and their culture.
      c. Follow-up is easier for those who need second visits or who fail to show up for appointments.
      d. Utilization of existing personnel is easier.
   2. The problems inherent in in-house programs include:
      a. Staff may be so busy with current job duties that they have little energy or motivation to take on additional program activities.

    b. Space for programs is often limited, and finding additional room may prove difficult.

    c. Existing personnel may lack the expertise, experience, or motivation required to conduct educational programs or to provide administration of broader health and safety programs.

  3. The "pros" of outsourcing health and safety programs include:

    a. Confidentiality (or the perception of it) may be easier to maintain, especially when there is a concern that assessment, utilization, or outcome data may endanger employees' job security.

    b. Interference with existing health services activities and setting priorities is less likely.

    c. Scheduling offsite programs, such as exercise programs, closer to workers' homes could improve program attendance.

  4. The problems inherent to outsourcing programs include:

    a. Extra costs may include contractor's travel time, overhead for employees, and nonproductive time spent in setting up programs.

    b. Contract employees do not share same loyalty to the company as in-house workers and thus are not as vested in program outcomes or overall program success.

D. *Policies* and *procedures* serve as guides to assist in achieving the goals and objectives of the health and safety programs.

  1. Program policies and procedures provide direction and consistency for the implementation phase and can serve as the basis for program evaluation.

  2. Compliance with company and regulatory guidelines should be maintained with well-developed, well-written, and updated procedures.

    a. Procedures define specific steps or activities that must be followed, provide an excellent avenue for staff orientation, and assure compliance with protocols and other activities.

    b. Procedures also provide legal backup for both nurse and company should a question arise regarding whether programs/activities are within the scope of practice, consistent with company policy, or compliant with national standards and expectations.

  3. Resources for policies and procedures are available through various agencies and organizations and are useful guidelines; however, these guides should be customized to reflect the goals and priorities of the company and its clients.

E. Barriers to implementation may include the following:

  1. Political considerations

  2. Seasonal variations in production and weather

  3. Union strikes and bargaining or territorial turfs

  4. Personnel changes or availability

  5. Management changes leading to direction shifts

  6. Equipment delays, availability, or design flaws

  7. Lack of resources

Program Evaluation

The Evaluation Process

    The *evaluation process* is used as an opportunity to identify and improve services provided by the occupational health nurse for the company.

A. Evaluation is an integral component of all phases of development and implementation of occupational health and safety programs.

B. Methods of evaluation should be appropriate to program goals and objectives as they have been defined.

$\overline{V}$

Structure, Process, and Outcome

Donabedian (1966) developed a three-pronged approach to evaluation that provides an excellent framework for occupational health; the three prongs are *structure, process,* and *outcome* (see Table 8-1).

A. *Structural elements:* Examples include management support; physical facilities; supplies and equipment; staff and health resources; worker demographics; and the mission, goals, and objectives to meet the health and safety needs of the worksite community.

  1. Review the management reporting structure and support for the occupational health program. Ask the following questions:
     a. Who does the nurse report to, administratively and professionally?
     b. Does the nurse participate in the formulation and implementation of administrative procedures?
     c. Does the nurse participate in developing policies and procedures applicable to the health issues of the company (e.g., return to work, case management, fitness for duty)?
     d. Who develops the philosophy and the written goals and objectives for the occupational health program?
     e. Does the occupational health nurse conduct periodic reviews of the occupational health program to assure that goals and objectives are being met?
     f. Does the occupational health staff participate in meetings that address health issues (e.g., safety, management staff, department, and human resource meetings)?

TABLE 8-1

Structure, Process, and Outcomes:
Evaluative Elements in Quality Assurance

Structural Elements	Process Elements	Outcome Elements
Physical setting	Management of the operation	Improved health
Philosophy of health by management, employees, health care professionals	Decision-making processes	Compliance with treatment regimens
Organizational mission and structure	Collaboration	Reduced morbidity and mortality
Unit goals and objectives	Nursing interventions/ monitoring	Positive changes in knowledge and attitudes about health
Human and financial resources	Services provided	Satisfaction with service quality
Operational resources	Development of records and reports	

Source: Rogers, B. (1994).

g. Does the occupational health nursing staff communicate clearly and in writing with management and department heads as needed?

h. Does the occupational health staff demonstrate the effectiveness of the health services department in terms of cost, productivity, and return on investment?

i. Is workplace information—distribution lists, upcoming events, and future plans—communicated to the occupational health staff?

2. Evaluate the physical facilities provided for the occupational health program.
   a. Office for nurse and related space
   b. Worker/client waiting area
   c. Treatment area
   d. Recovery (quiet) area
   e. Space for education/teaching
   f. Toilet facilities
   g. Supply/storage
   h. Health record storage

3. Identify supplies and equipment utilized by the occupational health program.
   a. Supplies and medications appropriate for the practice are maintained in adequate supply, stored under proper conditions, and not kept beyond expiration dates.
   b. Appropriate medical equipment is available and in good working condition. Examples: Refrigerator, oxygen, otoscope, sphygmomanometers
   c. Equipment used in performing exams required by OSHA is maintained and calibrated according to federal standards. Examples: Audiometric booths, spirometer
   d. Laboratory tests are conducted in accordance with state health departments. Examples: Cholesterol tests, Strep A tests

4. Identify staffing requirements, qualifications, and professional development recommendations.
   a. Copies of professional licenses and required certifications are kept for all staff.
   b. Copies of updated curriculum vitae are kept on file.
   c. Occupational health staff takes advantage of opportunities to grow professionally and to advance the specialty of occupational health nursing.
   d. Occupational health nursing certification is supported and encouraged.
   e. Nursing staff's active membership and involvement in AAOHN, including attendance at the annual American Occupational Health Conference, is encouraged and supported.
   f. Nursing staff's participation in professional development seminars designed to advance individual practice in occupational health nursing is supported and encouraged.
   g. Occupational health staff is encouraged to continue formal and informal education.
   h. Professional nursing journals and resources are available.
   i. Nursing responsibilities are defined in a position description.

5. The worksite community should be assessed and programs, including those required by OSHA, should be available to meet the needs of the workers.
   a. Work force analysis: Number of workers and managers, median age of population, approximate distribution of population by gender, number of disabled (ADA-placed) associates on property, and health status of worker population

    b. Health and safety hazards, exposures, and OSHA-required programs are identified. Examples: Bloodborne pathogens, hearing conservation, respirator usage

  6. Mission, goals, and objectives are developed to meet the health and safety of the workers as well as the business needs of the company.

    a. Goals and objectives need to be are revised and updated on a regular basis.

    b. Mission, goals, and objectives should reflect current issues and practices in occupational health.

B. *Process elements:* Examples are the delivery of nursing clinical practice; scope of services and programs; and documentation and recordkeeping abilities.

  1. Nursing clinical practice is appropriate for the occupational health setting.

    a. Clinical practice is consistent with:
- State Nurse Practice Act
- Pharmacy and Medical Practice Acts
- AAOHN Standards of Practice

    b. A policy and procedure manual is written and reflects current occupational health practice.

    c. Occupational health nursing resources are used to guide clinical practice.

  2. The scope of clinical services and programs are designed to meet the needs of the worksite community.

    a. Injury and illness management services include:
- Care and treatment of occupational injuries/illnesses
- Care and treatment of nonoccupational illnesses/injuries
- Emergency care for workers and visitors at the facility
- Supervision by a registered nurse over the nursing care of all workers

    b. Health promotion and screening program
- Identify the health promotion programs that have been successfully delivered at the worksite. Examples: Back care, ergonomics, hearing/sight conservation, occupational dermatitis, self-care, hypertension screening
- Evaluate formats used to offer programs. Examples: Formal lecture, management meetings, informational pamphlet distribution, poster and bulletin board displays

    c. Case management (including absenteeism) of both occupational and nonoccupational injury and illness
- The nurse collaborates with managers, claims administrators, workers, and medical providers to facilitate appropriate, safe, and timely return to work.
- The nurse is familiar with the state's workers' compensation laws.
- The nurse reviews health care and response to treatment.
- The nurse recommends an independent medical evaluation (IME) when appropriate.
- The nurse has a working knowledge of medical and health benefit programs offered by the employer.
- The nurse, together with the manager, develops transitional duties or jobs that support treatment goals.
- The nurse maintains contact with workers who have sustained an injury or illness.
- The nurse evaluates workers who are absent from work for more than 5 days with non-work-related illness or injury.

   d. Worksite tours for health and safety evaluation are conducted on regular basis.
   - Health and safety reports are utilized.
   - Nurse attends meetings of the safety committee to present findings.
   e. OSHA programs, other required programs, and training sessions are completed. Examples: Drug testing for the Department of Transportation (DOT), hearing conservation, respirator approval
   f. Employee assistance program (EAP) and/or referrals are available to workers.
   - Identify how EAP services are provided at the worksite.
   - The nurse is responsible for assessing workers and referring them for appropriate treatment.
   g. Identify the types of immunization programs offered for prevention, postexposure, and travel. Examples: Hepatitis B, influenza vaccine, tetanus
   h. Ensure that an emergency response plan is available.
   - Identify the person(s) responsible for the coordination and implementation of the disaster plan within the facility.
   - The disaster plan is revised and tested as needed.
   - The nurse is included in the planning and implementation procedure of the disaster plan.
   - Written procedures and defined functions are incorporated into the disaster plan.

3. Evaluate the documentation and recordkeeping system.
   a. Evaluate the quality of documentation and recordkeeping to be sure records are appropriate and clear and that they meet legal reporting requirements.
   b. Identify system used for documentation (manual or computer)
   - Documentation is timely and complete.
   - Entries on the OSHA daily log reflect accurate documentation in the health record.
   - Daily logs are utilized to summarize clinical activity and trends to report to management.
   - All health records are secured in a locked cabinet.
   - Computerized records are secured by passwords, limiting access to occupational health staff only.
   - Health records are retained according to federal law (exposure records are to be retained for 30 years; health records are retained for the duration of employment plus 30 years).
   - Disclosure of information from a worker's health record is made only with written informed consent of the individual.
   - Work-related injuries and illnesses are shared with the employer only on a need-to-know basis.
   c. Review OSHA forms, training logs, and other management reports.
   - Bloodborne pathogens training
   - Hearing conservation
   - Respirator fit testing and exams
   - OSHA logs

C. *Outcome elements:* Evaluate if the care provided to a single worker or population of workers achieved expected outcomes or that the processes used are likely to lead to positive outcomes.

1. The occupational health nurse should utilize clinical practice guidelines as a basis for practice.

2. Health outcomes include:
    a. Prevention of preventable illness and injury
    b. Increased compliance with treatment regimens
    c. Increased worker knowledge about self-care
    d. Restoration of function
        • Physical functions—ambulation, lifting, etc.
        • Psychological functions—memory, cognition, or mood
        • Social function—interpersonal relationships, communication
        • Role function—worker, parent, etc.
    e. Cure or retardation of disease, such as an infection or hypertension
    f. Relief of discomfort
        • Physical discomfort, such as pain
        • Psychological discomfort, such as depression

3. Health care outcomes are compared with the cost of health services so that judgments about the value of the health care services can be made for the company. Some examples follow:
    a. Back injury prevention program provided to prevent the incidence of back injury.
        • *Health outcome:* Workers who participate in the program will have a decreased incidence of back injury.
        • *Cost:* The company will experience decreased cost associated with this type of injury.
    b. Heart disease awareness program provided to educate workers about the importance of compliance with blood pressure medications and evaluation of blood pressure.
        • *Health outcome:* Workers with hypertension will increase compliance with therapeutic regimens including exercise, weight control, and taking medication; the result will be an increased number of workers who are normotensive.
        • *Cost:* The company will have a healthier workforce resulting in less absenteeism and improved productivity among these workers.

4. The measurement of health outcomes begins at the individual level; many individual outcomes may be pooled to assess factors of interest across worker groups.

5. The relationship between good health outcomes and interventions is complex.
    a. What nurses do and how well they do it only partially account for a worker's health outcome.
    b. It is often impossible to definitively attribute a specific outcome to the performance of the nurse.
    c. Other worker-related and community-related factors affect outcomes.
    d. The closer in time the measured outcome is to the provided treatment, the more likely it is attributable to the nurse.
        • Outcomes that occur immediately after an intervention are the most likely to be attributable to the treatment (immediate).
        • Outcomes that occur following the nursing intervention, though not immediately, may be related to the treatment (intermediate).
        • The ultimate outcome of a nursing intervention, which may occur 2 to 5 years following the initial episode of injury or illness, is the most difficult to attribute to that treatment (long-term).

VI
Methods of Evaluation

A. Techniques for gathering information
1. Retrospective chart audit
   a. Focuses on documented evidence of nursing care provided
   b. Assumes that what is documented is what has been performed
2. Concurrent document review
   a. Critical examination of case management while care is in progress and of client outcomes
   b. Review of chart, plans for care, immediate feedback
3. Interviewing
   a. Verbal interaction: clarifying questions, attitudes, opinions, client satisfaction, and management understanding of health care
   b. Important to word questions consistently from worker to worker to decrease bias
4. Questionnaire
   a. Most frequently used tool for program evaluation
   b. Important to write questions clearly and to provide clear directions for completion
5. Observation
   a. Observation of nursing practice related to physical assessment skills, such as occupational history taking, medication administration practices, and treatment plans
   b. Opportunity to provide immediate feedback and validate procedure manual for appropriateness and to determine the relationship of outcomes to actual nursing practices

B. Conducting a quality review
1. In corporate settings with a number of nurses, a quality-assurance program can be developed by this group and utilized at several different sites.
2. In settings where nurses work alone, develop a quality-review team of interested peers located nearby or form a team of occupational health nurses representing local AAOHN constituencies.
3. Develop and customize an evaluation tool to identify the specific needs of your company's occupational health program.
4. Utilize an evaluation tool that reflects current practice in occupational health as a framework to develop your own evaluation tool; consult, for example, AAOHN's "Guidelines for an Occupational Health and Safety Service" (Travers & McDougall, 1995), which provides a quality assurance audit.

VII
Cost-Effective and Cost Benefit Programs

A. Purposes of Cost Evaluation
1. Management's goal for developing or maintaining occupational health services and programs is often to contain costs.
2. Cost-benefit and cost-effectiveness analyses can be used to demonstrate the cost-effectiveness of the overall program as well as the cost-benefit of its specific components.
3. Health conditions and safety problems that are having a significant impact

on the company's "bottom line" should be targeted for program development, followed by cost-benefit analyses.

B. Definition of terms
1. "Cost-benefit analysis looks at return on investment" (AAOHN, 1996). A *cost-benefit analysis:*
   a. Considers both costs and benefits (or outcomes) of a program in monetary terms
   b. Permits a comparison between unlike elements
   c. Yields a benefit-to-cost ratio
2. *"Cost-effectiveness analysis* is used to determine which activities or interventions, given alternative approaches, will achieve the program objective and yield the most value or greatest impact on cost" (AAOHN, 1996).

C. Why do a cost analysis?
1. Cost-benefit and cost-effectiveness analyses will help determine which programs or services can produce a benefit that is greater than the cost, since many administrators are not aware of the true potential of health services or programs for the company or their workers.
2. Demonstrating short- and long-term costs and benefits:
   a. Find cause-and-effect relationships between programs and benefits as noted above, and project how the organization can gain from effective programming in these areas.
   b. Categorize, quantify, and compare benefits and costs.
   c. Short-term *benefits* may include increased morale, productivity, and corporate image.
   d. Long-term *benefits* may include decreased health and life insurance costs, decreased workers' compensation claims, and decreased employee turnover.
   e. Short-term *costs* involve commitment of space, resources, supplies, and equipment, as well as organizational time and involvement.
   f. Long-term *costs* can include time for participation of management and workers as well as the ongoing cost of utilities and program maintenance expenses.
   g. Determine the areas of greatest program impact, such as physical impairments, workers' compensation claims, or public relations.
   h. Compare the program costs to those of other current company programs and determine how this program compares with their costs and benefits.
   i. Ask whether the proposed health and safety program is a good investment and worthy of everyone's time and effort.
   j. A documentation of workers' compensation costs may help to demonstrate the need for work-related programs in the organization.

D. Steps in conducting cost-benefit and cost-effectiveness analyses
1. "Determine the program/service for financial analysis;
2. Formulate the objectives and goals of the program/service;
3. List alternative ways objectives and goals can be achieved;
4. Determine costs/benefits for all alternatives;
5. Determine monetary values for costs/benefits, or determine outcome measures" (i.e., absenteeism rates; health services utilization; changes in risk behaviors) (AAOHN, 1996).
6. Calculate discounting
   a. Discounting reduces future costs to their present worth.
   b. It answers the question: "What is the cost of providing this service now compared to what it will cost in the future?" (AAOHN, 1996).

E. Resources
  1. See Guidelines for Occupational Health and Safety Service (Travers & McDougall, 1995) for a case study on cost effectiveness.
  2. See Davidson, Widfeldt, & Bey (1992a and 1992b) for additional information about estimating cost savings for on-site occupational health nursing services.

Overall Health and Safety Program Considerations
VIII

Conclusion

Occupational health nurses who are actively involved in planning and developing health and safety programs will need to explore many issues to ensure program success and participation.

A. Issues that should be addressed in health and safety programs include confidentiality, legal aspects, involvement of advisory committees, and management support.
  1. Confidentiality of information collected from and/or about employees is a major concern, especially as it relates to personal health data, because employees often fear that these data may be used to punish, dismiss, or otherwise endanger their employment.
  2. Legal concerns include the company's liability for employees if they become injured when participating in company-sponsored health programs such as Fun Runs and Health Fairs.
  3. The involvement of a health and safety advisory committee in program planning, implementation, and evaluation is mandatory.
      a. Labor *and* management representation, input and viewpoints are necessary to assure success of programs.
      b. A committee is instrumental in suggesting topics, obtaining peer support, identifying barriers, and identifying resources.
  4. Management support must be garnered early in the planning stages to approve the program's financing, workers' involvement, the program's relevance for the workplace, as well as to take into account other political and philosophical considerations.

B. Occupational health nurses should consider using a business approach to health and safety program development since the language of business is more easily understood by management; additionally, a *business plan* is helpful in setting up programs and their monitoring success.
  1. A business plan can serve the following functions:
      a. Provide an overview of the services included in the comprehensive occupational health and safety program
      b. Serve as an operating tool to help guide the program in its implementation and evaluation
      c. Provide guidelines for identifying resources required to implement a program
      d. Serve as a means of communicating ideas and approaches to management and unions
  2. A business plan should be tailored to the individual needs of the organization and the program; the basic components of a business plan are (Helmer, Dunn, Eaton, Macedonio, and Lubritz, 1995):

a. *Executive summary:* includes a summary of the plan, including the projected return on the investment
b. *Purpose of plan:* explanation of what is to be accomplished with the plan
c. *Ground rules:* guidelines for the plan through the identification of constraints, limitations, and resources; terminology is defined so there is a common understanding
d. *Approach:* description of how and when the plan will be implemented
e. *Requirements:* description of the specific outcomes that must be accomplished as a result of the plan
f. *Scope of work:* specific description of the nature of tasks related to the plan, including who is responsible for each task
g. *Schedule:* the development of timelines to serve as target dates for each stage of the implementation of the plan
h. *Financial:* may be framed as a profit and loss statement; "An accurate projection of costs . . . strengthens the plan and demonstrates to key decision makers that one is serious about the company's 'bottom line.'" (Helmer et al., 1995, p. 562)

BIBLIOGRAPHY

American Association of Occupational Health Nurses. (1994). *Standards of occupational health nursing practice.* Atlanta: AAOHN Publications.

American Association of Occupational Health Nurses. (1996). *Cost benefit and cost effectiveness analyses. AAOHN Advisory.* Atlanta: Author.

Davidson, G., Widfeldt, A., & Bey, J. (1992a). On-site occupational health nursing services: Estimating the net cost savings. Part I. *AAOHN Journal, 40*(4), 172–181.

Davidson, G., Widfeldt, A., & Bey, J. (1992b). On-site occupational health nursing services: Estimating the net cost savings. Part II. *AAOHN Journal, 40*(5), 242–249.

Dees, J. P., & Garcia, M. (1995). Program planning: A total approach. *AAOHN Journal, 43*(5), 239–244.

Donabedien, A. (1966). Evaluating the quality of medical care. *Milbank Fund Quarterly, 44*(3), 166–206.

Fefer, M. D. (1992). What to do about worker's comp. *Fortune, 125*(13) 80–83.

Filios, M. S., Travers, P. H., & Summers, V. (1991). Quality assurance through use of a self-evaluation tool. *AAOHN Journal, 39*(1), 20–23.

Green, L. W., & Kreuter, M. W. (1991). *Health Promotion Planning: An Educational and Environmental Approach.* (Chapter 9: Applications in Occupational Settings (pp. 308–348). Mountain View: Mayfield Publishing.

Helmer, D. C., Dunn, L. M., Eaton, K., Macedonio, C., & Lubritz, L. (1995). Implementing corporate wellness programs: A business approach to program planning. *AAOHN Journal, 43*(11), 558–563.

National Safety Council. (1990). *Starting an occupational health nursing service.* Chicago: Author.

Occupational Safety and Health Administration. (1989). *Occupational Safety and Health Administration Guidelines on Workplace Safety and Health Program Management,* 54 FR 3904, January 26, 1989: Washington DC: Author.

O'Donnell, M. P., & Ainsworth, T. (Eds.). (1994). *Health Promotion in the Workplace.* Albany, NY: Delmar.

O'Donnell, M. P. (1987). *Designing Workplace Health Promotion.* (2nd ed.). New York: Wiley.

Parker-Conrad, J. E. (1991). Designing data-based programs. *AAOHN Update Series IV: Cost Containment Issues in Occupational Health Nursing, 4*(11), 16–22.

Parker-Conrad, J. E. (1993). Hiring practices and the occupational health nurse manager. *AAOHN Journal, Management File, 41*(3), 1–4.

Rogers, B. (1994). *Occupational health nursing: Concepts and practice.* Philadelphia: W. B. Saunders.

Rogers, B., Randolph, S. A., & Mastroianni, K. (1996). *Occupational health nursing guidelines for primary clinical conditions* (2nd ed.). Boston: OEM Press.

Rooney, E. (1990). Corporate attitudes and responses to rising health care costs. *AAOHN Journal, 38*(7), 304–11.

The State Medical Society of Wisconsin. (1992). *Occupational health guide for medical and nursing personnel.* Madison: Author.

Travers, P. H., & McDougall, C. (1995). *Guidelines for an occupational health and safety service.* Atlanta: AAOHN Publications.

U.S. Department of Health and Human Services. (1989). *Guide to clinical preventive services: An assessment of the effectiveness of 169 interventions.* Baltimore: Williams & Wilkins. (Report of the U.S. Preventive Services Task Force).

U.S. Department of Health and Human Services, Agency for Health Care Policy and Research, 1995. *Using clinical practice guidelines to evaluate quality of care.* AHCPR Pub. No. 95-0046, Vol. 1 and 2. Washington DC: Author.

U.S. Department of Health and Human Services, PHS, CDC, NIOSH. (1988). *Guidelines for protecting the health and safety of health care workers.* Atlanta: Author

Wachs, J. E., & Parker-Conrad, J. E. (1990). Occupational health nursing in 1990 and the coming decade. *Applied Occupational and Environmental Hygiene, 5*(4), 200–204.

9

Prevention of Occupational Injuries and Illnesses

MAJOR TOPICS

- *Recognition and anticipation*
- *Methods of hazard identification*
- *Exposure monitoring*
- *Ergonomic analysis*
- *Occupational surveillance*
- *Elimination and substitution*
- *Engineering controls*
- *Work practices*
- *Administrative controls*
- *Personal protective equipment*

The prevention of occupational illness and injury requires an in-depth knowledge of the work environment as well as the appropriate skills to recognize and identify actual and potential hazards. This chapter provides a broad overview of techniques and strategies that can be adapted for a variety of health and safety programs. It is the responsibility of occupational health nurses to determine the particular needs of their organizations and to tailor those programs to their setting.

Recognition and Anticipation

In order to recognize and anticipate occupational health and safety hazards, occupational health nurses must know their workplaces and the nature of the work performed; they also need to appreciate the unique attributes, including the risk factors, that may characterize the worker population.

$\bar{\text{I}}$

First Steps in a Prevention Program

The first two steps in a worksite program to prevent illness or injury of the workers are: 1) the recognition of existing hazards and 2) the clear identification of potential hazards.

A. *Recognition* is the process of identifying and describing existing workplace hazards.

1. *Hazard* is "the potential for harm or damage to people, property, or the environment" (Manuele, 1994, p. 72).
2. Recognizing hazards requires knowledge of the workers, the worksite, the work practices and processes, and the industrial materials used.
3. Resources of information include: knowledgeable company representatives; health and safety professionals; professional publications and courses; and direct observation of workers' activities.

B. *Anticipation* is the foresight to recognize hazards in equipment and processes during the planning stages so they can be eliminated from the design (Manuele, 1994).

II

Methods of Identification of Hazards

A. A *site survey,* or *walk-through,* is a worksite inspection not related to any particular incident or concentrated area or piece of equipment (Travers & McDougall, 1995).
1. Purpose: to identify unsafe conditions and practices, including items out of compliance with Occupational Safety and Health Administration (OSHA) standards (see Table 9-1)
2. Types of walk-through inspections
   a. *Informal inspection:* focuses on routine work, such as inspecting and testing equipment at the beginning of each shift
   b. *Formal inspection:* performed periodically by a team of occupational health and safety professionals; scheduled at convenient times; includes a written report of findings
   c. *General inspection:* may be conducted to assure compliance with legal

---

TABLE 9-1

A Few Examples of What to Inspect

- **Atmospheric conditions**—dusts, vapors, odors
- **Illumination**—general and workstations
- **First aid and emergency units**—eye-wash stations, deluge showers
- **Containers**—labeling, flammable liquid, waste
- **Supplies and materials**—caustics, acids, poisons, compressed gases, cryogenics, oxidizers, flammable or spontaneously combustible materials
- **Buildings and structures**—windows, aisles, floors, stairs, exit signs
- **Electrical**—extension cords, outlet usage, cord condition, electric gear clearance, shock hazards
- **Fire fighting equipment**—fire extinguishers, sprinkler systems, standpipes, accessibility, alarms and testing
- **Machinery**—guarding of moving parts and pinch points, barrier safety shields, proximity switches, automatic shutoffs
- **Material handling**—lifting devices, conveyors, lift truck operations, cranes, hoists
- **Personal protective equipment**—clothing, safety glasses, chemical goggles, gloves, safety shoes, hard hats
- **Work practices**—eating at the workstation, personal hygiene, adherence to safe operating procedures, housekeeping

Source: National Safety Council, 1992

   requirements or for insurance purposes, corporate or union audits, and fire code compliance

3. A *site survey* follows the flow of work from the beginning to end.

4. A checklist is used to guide the inspection: inspection checklists should be site specific rather than generic.

5. Pre-inspection activities may include:
   a. Determination of inspection time
   b. Pre-inspection meeting with managers and supervisors
   c. Review of previous inspection and accident reports, material safety data sheets, and other relevant records and reports
   d. Gathering of essential protective equipment used at site
   e. Gathering of checklists, sampling devices, and other items needed for the inspection

6. Inspection activities may include:
   a. Explanation of procedure to supervisors at inspection sites
   b. Observation of employees' work practices
   c. Recording of unsafe conditions and practices, including items out of compliance with OSHA standards
   d. Identification of not only the problems but their causes
   e. Commendation of supervisor and workers when conditions are noted to be safe

7. Post-inspection activities may include:
   a. Post-inspection meeting with managers and supervisors
   b. A long-term analysis based on data from both current and previous inspections
   c. Preparation of report
   d. Circulation of report, which should include recommendations for possible solutions and correction priorities

8. Establish an audit system to periodically check for both corrected and unresolved problems.

B. Focused inspections are conducted periodically for the following purposes: to target specific processes, equipment, or areas; to investigate an accident; to evaluate a reported health or safety hazard; or to respond to complaints of such things as a strange odor or loud noise.

1. A multidisciplinary team of trained specialists/professionals with in-depth knowledge of the process or area should conduct the inspection (National Safety Council, 1995a).

2. Critical parts or operations usually require more frequent inspections; examples are light switches, safety valves, cables, belts, fire extinguishers, eyewash stations, or exhaust hoods.

3. Some focused inspections are legally mandated, such as elevator inspections, autoclave inspections, and boiler inspections.

4. A checklist can serve as a useful guide to a focused inspection (see Table 9-2 for an example).

C. A records review or audit may be done alone or as a supplement to other methods of hazard identification (Travers & McDougall, 1995).

1. Purposes of record audits are to:
   a. Identify worksite hazards
   b. Better acquaint the occupational health nurse with the site
   c. Provide historical data for trend analysis and epidemiological study
   d. Assure compliance with OSHA standards

TABLE 9-2

Focused Checklist for Electric Forklift

ELECTRIC FORKLIFT DAILY CHECKLIST Truck No.: Ser. No.: Check before each shift.										
Date:										
Hour Meter:										
Driver:										
Visual/Operation Checks	OK	Not OK	OK	Not OK	OK	Not OK	OK	Not OK	OK	Not OK
Obvious Damage/Leaks										
Tire Condition										
Battery Plug Connect										
Warning Lights										
Battery Discharge Meter										
Horn										
Steering										
Foot Brake										
Parking Brake										
Hydraulic Controls										
Fork Operation										
Battery Water Level										
Seat Belts										
Fire Extinguisher										
Repairs Needed:										
Comments:									Add additional comments on the back	

Source: Adapted from Ohio Division of Safety and Hygiene. (1995). Forklift truck driver's daily checklist electric. *Industry basic safety and health manual.* Columbus, OH.: Bureau of Workers' Compensation, Division of Safety and Hygiene, 80.

2. While records may indicate the absence or inadequate control of worksite hazards, the recorded information may not reflect the actual circumstance.
3. Records that may be helpful are:
   a. Records concerning production and quality-control problems
   b. Workers' compensation claims
   c. Employee assistance program utilization reports
   d. Personnel records, including absentee records and job histories
   e. Written hazard-control programs, training records, and records concerning fit testing and distribution of personal protective equipment
   f. Safety surveys, inspection reports, and exposure monitoring reports
   g. Machine and equipment maintenance logs
   h. Emission and process upset records
   i. System monitoring and alarm test records
   j. Plans for disaster preparedness and emergency response
   k. Designs and reviews of new or planned facilities, processes, materials, or equipment
   l. Written complaints from workers and minutes of the safety committee
   m. Occupational Safety and Health Administration (OSHA) recordkeeping forms
   n. Other site-specific records that may be identified and examined if deemed appropriate

D. *Job hazard analysis,* also called *job safety analysis,* is the process of studying and recording each step of a job to identify existing or potential health and safety hazards and to determine the best way to perform the job in order to reduce or eliminate these hazards (National Safety Council, 1995b).
1. Set Priorities: Begin with the jobs with the highest rates of accident and disabling injuries, jobs where "close calls" have occurred, new jobs, and jobs where changes have been made in processes and procedures (Vogel, 1991).
2. Assess the general conditions under which the job is performed, using a checklist if applicable. Then:
   a. List each step of the job in order of occurrence as you watch the worker performing the job, recording enough information to describe each job action
   b. Examine each step to determine the existing or potential hazards.
   c. Repeat the job observation as often as necessary until all hazards have been identified.
   d. Review each hazard or potential hazard with the worker performing the job to determine whether the job could be performed in a safer way or whether safety equipment and precautions are needed.
   e. List exactly each new step or method, and identify exactly what the worker needs to know to perform the job safely.
   f. Avoid general warnings such as "Be careful."
3. Recommend safe procedures and corrections, these include:
   a. Developing a training program
   b. Redesigning equipment, changing tools, adding guards, improving ventilation, or using personal protective equipment
   c. Reducing the necessity or frequency of performing the job
4. Repeat and revise the job hazard/job safety analysis periodically and after an accident or injury. (See Table 9-3 for an example.)
5. Benefits of a job hazard/job safety analysis include (National Safety Council, 1992):
   a. Worker overall hazard awareness is improved.
   b. Worker safety training and supervisor/worker communication is increased.

TABLE 9-3

Job Safety Analysis

JOB SAFETY ANALYSIS	Job:		Date:
Title of Worker Who Performs Job:	Foreman/Supervisor:		Analysis By:
Specific Work Location:	Section:		Reviewed By:
Required and/or Recommended Personal Protective Equipment:			

Sequence of Basic Job Steps	Potential Accidents or Hazards	Recommended Safe Job Procedures

Source: Ohio Division of Safety and Hygiene. (1995). *Industry basic safety and health manual.* Columbus, OH: Bureau of Workers' Compensation, Division of Safety and Hygiene.

    c. Identification of root causes of accidents is enhanced.

    d. It serves as a valuable tool for ergonomic studies (Hall, 1992).

    e. Machines are more closely inspected.

    f. It is helpful in training new supervisors in unfamiliar jobs.

    g. It determines physical and mental requirements necessary for job performance in the evaluation of job candidates with disabilities.

E. *Accident investigations* are fact-finding procedures to identify the pertinent factors that allow accidents to occur so that similar future accidents can be prevented (Travers & McDougall, 1995).

1. The first step in an investigation is to identify immediate causes by:

    a. Interviewing workers and collecting physical evidence, including results of any applicable drug screening and/or alcohol testing, as soon as possible after the accident

    b. Inspecting the scene of the accident and recording relevant details, using photographs, drawings, and measurements

    c. Interviewing witnesses in private

    d. Being alert to the possibility of attempts to hide injuries or facts because of fear of reprisal, poor evaluations, ruining safety records, discovery of substance abuse, embarrassment, or fear of implicating others (American Association of Occupational Health Nurses [AAOHN], 1995)

    e. Using the company's accident investigation form to avoid omitting information

    f. Trying to quote workers' statements in their exact words

    g. Staying objective, avoiding biased statements or questions

2. "Some of the root causes (of accidents) may be:

    • Lack of management support for safety

    • Failure to positively reinforce or reward safe behaviors

    • Lack of preventive maintenance programs

    • Production output stressed over safety

    • Low worker morale

    • Unqualified trainers

    • Lack of job safety analysis

    • No assigned responsibility for a function

    • Unsafe work behaviors without accident experience

    • Peer values

    • Poor supervisor/management example" (AAOHN, 1995)

3. Factors that exist in workplace environments often contribute to accident occurrence; these include procedures, facilities, communication patterns, and behaviors (see Table 9-4).

4. Benefits derived from accident investigations include:

    a. An increase of health and safety awareness for workers and supervisors

    b. Better rapport between the occupational health nurse, the supervisor, and the injured or ill worker

    c. Provision of data that can be used for an overall safety program evaluation and control of future incidents

F. An *incident historical review* is the compilation and analysis of accidents and near misses that have occurred over a selected period of time.

1. Categories of incidents include:

    • Accidents related to specific seasons

    • Accidents occurring on a particular shift

    • Accidents occurring to a specific group of workers

TABLE 9-4

Examples of Immediate Causes of Accidents

- **Procedures**—nonexistent, not followed, not trained in, not understood, not accurate, impossible to follow

- **Facilities/tools/equipment**—personal protective equipment failure, improper design, nonergonomic design, wear/deterioration, lack of proper equipment, poor housekeeping, process equipment failure, missing guards or safety devices

- **Hazards**—manmade, natural source, documented but not repaired, unidentified, identified but accepted, deficiently repaired, presenting a "challenge" to workers

- **Communication**—inadequate planning; breakdown in communication between co-workers, between workers and supervisors, or between contractor and company; confused communications; lack of warning signs; language barriers; illiteracy

- **Behavior**—rushed by supervision, coworker competition, motivation to finish early, taking shortcuts, no teamwork, heavy client workload, bonus incentives, medication effects, boredom, fatalistic "It can't happen to me" attitude, unauthorized smoking/eating, inattention/distraction, fear of asking for help

- **Training**—none, insufficient, safe work practices not addressed in training, training applied incorrectly, no hands-on training, inadequate follow-up, need for refresher training, training not site-specific

- **Other factors**—fatigue, lack of sleep, illness, physical stress, repetitive motion, fright, physical incapability, disrupted circadian rhythms due to shift work

Source: AAOHN, 1995

2. The method of investigation begins with an analysis of accidents and trends in accidents through review of relevant records, including:
   - OSHA forms
   - Safety committee minutes
   - Accident, incident, or near-miss reports
   - Logs of daily health service visits
   - Other periodic reports and records of the health and safety service
   - Comparison of accident rates with those in other similar industries (See Figure 9-1 for incident rate calculation.)
3. Factors to consider when evaluating accident trends include:
   a. Worker's attitudes and/or behavior: impatience, boredom, recklessness, feeling rushed (as those paid for piecework), insufficiently trained, upset by shiftwork
   b. Management's attitudes and/or behavior: emphasis on production over safety, failure to ensure hazard identification and perform corrective actions, failure to enforce safe behavior
   c. Work environment deficiencies: poor lighting, inadequate ventilation, obsolete equipment

G. Chemical Inventories and Material Safety Data Sheets
   1. Required by the OSHA 29 CFR 1910.1200 Hazard Communication Standard
   2. Useful for estimating potential hazards associated with raw materials, products, and other hazardous substances present in the facility (Certain laboratories are required to comply with a similar standard: 29 CFR 1910.1450, which is specific to laboratories.)

FIGURE 9-1 *Incidence Rate Calculation*

$$\text{Incidence rate} = \frac{\text{Number of new cases/year} \times 200,000 \text{ work hours per facility*}}{\text{Number of hours worked at facility/year}}$$

*200,000 work hours is equivalent to 100 employees working 40 hours per week, 50 weeks per year. (Multiplying by 200,000 allows one to compare rates to other companies and is a more readily understood number.)

or

$$\begin{array}{l}\text{Incidence rate} \\ \text{per 100 workers}\end{array} = \frac{\text{Number of new cases/year} \times 200,000 \text{ work hours}}{\text{Number of people at facility} \times 2000 \text{ hours}^\dagger}$$

†2000 hours = 40 hrs/wk × 50 wks of work/yr

III

Exposure Monitoring

Exposure monitoring is the quantitative assessment of worksite exposures to hazards that are recognized, suspected, or reasonably predictable, based on other preliminary hazard identification methods (Weeks, Levy, & Wagner, 1991).

A. Sampling for chemical exposures
   1. A sample should represent worker's exposure or condition to be evaluated.
   2. Considerations when sampling include:
      a. Whom to sample (those directly or indirectly exposed)
      b. Where to sample (breathing zone, room air, point of operation)
      c. Sampling duration or volume needed
      d. Number and types of samples needed
      e. Sampling period (i.e., day or night, summer or winter)
   3. Compare findings to occupational health standards such as OSHA's Permissible Exposure Limits (PEL) or the Threshold Limit Values (TLV) of the American Conference of Governmental Industrial Hygienists.
   4. Interpretation of results must also take into account (Burgess, 1995):
      • Exposure levels versus absorbed dose
      • Sites of entry versus sites of action
      • Combined effects of two or more substances
      • Individual susceptibility
      • Conditions of use in the work environment, including worksite controls in place
      • Individual worker practices
   5. Examples of sampling and analysis problems include:
      a. Air pumps and sound-level meters that are not accurately calibrated or that spontaneously change flow rates
      b. Flow rates or exposure circumstances intentionally altered by the subject worker
      c. Color shade changes
      d. Fluctuating environmental conditions
      e. Problems in quality control, such as failure to perform instrument calibrations or to properly store and analyze samples (Johnson & Bell, 1991; Coffman, 1992)

B. Assessment of noise exposure
   1. Measurements of sound-pressure levels are expressed in terms of decibels (dB).
   2. An A-weighted scale combines frequency with intensity to yield dBA measurement (Dobie, 1995).
   3. Potential hearing damage can be estimated with a knowledge of the dBA sound level, the duration of exposure during a work day, and the total work-life exposure (Plog, 1996).
   4. Personal dosimeters provide an integration of time and noise exposure (Plog, 1996).
   5. For engineering controls of noise, sound-pressure levels throughout the frequency spectrum must be measured using an octave band analyzer (Plog, 1996).

(See Chapter 12 for an example of a hearing conservation program.)

C. Atmospheric monitoring
   1. The purpose of atmospheric monitoring is to evaluate, over a given period of time, the presence and concentration of airborne contaminants to which the worker is being exposed (Ness, 1991).
   2. Various methods used to sample gases, vapors, and particulates include:
      a. Dosimeter badges
      b. Detector of colorometric tubes with a pump to draw air samples
      c. Electronic direct-reading instruments with sensors
      d. Filters or other entrapment methods
   3. Types of sampling procedures
      a. Instantaneous, or "grab," sampling collects an air sample over a short period of time ranging from a few seconds to less than two minutes.
      b. The integrated, or long-term, sample consists of drawing a known volume of air through an appropriate medium for a sampling period of from one to eight hours.
      c. An area sample determines the location of contaminants by creating a "map" of levels present (Ness, 1991).
      d. Air, chemicals, water, and soil are monitored by bulk sampling.
      e. Bioaerosol monitoring for bacteria, viruses, fungi, and other biologicals is performed by methods similar to airborne chemical contaminant monitoring (Ness, 1991).
      f. Combustible gas indicators are direct-reading instruments used to measure explosive levels of gases in confined spaces (Ness, 1991).
      g. Oxygen detectors are direct-reading instruments used to evaluate the percentage of oxygen in the air, especially in confined spaces. (Safe levels established by U.S. standards are from 19.5 % to 23.0% oxygen in air.) (Ness, 1991)
   4. The sense of smell and/or irritation of the skin, eyes, and upper respiratory system can provide valuable clues to the levels of concentration of the contaminant, but these sensory indicators are unreliable for actual concentration or presence determinations.

D. Ionizing radiation monitoring is best carried out by personal dosimetry.
   1. Thermal-luminescent dosimeters (TLDs) or the older, less used film badges are worn by workers, with collection and reading at periodic intervals based on the extent of potential exposure (Breitenstein, Jr., & Spickard, 1995).
   2. Swipe samples, consisting of a wet surface wipe-down and analysis, are

taken for evidence of surface contamination by radionucleides (Breitenstein, Jr., & Spickard, 1995).

3. Area monitoring is accomplished by measuring Roentgens per day with the Geiger-Mueller instrument ("Geiger Counter").

4. Results of radiation measurement are compared against allowable dose standards from the EPA, OSHA, and other radiation protection and measurement agencies.

E. Temperature monitoring identifies hazardous extremes in hot or cold environments.

1. Potential for heat stress requires measurement of air temperature by dry-bulb measurement, humidity by natural wet-bulb measurement, and radiant heat by black-globe temperature (American Conference of Governmental Industrial Hygienists [ACGIH], 1994).

2. Other considerations when measuring for heat stress include fluid and electrolyte balance, training for heat tolerance, drugs, alcohol consumption, age, obesity, and extent of clothing.

3. Proposed occupational health standards of exposure to heat consist of a sliding scale based on the wet-bulb globe temperature, differing for acclimatized and unacclimatized workers.

4. Potential for cold injury requires measurement of air temperature by dry-bulb method plus measurement of wind speed to arrive at a wind-chill factor.

5. Other considerations when measuring for cold injury include exposure to wet, extent of clothing, and level of exhaustion.

6. Surface sampling, or wipe sampling, can be performed to evaluate external surfaces and the worker's skin and clothing for chemical, radiation, and biological contaminations.

F. Continuous monitors are alarm units used primarily to detect emergency conditions and trigger evacuation rather than to measure worker exposure (Ness, 1991).

1. Monitors may detect high radiation levels, fire, smoke, flammable atmospheres, oxygen-deficient air, and toxic levels of poisonous gases, such as hydrogen sulfide or carbon monoxide.

2. Stationary systems may provide real-time alarm warnings to workers in the area of a hazardous environmental condition.

3. Personal continuous monitors may be worn by workers in areas where potential releases could reach evacuation levels, such as in confined spaces.

4. Portable continuous monitors are similar to personal monitors but may have more display capability and can collect data over a period of time for a specific chemical.

IV

Process Safety Reviews

A. *Process Safety Reviews* consist of evaluations performed on activities involving chemicals, including using, storing, manufacturing, handling, or moving chemicals at the site.

B. Information is gathered on the hazards of the chemicals, the technology, and the equipment used in a process. This information:

1. Identifies the hazards of new and changed processes

2. Evaluates processes reviewed within the past 5 years

3. Reviews processes related to incidents that had a potential for catastrophic consequences

C. These reviews serve as a means of determining what could go wrong and what safeguards must be implemented to prevent hazardous chemical releases.

D. The reviews are mandated by the EPA 40 CFR* Part 68: "Worst Case Scenario" section and/or the OSHA 29 CFR 1910.119: Process Safety Management of Highly Hazardous Chemicals for:

1. Industries using any of more than 130 chemicals in listed quantities
2. Industries using flammable liquids and gases in quantities of 10,000 pounds or more

Note: CFR refers to the Code of Federal Regulations, a compilation of final rules and regulations that are originally published in the Federal Register. The CFR is divided into 50 titles representing broad areas subject to federal regulation. Title 29 is labor; Title 40 is protection of the environment.

E. Methods to determine and evaluate the consequences of failure of engineering and administrative controls include (National Safety Council, 1992; Gressel & Gideon, 1991):

1. "What-if" is a method of thinking in which failure potentials are brainstormed and their cause and effects analyzed.
2. Checklists identify the major hazards and nuisances associated with a particular material.
3. A hazard and operability study (HAZOP) is a formal systematic study of a newly designed facility or operation to assess the potential of individual equipment components to fail, resulting in consequential effects on the overall facility.
4. Failure mode and effects analysis (FMEA) is a "bottom-up" technique in which the failure of a particular process component is assessed for its effects on other components and on the process system as a potential source for accidents.
5. Fault tree analysis is a formalized deductive technique that works backward from a defined accident to identify and graphically display the combination of equipment failures and operational errors that can lead up to the accident.

F. Worker health and safety information, including the health effects of chemicals and the possible need for specific first aid planning, should be evaluated.

$\overline{V}$

Ergonomic Analysis

A. The purpose of the ergonomic analysis is to evaluate stresses related to the performance of work so that strategies for prevention can be developed; preventive strategies include (Keyserling, Stetson, Silverstein, & Brouwer, 1993):

1. Redesigning work stations and work equipment (i.e., machine guards)
2. Improving work environment (i.e., developing a work-rest schedule to prevent heat stress)
3. Designing warning signs for hazardous equipment and/or locations

B. The National Institute for Occupational Safety and Health (NIOSH) Equation for Manual Lifting is a guide that can be used to evaluate tasks to prevent or reduce the occurrence of overexertion injuries and low back pain due to lifting and lowering.

1. The guidelines describe an equation that is based on the following variables: horizontal distance; vertical distance; distance of lift; asymmetry of lift; coupling; frequency of lifting (see Table 9-5).
2. The goal is to design the task so that the lifting index is at or below 1.0.

TABLE 9-5

NIOSH Lifting Guidelines

- NIOSH lifting guidelines use a recommended weight limit (RWL) that healthy male workers and 75% of female workers could perform for up to 8 hours without adverse health effects.
- NIOSH lifting guidelines are based on multipliers that assess the following task variables:

  H   horizontal location (distance of the hands away from the midpoint between the ankles)

  V   vertical location (vertical heights of the hands above the floor)

  D   travel distance (vertical travel distance of the hands between the origin of the lift and the highest point during the lift—often the destination)

  A   asymmetrical angle (lifts that involve twisting outside the midsagittal plane or neutral body position)

  C   couplings (gripping methods, object interface)

  L   lifting frequency (number of lifts per minute)

  LC load constant = maximum recommended load weight under ideal lifting conditions, defined as 51 lbs.

- The lifting index (LI) provides an estimate of the degree of physical stress associated with a lifting task. The formula is LI = Load Weight (lbs.) divided by RWL (lbs.) = L. An LI of 1.0 or less implies a safe job (Garg, 1995).
- Additional analyses take into account rest allowances, task variables such as grip changes, and multiple tasks.

Source: Waters, Putz-Anderson, & Garg (1994). Details regarding performing this analysis according to the revised lifting equation can be found in Garg (1995).

C. Effective ergonomics programs include the following (Keyserling et al., 1993):
1. Surveillance strategies to assess patterns of exertion injuries
2. Job hazard analysis/job safety analysis to identify workers at risk
3. Job design or redesign that considers ergonomic factors
4. Management and worker training related to the recognition and control of biochemical hazards
5. Protocol for health management of injured workers

VI

Occupational Health Surveillance

A. *Occupational health surveillance* consists of the "process of monitoring the health status of worker populations to gather data on the effects of workplace exposures and using data to prevent injury and illness" (AAOHN, 1996).

B. Surveillance terminology
1. Surveillance applied to populations is called *public health surveillance;* occupational health surveillance is a subset (Levy & Wegman, 1995).
2. Surveillance of individuals, which is sometimes called *medical surveillance,* includes history taking, examination, and monitoring of an individual.
   a. *Medical surveillance* may include activities performed by occupational health nurses; thus the term *health surveillance* "is more accurate and reflective of the nature of the activity" (Rogers, 1994, p. 229).
   b. Biological monitoring and worker surveillance requirements in OSHA standards for specific chemical hazards are listed under "Medical Surveillance."

C. Primary goals of occupational health surveillance are as follows (AAOHN, 1996: Levy & Wegman, 1995):

1. Identify the occurrence of injuries and illnesses related to hazard exposure in the worksite.
2. Define the magnitude and distribution of occupational disease and injury occurrences.
3. Identify and track trends in disease and injury occurrence as a means of assessing effectiveness of prevention strategies.
4. Describe specific occupations or industries that would benefit from prevention strategies.
5. Guide the development of engineering and administrative strategies for prevention and control.

D. Other benefits to health surveillance include:

1. More appropriate therapeutic and rehabilitation activities
2. Appropriate compensation for workers with illnesses resulting from occupational exposures
3. Discovering new relationships between work exposure and disease

E. Challenges to the identification and recognition of occupational illness

1. Occupational illnesses often have long latency periods; years and even decades may elapse between time of exposure and occurrence of symptoms.
2. Occupational illness may be indistinguishable from nonoccupational illness (i.e., occupational asthma resembles nonoccupational asthma)
3. Causes of occupational illness are multifactorial; it is difficult to determine the exact cause of illness.
4. Americans are on the move, making it difficult to track exposures.

F. The occupational health nurse is key to providing a quality health surveillance program because the occupational health nurse (AAOHN, 1996):

1. Is the most frequently available occupational health professional at the worksite
2. Is knowledgeable about health surveillance and other occupational health and safety programs
3. Is familiar with the health status of workers
4. Provides cost-effective care

G. Occupational health nursing roles related to occupational health surveillance (AAOHN, 1996):

1. Work with company representatives and other occupational health and safety professionals to plan, conduct, supervise, and evaluate the occupational health surveillance program.
2. Conduct and interpret results of the tests required for occupational health surveillance, and refer employees for additional tests as necessary.
3. Recommend identification, prevention, and control strategies based on test results.
4. Establish and maintain a system of recordkeeping.
5. Evaluate a program's effectiveness; modify the program as needed.
6. Ensure compliance with Occupational Safety and Health Administration regulations.
7. Select, manage, and evaluate vendor-provided health services.

VII

Analysis of the Hazards

A. Types of industry standards for hazard exposure

1. Mandatory standards that establish maximum levels of permitted exposures are required and enforceable by government agencies, such as the Occupational Safety and Health Administration (OSHA) and the Environmental Protection Agency (EPA).

2. Consensus standards are voluntary and adopted by agreement with participating members.

   a. They can serve as professional yardsticks against which to measure hazard identification and prevention activities.

   b. Occasionally mandatory standards quote consensus standards as their requirements.

   c. They can carry heavy weight in issues such as insurance company coverage, legal actions, and other issues in which competency and compliance issues are involved.

   d. Trade associations, scientific and technical societies, and insurance companies may have certification or compliance requirements that industry can use as a yardstick for hazards and preventive measures

B. Limitations of standards

1. Some standards are inadequate.

2. Standards can conflict with each other in their requirements, such as the labeling requirements of the Department of Transportation versus those of OSHA.

3. Standards in the United States may differ from those of other countries, thus affecting international corporations.

4. "Regulatory compliance does not actually address an organization's principal risks or lead to effective hazards management" (Manuele, 1994, p. 73).

C. Evaluating the significance of hazard identification

1. "Low numbers of incidents and injuries do not necessarily mean a hazard-free worksite" (Manuele, 1994, p. 72).

2. A hazardous event may be rated as: catastrophic, critical marginal, or negligible in its severity; these are subjective categories based on fatalities, injury severity, and/or damage in financial terms (Manuele, 1994).

3. The likelihood of a hazardous event is estimated subjectively as frequent, probable, occasional, remote, or improbable.

4. Risk analysis should address both the probability of an incident occurring and the expected severity of adverse results, thus ranking the risks. (See Figures 9-2 and 9-3.)

5. Risk analysis should define the people, property, and environment that identified hazards may affect.

D. Analysis and evaluation strategies serve as guides for program implementation.

1. When exposure monitoring indicates that agent action levels have been reached, a worker health surveillance program should be implemented.

2. When worker health data suggest adverse worksite exposures, exposure monitoring may be indicated.

3. Elevated exposure results and/or biological monitoring results may indicate the need for additional engineering and administrative control measures or for additional training in the proper use of personal protective equipment.

FIGURE 9-2 *A Formula for Estimation of Risk Score*

$$R = S \times E \times P \quad \text{where}$$

$$R = \text{Risk Score}, \; S = \text{Severity}, \; E = \text{Exposure}, \; P = \text{Probability}$$

Risk scores can be used to rank the priority of hazards. Assign a value to each variable (for example, by using a scale from 1 to 5); then multiply the potential severity of injury by the frequency of exposure by the probability of exposure to obtain a risk score estimate. (Perkinson, 1995)

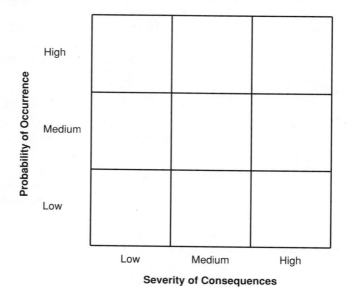

FIGURE 9-3 *Risk Analysis Matrix*

VIII

Worker Populations Analysis

Worker populations should be viewed not just as a collection of individuals but as a single entity; worker populations include communities and subgroups of workers.

A. Analyzing groups, not just individuals, can detect patterns, trends, changes and commonalties (Travers & McDougall, 1995).

　　1. Population data can be used to describe injury and illness trends over time, so that patterns with common causes can be identified and prevented.

　　2. Occupational health nurses should be alert to group patterns of injury and illness, as follows:

　　　　a. If health visits reveal a cluster of illnesses or injuries, visit the worksite to get an understanding of how and why these events may be happening (Weinstock, 1993).

　　　　b. Attempt to identify whether workers with similar complaints perform the same job, work in the same area, or have something else in common (Barnes, 1992).

    c. Monitor trends that may suggest new hazards or the breakdown of prevention and control measures.

    d. Determine whether conditions are improving or worsening (Weinstock, 1993).

    e. Identify the worksite locations involved.

    f. Enlist colleagues from other disciplines (i.e., industrial hygiene, engineering), as appropriate.

B. *Epidemic events* are any marked upward fluctuation in disease incidence.

1. Epidemics are verified when the incidence of a disease or injury exceeds what normally would be expected.

2. An epidemic must have an agent as well as individuals who are susceptible to infection by the agent.

3. Epidemics are categorized according to their mode of transmission as follows:

    a. Common source epidemics occur when the mode of transmission of the causal agent is from a common source, such as food, air, or water.

    b. Propagated or progressive epidemics occur when the mode of transmission is from person to person, such as influenza.

4. Management of an epidemic in the work setting should follow these steps:

    a. Identify and arrange for treatment of clients.

    b. Institute control measures to decrease spread of contamination and prevent recurrence.

    c. Provide workers with appropriate health education.

    d. Establish a program of continued surveillance and monitoring for infection.

    e. Establish a program to prevent recurrence.

C. *Epidemic (mass) hysteria* (also called mass psychogenic illness) is an event in which group of workers exposed to the same stimulus exhibit common physical symptoms of psychological origin (Kahn, 1993).

1. Characteristics of exposure:

    a. This illness occurs most frequently in work settings with physical and emotional stressors, such as boring, repetitive tasks and poor rapport between the workforce and company management.

    b. A noxious odor, a substance perceived as toxic, extreme heat, or loud, repetitive noises may serve as triggers (Kahn, 1993).

    c. Transmission of symptoms occurs by sight, sound, or word of mouth rather than by simply being in a common exposure area.

2. Symptom development includes:

    a. An explosive onset of symptoms whose severity is out of proportion to the apparent cause and that can disappear and return rapidly.

    b. A range of symptoms, including headache, nausea, dizziness, chills, difficulty in breathing, and other vague, subjective complaints, divert the worker's attention from hidden stress to external worksite factors (Kahn, 1993).

3. Recognition is achieved through:

    a. Careful complaint investigation and exposure analysis of all potential toxicological and biologic causes in order to rule out a physical basis

    b. Evaluation of the worksite for psychosocial stressors

    c. Identification of workers at high risk for somatoform disorders

4. Other considerations:

    a. A careful worksite analysis should be performed; the possibility of physical symptoms must be considered even in the absence of objective findings.

b. "Hysteria" reactions may be the result of psychosocial stressors in the workplace; this possibility should be investigated.

c. Treatment consists, firstly, of establishing and communicating the lack of connection between the symptoms and the "trigger"; and, secondly of taking measures to reduce occupational stressors.

D. Sentinel health event-occupational (SHE-O)

1. *SHE-O* is a disease, disability, or untimely death that is work-related and whose occurrence may:

   a. Provide the impetus for epidemiologic or industrial hygiene studies (Weeks, Levy, & Wagner, 1991)

   b. Serve as a warning that prevention and control strategies are needed

2. The occurrence of sentinel health events may serve as the stimulus for:

   a. The development of epidemiologic or industrial hygiene studies

   b. Hazard evaluation and reassessment of control measures

   c. The implementation of prevention or control activities

3. The occupational health nurse may play a key role in identifying sentinel health events; it is essential that the occupational health nurse:

   a. Have a thorough knowledge of the worksite and its hazards

   b. Collaborate with professional colleagues within the company when a sentinel health event is suspected

   c. Participate in continuing education efforts

   d. Maintain a high index of suspicion for the possibility of a sentinel health event ("gatekeeper" role)

   e. Refer all potentially exposed workers for further evaluation when a work-related problem is suspected (Hau, 1993)

E. Multiple chemical sensitivity (MCS)

1. *Multiple chemical sensitivity* has been described as a syndrome that may develop in one or many workers and "affect(s) multiple systems and occur(s) in multiple unrelated environments" (Levy & Wegman, 1995, p. 67).

   a. Common symptoms are fatigue, headache, frequent colds, dizziness, nausea, lack of concentration, memory loss, menstrual irregularities, and visual problems (Voelker, 1994).

   b. Often the symptom pattern changes, with some symptoms disappearing and new ones occurring; symptoms can produce total disability

2. MCS is poorly understood; hence it is a highly controversial phenomenon.

   a. Symptoms are subjective, with no objective evidence of organ system damage or dysfunction.

   b. Health effects described as MCS are related to documentable environmental exposure.

   c. MCS symptoms are elicited by extremely low exposures to chemicals.

   d. MCS symptoms seem to have a predictable return with environmental stimuli (Sparks, et al., 1994).

3. There is a need for epidemiological studies and for careful environmental and occupational history-taking in order to better understand multiple chemical sensitivity.

F. Worksite violence and homicide

1. Because of epidemic growth, workplace violence is creating a new form of job hazard and an increased sense of worker vulnerability.

2. Workplace violence includes harassment, threats, and actual physical assaults in the worksite.
3. High-risk industries: public service establishments; public transportation services; detective and protective services; and hotel, motels and lodging places (Castillo, 1994).
4. California OSHA has identified three types of violent worksite offenders (California, Worksite Violence Safety Act of 1994):
   a. Type I: No legitimate relationship to the worksite; enters to commit a robbery or other criminal act
   b. Type II: A recipient or the object of a service provided at the site—a client, customer, or passenger
   c. Type III: Involvement with the worksite as a co-worker, worker, or as the spouse, relative, or friend of a worker
5. The profile of a Type III perpetrator has been described as follows (Kinney, 1993; Gates, 1995):
   a. Typically, a disgruntled worker with very little social support who projects personal problems onto others
   b. Usually a young white male with a preoccupation with weapons
   c. A person with predisposition to resolving difficulties through violent, aggressive behavior
   d. A person whose behavior may be triggered by threatening events such as job termination, job discipline, an autocratic management, and worker-supervisor disputes
6. Decisions regarding return to work, time off, and other occupational health services activities place the occupational health nurse and the occupational health physician on the list of potential targets (Olson, 1994).
7. Recognizing and understanding the potential hazard of worksite violence is a new essential assessment in industry (Gates, 1995).

Prevention and Control

The prevention and control of occupational hazards is central to occupational safety and health nursing practice. Several approaches can be used to achieve this objective, including elimination or substitution of materials, engineering controls, modification of work practices, administrative controls, and/or the use of protective equipment. The choice of control strategy depends on the nature of the workplace, the work tasks, and the workers. Oftentimes, more than a single approach is required to achieve optimal safety and health.

$\overline{IX}$

Approaches That Focus on the Workplace

 Elimination of or *substitution* of hazardous materials is intended to minimize the source of potential exposure through either the complete removal or the replacement of the hazardous material with a less toxic substitute.
   1. Elimination (or substitution) is the most preferred strategy for control and the method of choice whenever possible.
      a. The benefits to health and safety of elimination and substitution often have to be weighed against the technological and economic consequences.
      b. When using substitution, care must be taken to assure that the replacement product does not pose other health or safety risks.

2. Examples of elimination or substitution include:
  a. Removing insulation that contains asbestos fibers
  b. Using mechanical or vacuum lifting devices to replace manual lifting
  c. Using a dipping method to coat an object rather than spraying, thus reducing the danger of inhalation by workers
  d. Substituting unbreakable Plexiglas for breakable glass
  e. Using a less toxic and less flammable chemical than one in current use

B. *Engineering controls* are intended to stop hazards at their source or in the path of their transmission and are the preferred strategy when elimination or substitution is not possible.
  1. Characteristics of workplace designs that promote occupational health and safety include:
    a. Appropriate lighting to enable workers to perform their tasks safely
    b. Workstations that are ergonomically designed to reduce the risk factors of repetitive motions, static or awkward postures, forceful exertions, and mechanical pressure on soft tissues
    c. Stairs or platforms with railings, guarded floor and wall openings, and proper floor finishes to reduce slips, trips and falls
    d. Mats that are specially designed to reduce safety hazards (see Box 9-1)
    e. Security designs to reduce the potential for worksite violence (i.e., bullet-proof glass, silent alarms, well-lit parking lots)
    f. Designs that consider the personal comfort of workers; well-designed workstations can reduce worker stress (see Box 9-2)
  2. Examples of beneficial workplace designs
    a. *Isolation:* provides a barrier between a hazard and those who might be affected by that hazard.
      1) Process isolation: operations handled through remote computer applications in a control room
      2) Underground tanks and isolated storage buildings for hazardous materials
      3) Noise barriers
      4) Shields that prevent exposure of nearby persons to welding arcs
    b. *Time-distance-shielding* is the most common approach to protecting workers from ionizing radiation (National Safety Council, 1992)

BOX 9-1

Examples of Mats Designed to Reduce Safety Hazards

- **Fatigue-reducing mats:** lessen muscular fatigue and often reduce noise

- **Slip-resistant mats:** protect against slipping on water, oil, ice, or mud underfoot

- **Conductive mats:** dissipate static electricity in rooms with high oxygen content, sensitive electronic components, explosives, or volatile liquids

- **Nonconductive rubber mats:** used in front of switchboards and other hazardous locations to insulate against high voltages

---

BOX 9-2

Stress-Reducing Workplace Designs

- Informal and formal meeting places
- Enclosures accommodating the need for personal space
- Permission to personalize spaces
- Access to daylight/sunlight
- Incorporation of variability through artifacts and cultural symbols, colors, and textures
- Freedom from distractions; visual and auditory privacy

---

    1) *Time*: controlling the amount of time exposed to the radiation source, measured in mR/hr.

    2) *Distance*: remaining as far away from the radiation source as possible

    3) *Shielding*: placing a barrier impenetrable to radiation between the worker and the source

  c. Avoiding ingestion and inhalation of radioactive particulates is also a protection measure, most applicable in the event of radioactive fallout.

  d. *Automatic systems* which shut down processes or issue warnings when hazardous conditions develop (Cote, 1995):

    1) Fire detectors/alarms, water sprinkler systems, and gas extinguisher systems, such as Halon, in computer rooms

    2) Safety valves, fusible plugs, and rupture discs in boilers and pressure vessels to permit excess pressure relief

    3) Automatic fall-protection devices that allow normal descent by a worker in the device, but lock in the event of a rapid descent or fall

    4) Circuit breakers, fuses, and other electrical current interruption devices that respond to overcurrents or overloads

    5) Explosion detectors that release a suppressant to inhibit further reaction

  e. *Ventilation* captures or dilutes airborne contaminants, cleaning the air before or after release (Burton, 1995).

    1) Local exhaust systems: Remove contaminated air from the point of origin, away from the worker's breathing zone, through a scrubber or cleaning system to the outside (Burton, 1995)

    2) Dilution ventilation: Circulates fresh air into the worksite to dilute the contaminant air to an acceptable exposure level (Burton, 1995)

    3) Filtration: Used to clean the air prior to release back into the general ventilation or release to the outside

    4) Other air cleaning methods: electrostatic precipitators, scrubbers, absorbers, and chemical reactors (Burgess, 1995)

3. Storage of hazardous materials

  a. Flammable liquids are stored using bonding and grounding to dissipate static electricity, which could ignite their vapors.

  b. Special lead containers are used to store radioactive materials.

  c. Refrigerators are used to store heat-sensitive or heat-reactive chemicals.

  d. Air-reactive chemicals are stored under water.

  e. Special storage cabinets and safety cans are used to store small amounts of flammable liquids, such as hydrocarbons, gasoline, and kerosene.

      f. Puncture-proof sharps containers are used to store contaminated needles and sharps awaiting disposal as hazardous health waste.

      g. Cylinders of compressed gas, including the oxygen cylinders used by the occupational health nurse, must be kept upright and secured.

      h. Certain highly toxic specialty gases, such as silane, must be kept in special gas cabinets.

      i. Only the amount of hazardous substance that will actually be needed to be consumed in a reasonable time during the manufacturing process should be kept.

4. *Hazardous energy control* is used to prevent contact between the worker and hazardous energy sources.

      a. Hazardous energy sources include electrical energy, chemical reactivity, thermal extremes, mechanical energy, and physical energy.

      b. Machine safeguarding to eliminate machine hazards

          1) All moving parts on machines (pulleys, belts, chains, etc.), should be guarded at all times.

          2) Portable power tools, lawnmowers, and grinders should also be guarded (OSHA 3067, 1992).

          3) Methods of machine safeguarding are based on the type of operation, stock size and shape, handling method, and physical layout of the area (OSHA 3067, 1992).

              • Guards are barriers that prevent access to danger areas (see Figures 9-4 and 9-5).

              • Devices such as restraints, gates, presence-sensing (optical) devices, and trip controls stop the machine if a hand or other body part is inadvertently placed in the danger area.

      c. Electrical shock control is accomplished through:

          1) Proper initial installation

          2) The use of grounded outlets, circuit breakers, and disconnects (devices that interrupt current flow when it exceeds the wire's capacity)

          3) The use of ground fault circuit interrupters

          4) Proper insulation

      d. Robots are used to perform unsafe, hazardous, highly repetitive, and unpleasant tasks.

      e. Lockout/Tagout is used to control hazardous energy sources during the service and maintenance of machinery or equipment when unexpected energization, startup, or stored energy release may occur (National Safety Council, 1992).

          1) OSHA 29 CFR 1910.147 Control of Hazardous Energy requires:

              • Employee training

              • Periodic inspections of the energy control program

              • Written procedures for identifying all energy sources

              • A tag warning system (see Figure 9-6)

              • Periodic review/revisions

          2) All energy control devices are placed in the "off" or "safe" position, locked in that position, and tagged with a warning tag.

          3) Chemical process lines are bled out and disconnected or have a line block, called a "blank," inserted.

          4) Upon work completion, the authorized employee will verify that the equipment has been returned to a safe state of operation before lockout/tagout devices are removed.

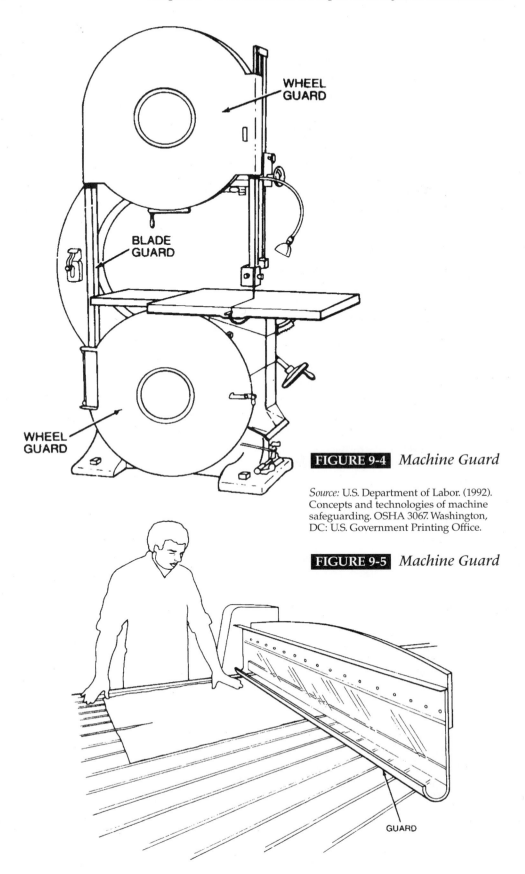

WHEEL
GUARD

BLADE
GUARD

WHEEL
GUARD

FIGURE 9-4 *Machine Guard*

Source: U.S. Department of Labor. (1992).
Concepts and technologies of machine
safeguarding. OSHA 3067. Washington,
DC: U.S. Government Printing Office.

FIGURE 9-5 *Machine Guard*

GUARD

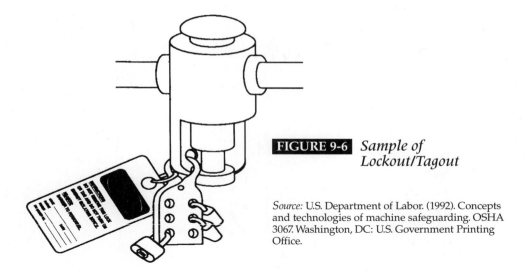

FIGURE 9-6 *Sample of Lockout/Tagout*

Source: U.S. Department of Labor. (1992). Concepts and technologies of machine safeguarding. OSHA 3067. Washington, DC: U.S. Government Printing Office.

$\overline{\text{X}}$
Approaches That Focus on Work Tasks

Changing work practices (the manner in which work is performed) is often an important strategy that can limit or reduce a worker's exposure to workplace hazards.

A. Characteristics of work practices
  1. Work practices, as control strategies, may include elements of engineering controls, administrative controls, and protective equipment usage.
  2. Changes in work practices should be accompanied by on-site evaluations in order to:
     a. Characterize the risks inherent to the tasks
     b. Assure that the work practice is appropriate to the task
     c. Analyze individual work tasks and identify those that may contribute to exposure
  3. It is essential that the workers performing the job participate in the development of safe work practices in order to maximize the effectiveness of these strategies.

B. Barriers to the implementation of safe work practices
  1. Piecework production practice as a payment mechanism encourages workers to cut corners for the sake of production output, often sacrificing safe work practices.
  2. Refusing to provide support and funding to safety programs undermines their effectiveness.
  3. Fear of harassment or violence can prevent the adoption of safe work practices.
  4. Incentives that reward productivity may lead to unsafe work practices.

C. Examples of work practice modifications
  1. Vacuuming with equipment which has high-efficiency particulate (HEPA) filters can keep hazardous dusts from being resuspended.
  2. Wet mopping instead of sweeping is another method of minimizing contamination from hazardous dusts and particulates.

3. Using proper body mechanics when bending or lifting can prevent strains and sprains.

D. Assuring safety through work practices

1. The role of safety committees in assuring safe work practices includes (National Safety Council, 1992):
   - Evaluating worker suggestions
   - Individually promoting accident prevention and safe work practices within each member's own work area
   - Investigating reported safety deficiencies or assisting in the investigation
   - Reviewing accidents and identifying root causes and prevention methods
   - Performing walk-through surveys and safety inspections
   - Making recommendations on company safety rules
   - Assisting in safety training programs
   - Voting on safety awards recipients
   - Suggesting and promoting safety incentive programs

2. Safety training provides specific knowledge, instructions, and skills to enable workers to perform jobs safely while optimizing productivity.

3. Safety committees are required in certain regulatory standards, such as team hazard evaluations in the Process Safety Standard. 29 CFR 1910.119. (Warren & Amundson, 1995).

E. *Administrative controls* are supervisory and management practices to promote safe work behaviors that eliminate or limit hazard exposures.

1. Mechanisms for implementing administrative controls
   a. Proper scheduling can reduce the amount of time any worker is exposed to a hazard or in controlling the timing of the work to avoid the hazard; examples are:
      1) Scheduling work activities that can produce heat stress so that they are performed during cooler parts of the day
      2) Scheduling rotations among various job assignments, limiting exposure associated with a single job
      3) Not scheduling new workers to perform a job assignment alone until they have demonstrated adequate job knowledge and performance
   b. Work permits are a system to evaluate projects for hazards, specify safe work practices, identify essential personal protective equipment and other safety measures, and provide authorization before any work is done (National Safety Council, 1992).
      1) A Hot Work Permit is used for activities that produce sparks or flames, referred to as "hot work."
      2) A Confined Space Entry Permit is required prior to work in areas defined as confined spaces.
         - A confined space is an area that has limited means of access, is not designed for continuous worker occupancy, and may have little or no natural ventilation.
         - Hazards associated with confined spaces that must be evaluated in the permitting process are hazardous atmospheres (oxygen-deficient, flammable, toxic), temperature extremes, engulfment hazards, noise, falling objects, and any other recognized serious hazard.
   c. Housekeeping practices that promote safe working conditions are: pest control; disposal of waste; keeping floors clear of oil, grease or water; preventing trip hazards; and properly storing materials, tools and equipment.

    d. Labeling, coding, and posting warning signs all assist in communicating safety throughout the worksite.

       1) Some OSHA standards require posting of warning signs in areas where hazards have been identified (i.e., noise or radiation)

       2) Fire response equipment and alarms are marked with signs and color coding to enhance visibility and rapid retrieval.

       3) Exits must be clearly identified with lighted signs; doorways that are not exits must be clearly labeled as such.

       4) Color, indicators of direction of flow, and other signs mark controls, piping outlets, and pipelines.

       5) A few standard color codes include:
- Red—fire protection equipment, danger, and "emergency stops" on equipment
- Yellow—trip hazards, flammable-liquid storage cabinets, materials-handling equipment, such as forklifts
- Green—location of first-aid and safety equipment
- Black on yellow—radiation hazard
- Bright blue—inert gases

       6) Signs and maps are posted throughout the facility to mark evacuation routes and shelters.

       7) General warning signs do not substitute for safe work practices but can serve as cautions and reminders (National Safety Council, 1992).

    e. Preventive maintenance is the planned, periodic scheduling of equipment and the refurbishing, refitting, inspection and/or overhaul of process units to prevent hazardous operating conditions from developing over time and after repeated use (National Safety Council, 1992).

    f. Safety newsletters are used to relate safety information directly to each worker.

       1) They impart information and help to boost morale.

       2) To be successful, they should put the spotlight on workers, balancing useful information with recognition of workers' accomplishments.

       3) They can run safety contests, provide a network for news, offer a management column, and report actual incidents (Willen, 1995).

2. Testing and certification are methods for determining competency and assuring safe performance of various job functions. The following are a few examples:

    a. Forklift operator training is often followed by written and performance testing to evaluate for proper, safe forklift operation.

    b. Boiler operators are licensed by the state.

    c. Drivers of certain types and sizes of vehicles must pass a Commercial Driver's License examination.

    d. Structural welders are usually certified in their skills by the Welder's Institute.

    e. Hazardous materials technicians are certified upon successful completion of the OSHA requirements under 29 CFR 1910.120.

3. Examples of programs for administrative control

    a. The two-man concept (or "buddy system") is a safeguard for workers involved in hazardous operations.

       1) Both persons are exposed to the same hazard simultaneously; each one monitors the other and provides assistance when needed, such as the mutual aid and surveillance employed by power company personnel on live high-voltage systems (National Safety Council, 1992).

2) One person is exposed to the hazard, while the other acts as an attendant to observe and summon help if an emergency develops (Terpin, 1992).

b. Health promotion programs target lifestyles to lessen workers' vulnerability to worksite exposures and to enhance their ability and capacity to perform job assignments more safely.

1) Back strengthening through exercise programs can help reduce the incidence of back strain during materials handling.

2) Smoking cessation programs can reduce risks of synergistic effects of cigarette smoke and asbestos exposure.

3) Stress management programs can assist workers in dealing with work-related stress.

c. Incentive programs are used to motivate workers to work safely and prevent accidents and injuries (Minter, 1995).

1) Examples of incentive programs include:
- Contests among departments for the best safety record
- Safety awards for companies and plants that are offered by organizations such as local safety councils
- Safety patches, pins, hard-hat stickers, ball caps, and other apparel bearing positive safety messages
- Bonuses to workers, supervisors, and/or managers when targeted safety goals are reached

2) Programs should be monitored so that workers, supervisors, and/or managers do not attempt to hide accidents, injuries, and other events in order to avoid being the cause of a lost record or award or to avoid losing a bonus or prize.

3) The primary focus of managers should not be numbers and statistics but rather acknowledging the excellent safety performance of workers.

d. Medical removal (removal from exposure for medical reasons) and restricted work programs

1) Some OSHA regulations have medical removal requirements, which require removal of a worker based on biological monitoring results prior to clinical health effects and organ system injury; these regulations include the lead and cadmium standards.

2) Some companies adopt light-duty programs to return workers gradually to the rigors of full work assignments.

e. Emergency preparedness planning and response operations

1) *Emergency preparedness* is a control measure intended to prevent or minimize harm to persons, property, systems, and environment in the event of a critical incident.

2) This strategy may be used for a medical emergency, fire, technological event (such as a hazardous materials release), and civil event (such as a bomb threat).

3) Processes include mitigation, planning, response, and recovery.
- In the mitigation phase, the attempt is made to identify and eliminate hazards that have a potential for generating an emergency.
- Planning is then conducted to respond effectively in coordination with community response agencies to bring emergency conditions under control and eventually return to normal operations, if possible. (See Figure 9-7.)

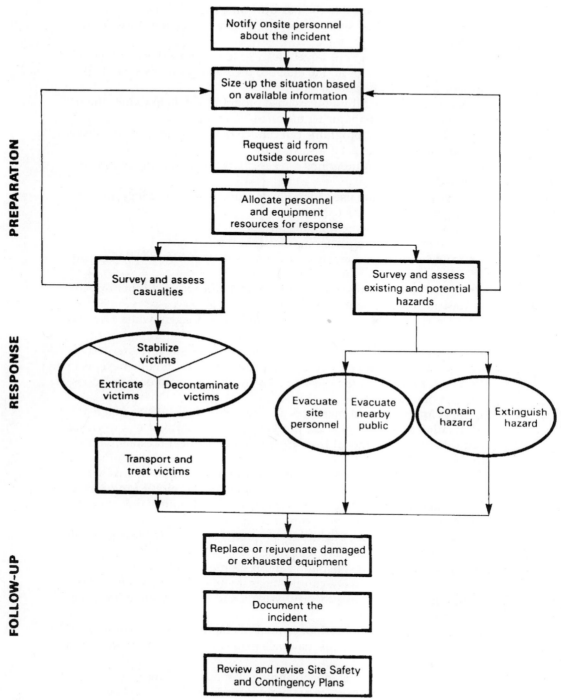

FIGURE 9-7 *Emergency Response Operations*

f. Critical-incident stress debriefing (CISD) is an administrative tool to prevent the development of critical-incident stress that typically affects the emergency response personnel of both an industry and a community (McNeely, 1991).
   1) Critical-incident stress can develop when providers do not allow themselves to react emotionally to an emergency event.
   2) Debriefing enables providers to come to terms with their thoughts and feelings by bringing them out in the open and expressing them.
   3) CISD should be conducted within 24 to 72 hours after the event in a nonthreatening environment, confidentially, by trained leaders (Mitchell & Resnick, 1981 cited by Hayes, Goodwin, & Miars, 1990).
   4) CISD teams can usually be found through community emergency response agencies, such as the local fire department.

XI

Approaches That Focus on Workers

Personal protective equipment (PPE) includes all clothing and other personally-worn work accessories designed to create a barrier against worksite hazards.

A. Characteristics of personal protective equipment
1. Workers must be trained in: the reasons for wearing PPE; what PPE to wear; how to don, use, and wear PPE; the proper care, maintenance, and useful life of PPE; and any other training requirement involving PPE.
2. The occupational health nurse should become familiar with the details of the specific PPE used at the facility and with the requirements of the applicable OSHA standard.
   a. Typical PPE dispensed by the occupational health nurse includes eye protection, hearing protection, and skin barrier creams.
   b. The occupational health nurse must take special care to review the research and professional recommendations regarding proper PPE selections.

B. Regulations related to personal protective equipment.
1. The company is required to have a written PPE program and to provide the PPE to the workers. (Exceptions are some companies that have workers contribute to the cost of prescription safety glasses and safety shoes.)
2. OSHA 29 CFR 1910.132 requires a hazard assessment of the worksite that (Roughton, 1995):
   a. Includes a walk-through survey
   b. Requires a written certification that the assessment has been performed
   c. Provides a mechanism for ensuring that the need for PPE has been determined and that the PPE selected is appropriate to the hazard

C. Examples of personal protective equipment:
1. Eye and face protection under 29 CFR 1910.133 requires protective eye and face equipment.
   a. Safety glasses with sideshields are used to protect against flying objects; they must be heat-treated and able to withstand the drop of a 5-lb. lead ball without shattering.
   b. Chemical goggles, of vented and air-tight varieties, protect against chemical splashes, vapors, and gases.
   c. UV light protection is used most frequently by welders to protect against the ultraviolet welding arc.

    d. Laser beam protection is necessary to prevent corneal and retinal injuries from exposure to laser beams.

    e. Face shields add further protection against splashes or sparks.

    f. The use of contact lenses, especially while wearing respiratory protection, is under evaluation; the concern exists that dirt or other debris can lodge between the lens and the pupil or that soft lenses will absorb chemical contaminants from the air.

2. Hearing protection under 29 CFR 1910.95 requires a written hearing conservation program, including hearing protection and annual audiometric testing for workers exposed to excessive noise. (See Chapter 12 for an example of a program.)

    a. Hearing protection devices include ear plugs, ear muffs, ear molds, and canal caps. (See Chapter 12 for description.)

    b. Hearing aids do not protect against the effects of loud noise, even when the worker cannot hear the noise.

    c. Workers must be shown how to wear hearing protection, told how to care for it, and observed to ensure that they are using it correctly.

    d. Changes in noise levels may require changes in hearing protection devices.

3. Hand/skin protection is required under 29 CFR 1910.138.

    a. Gloves are selected to protect against heat, cold, abrasion, and chemicals.

    b. Barrier creams are of two varieties, setting up a coating to shield the skin either against water-related exposures or against drying powder-type exposures.

    c. Tapes, similar to adhesive tape, have a gritty or rubbery external surface to protect fingers against abrasion from frequent rubbing or gripping and to aid in grip.

    d. UV radiation protection is sunscreen to protect workers from the sun and other UV sources.

    e. Glove boxes, although not strictly PPE, are also used to protect hand exposures, particularly against biological agents.

4. Foot protection under 29 CFR 1910.136 specifies safety shoes for protecting feet from being crushed and fractured.

    a. Boots are used to protect against water, chemicals, and fire response exposures.

    b. Steel-toed shoes protect the toes from hazards such as heavy rolling or falling objects.

    c. Metatarsal plates fit over the shoe and extend protection to the metatarsals from toe-injury hazards.

5. Torso protection is selected according to the specific type of hazard involved:

    a. Chemical protective clothing may consist of aprons, coveralls, hooded suits, fully encapsulated suits with self-contained breathing apparatus, sleeves, pants, or chaps and is selected to protect against heat, cold, abrasion, and chemicals.

    b. Radiation protection is provided through the use of lead aprons and protective suits.

    c. Thermal garments include heat-resistant firefighter gear, flash-protection garments, proximity suits for radiant heat, cooling garments and vests using ice packs or circulating cold water, and other garments to protect against extremely hot or cold conditions.

    d. Blast and fragmentation suits are used for protection against small detonations; they do not provide hearing protection.

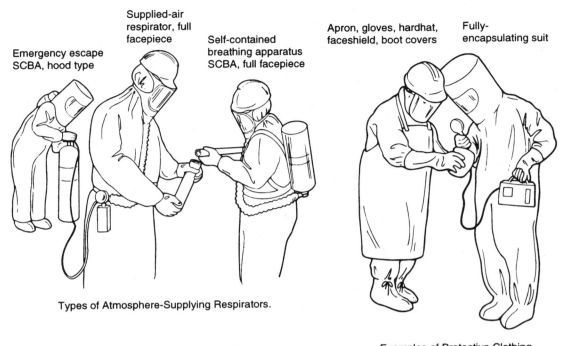

Emergency escape
SCBA, hood type

Supplied-air
respirator, full
facepiece

Self-contained
breathing apparatus
SCBA, full facepiece

Apron, gloves, hardhat,
faceshield, boot covers

Fully-
encapsulating suit

Types of Atmosphere-Supplying Respirators.

Examples of Protective Clothing.

Full-facepiece,
dual cartridge

Full-facepiece
chin-mounted canister

Full-facepiece
harness-mounted
canister

Powered air-purifying
respirator, half-mask

Half-mask,
facepiece-mounted
cartridge

Types of Air-Purifying Respirators.

FIGURE 9-8 *Examples of Respiratory Equipment*

Source: U.S. Department of Health and Human Services (1987).

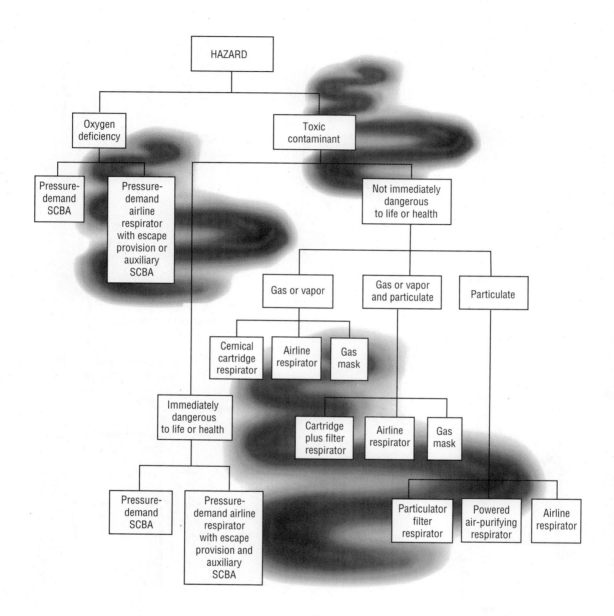

FIGURE 9-9   *Guidelines for the Selection of Respirators for Routine Use*

6. Head and neck protection under 29 CFR 1910.135 specifies head protection from impact and penetration from falling and flying objects and from limited electric shock and burn hazards.
   a. Hard hats are used in areas where falling and flying objects are a hazard.
   b. Heat-resistant and chemical-resistant hoods are also used.
7. Respiratory protection under 29 CFR 1910.134 is required when airborne contamination exceeds the TLV or PEL and cannot be engineered out.
   a. Requirements include a written comprehensive respirator program with annual fit testing and worker training.
   b. Respiratory protection is of two types: supplied air and air-purifying (NIOSH, 1987). (See Figure 9-8 for examples of respiratory equipment and Figure 9-9 for guidelines for selection of equipment.)
      • Supplied air respirators provide clean air from either a tank (a self-contained breathing apparatus or SCBA) or an air line connected to an air supply.
      • Air-purifying respirators use a filter or cannister to remove hazards from inhaled air; they may be full-mask or half-mask.
   c. Respirator face masks must form a tight seal against the face, requiring fit testing with isoamyl nitrate or irritant smoke as a fit check, prohibiting facial hair growth over 24 hours, and no eyeglass sidebars underneath the mask.
   d. Respirators must be tested for fit by the wearer before each use.
   e. After use, respirators must be properly stored, regularly inspected, and repaired as needed.
   f. A respirator wearer's health status must be reviewed periodically (usually annually) to assess physical and psychological fitness for using the respiratory protection equipment.
   g. "Criteria for respirator use are specific for each airborne hazard" (Weeks et al., 1991, p. 49). Respirator and cartridge selection is based on air sampling data performed in an exposure monitoring program.
   h. Only NIOSH approved respirators can be worn.
   j. Escape respirator devices allow a person working in a normally safe environment sufficient time to escape from suddenly occurring respiratory hazards. They should be used for escape purposes only.
   j. Because respirators are uncomfortable or unacceptable to some workers, they may not be worn properly and thus, not protect the worker from hazardous exposure.

BIBLIOGRAPHY

American Association of Occupational Health Nurses. (1995). Accident investigation. *AAOHN Advisory* Atlanta: AAOHN Publications.

American Association of Occupational Health Nurses. (1996). AAOHN position statement: occupational health surveillance. *AAOHN Journal, 44*(8), 407.

American Conference of Governmental Industrial Hygienists. (1994). *1994–1995 Threshold limit values for chemical substances and physical agents and biological exposure indices.* Cincinnati, OH: American Conference of Governmental Industrial Hygienists Technical Affairs Office.

Barnes, D. L. (1992). Analysis of group data helps identify subtle changes in health, hazard status. *Occupational Health and Safety, 69*(12), 30–34.

Breitenstein., B. D., Jr., & Spickard, J. H. (1995). Ionizing radiation. In P. H. Wald and G. M. Stave, (Eds.). *Physical and Biological Hazards of the Workplace.* New York: Van Nostrand Reinhold.

Burgess, W. A. (1995). *Recognition of health hazards in industry.* New York: John Wiley & Sons, Inc.

Burton, D. J. (1995). Indoor air quality cases require detective like analyses of facts. *Occupational Health and Safety 64*(3), 23.

Castillo, D. N., & Jenkins, E. L. (1994). Industries and occupations at high risk for work-related homicide. *Journal of Occupational Medicine. 36*(2), 125–132.

Clement-Stone, S., Eigsti, D. G., & McGuire, S. (1995). *Comprehensive family and community health nursing.* St. Louis, MO: C.V. Mosby Co.

Coffman, E. (1992). Sample integrity begins with knowledge of proper collection, storage methods. *Occupational Health and Safety.* Sept., 14, 29.

Cote, A., & Bugbee, P. (1995). *Principles of fire protection.* Quincy, MA: National Fire Protection Association.

Dessoff, A. L. (1995). Assess risks to control hazards. *Safety + Health, 152*(5), 62–65.

Dobie, R. A. (1995). Noise. In P. H. Wald & G. M. Stave (Eds.), *Physical and Biological Hazards of the Workplace.* New York: Van Nostrand Reinhold.

Eichenberger, J. (1995). How to achieve results through employee committees. *AAOHN Journal, 42*(7), 344–348.

Garg, A. (1995). Revised NIOSH equation for manual lifting: A method for job evaluation. *AAOHN Journal, 43*, 211–216.

Gates, D. M. (1995). Workplace violence. *AAOHN Journal, 43*(10), 536–543.

Gressel, M. G., & Gideon, J. A. (1991). An overview of process hazard evaluation techniques. *American Industrial Hygiene Association Journal, 52*(4), 158–163.

Group warned of increasing recognition of multiple chemical sensitivity as illness. (1995). *Occupational Safety & Health Reporter, 25*(24). Washington, DC: The Bureau of National Affairs, Inc.

Hales, T., Seligman, P., Newman, S., & Timbrook, C. (1988). Occupational injuries due to violence. *Journal of Occupational Medicine, 30*(6), 483–487.

Hall, S. L. (1992). Principles of risk management and loss control. *AAOHN Update Series, 4*(22). Skillman, NJ: Continuing Professional Education Center, Inc.

Hammer, W. (1989). *Occupational safety management and engineering* (4th Ed.). Englewood Cliffs, NJ: Prentice-Hall, Inc.

Hau, M. (1993). Prevention through sentinel health event recognition. *Preventing Occupational Injuries, Diseases and Disability: 1993 National Seminar.* Tampa, FL: Seak Legal and Medical Publishers, Inc.

Hayes, G., Goodwin, R., & Miars, B. (1990). After disaster. *American Journal of Nursing, 90*(2), 61–64.

Johnson, D. L., & Bell, M. L. (1991). Sources and control of error in industrial hygiene measurements. *AAOHN Journal, 39*(8), 362–368.

Kahn, Jeffrey. (1993). *Mental health in the workplace.* New York: Van Nostrand Reinhold.

Keyserling, W. M., Stetson, D. S., Silverstein, B. S., & Brouwer, M. L. A checklist for evaluating ergonomic risk factors associated with upper extremity cumulative trauma disorders. *Ergonomics, 36*(7), 807–831.

Kinney, J. (1993). Preventing workplace violence. Chicago, IL: National Safe Workplace Institute.

Kurtz, P.H., & Esser, T.E. (1989). A variant of mass (epidemic) psychogenic illness in the agricultural work setting. *Journal of Occupational Medicine, 31*(4), 331–334.

Levy, B. S., & Wegman, D. M. (1995). Occupational health: Recognizing and preventing work-related disease (3rd ed.) Boston: Little, Brown and Company.

Manuele, F. A. (1994). Learn to distinguish between hazards and risks. *Safety + Health. 150*(5), 70–74.

McNeely, Gail. (1991). Critical incident stress debriefing. *Texas EMS Messenger,* February/March, 6–9.

Minter, S. G. (1995). A safe approach to incentives. *Occupational Hazards, 57*(1), 171–172.

Mitchell, J., & Resnick, H. L. (1981). *Emergency response to crisis.* Bowie, MD: R. J. Brady Co.

Mullan, R. J., & Murthy, L. I. (1991). Occupational sentinel health events: An updated list for physician recognition and public health surveillance. *American Journal of Industrial Medicine,* (19), 775–799.

National Safety Council. (1992). *Accident Prevention manual for business & industry: Administration & programs* (10th Ed.), Itasca, IL: National Safety Council.

National Safety Council. (1995a). Principles of occupational safety & health for small business-es (POSH). *POSH for Small Business Course.* Itasca, IL: National Safety Council.

National Safety Council. (1995b). *Accident Prevention manual for business & industry: Engineering & technology* (10th Ed.), Itasca, IL: National Safety Council.

Ness, S. A. (1991). *Air monitoring for toxic exposures.* New York: Van Nostrand Reinhold.

Northwestern National Life. (1993). *Fear and violence in the workplace: A survey documenting the experience of American workers.* Minneapolis: Northwestern National Life.

Olson, N. (1994). Workplace violence, theories of causation and prevention strategies. *AAOHN Journal, 42,* 477–482.

Perkinson, L. (1995). JSA: A new look for an old friend. *Occupational Hazards, 57*(8), 63–66.

Plog, B. A., Benjamin, G. S., & Kerwin, M. A. (1996). *Fundamentals of industrial hygiene.* Itasca, IL: National Safety Council.

Recipe for an effective safety team. (1995). *Safety Management, 382,* 1–3.

Rempel, D. (1990). Medical surveillance in the workplace: Overview. *Occupational Medicine: State of the Art Reviews, 30,* 435–438. Philadelphia: Hanley & Belfus, Inc.

Robinson, S. (1990). Role of industrial hygiene in medical surveillance. In D. Rempel (Ed.), *Occupational Medicine: State of the Art Reviews—Medical Surveillance in the Workplace, 5*(3), pp. 470–471. Philadelphia: Hanley and Belfus, Inc.

Rogers, B. (1994). *Occupational health nursing concepts and practice.* Philadelphia: W.B. Saunders Co.

Rosenberg, J., & Rempel, D. (1990). Biological Monitoring. In D. Rempel (Ed.), *Occupational Medicine: State of the Art Reviews—Medical Surveillance in the Workplace, 5*(3), (July–September) (pp. 491–498). Philadelphia: Hanley & Belfus, Inc.

Roughton, J. E. (1995). Personal protective equipment: Complying with the standard. *Professional Safety, 40*(9), 27–30.

Rutstein, D. D., Mullan, R. J., Todd, M. F., Halperin, W. E., Melius, J. M., and Sestito, J. P. (1983). Sentinel health events (occupational): A basis for physician recognition and public health surveillance. *American Journal of Public Health, 73*(9), 1054–1062.

Saunders, G. T. (1993). *Laboratory fume hoods.* New York, N.Y.: John Wiley & Sons, Inc.

Senecal, P., & Burke, E. (1994). Root cause analysis: What took us so long? *Occupational Hazards, 556*(3), 63–65.

Siler, C. (1994). Chemical companies concoct formulas for safety. *Safety + Health, 150*(5), 50–53.

Smith, S. L. (1994). Near misses: Safety in the shadows. *Occupational Hazards, 56*(9), 33–36.

Sparks, P. J., Daniell, W., Black, D. W., Kipen, H. M., Altman, L. C., Simon, G. E., & Terr, A. I. (1994). Multiple chemical sensitivity syndrome: A clinical perspective. I. Case definition, theories of pathogenesis, and research needs. *Journal of Occupational Medicine, 36*(7), 718–730.

Stanevich, R. S., & Stanevich, R. L. (1989). Guidelines for an occupational safety and health program. *AAOHN Journal, 37*(6), 205–214.

Terpin, D. (1992). Taking the risk out of response—confined space entry and rescue. *Industrial Fire World, 7*(1), 16–18, 24.

Travers, P. H., & McDougall, C. (1995). *Guidelines for an occupational health & safety service.* Atlanta, GA: AAOHN Publications.

U.S. Department of Health and Human Services. (1987). *NIOSH Respirator Decision Logic.* Cincinnati, OH: DHHS (NIOSH) Number 87-108.

U.S. Department of Health and Human Services. (1994). *Workplace use of back belts—Review and recommendations.* Cincinnati, OH: DHHS (NIOSH) Number 94-122.

U.S. Department of Labor. (1985). OSHA 3071. *Job hazard analysis.*

U.S. Department of Labor. (1993). OSHA 3132. *Process Safety Management.*

Voelker, R. (1994). Does multiple chemical sensitivity exist? *Safety and Health, 150*(3), 54–58.

Vogel, C. (1991). Cut your losses with JSAs. *Safety & Health, 148*(10), 38.

Wachs, J. E. (1991). Levels of prevention: A framework for cost-effective occupational health programs. *AAOHN Update Series 4*(7), Skillman, NJ: Continuing Professional Education Center, Inc.

Waters, T. R., Putz-Anderson, V., & Garg, A. (1994). *Applications manual for the revised NIOSH lifting equation.* Cincinnati, OH: U.S. Department of Health and Human Services, National Institute for Occupational Safety and Health, Division of Biomedical and Behavioral Science.

Warren, S. B., & Amundson, R. M. (1995). Comprehensive baseline hazard assessments—a team approach. *Professional Safety, 40*(7), 26–29.

Weeks, J. L., Levy, B. S., & Wagner, G. R. (Eds.). (1991). *Preventing occupational disease and injury.* Washington, DC: American Public Health Association.

Weinstock, M. P. (1993). Chasing the missing link, *Occupational Hazards, 55*(9), 116–120.

Willen, J. (1995). How to produce an effective safety newsletter. *Safety and Health, 151*(1), 46–49.

CHAPTER

10

Direct Care in the Occupational Setting

MAJOR TOPICS
- *Primary care*
- *Health assessment*
- *Health history*
- *Physical examinations*
- *Management of injury and illness*

The previous chapter focused primarily on worker populations. This chapter discusses strategies for providing direct services to individual workers. These services include the important steps involved in conducting an exposure history and a physical examination. The last section presents an overview of approaches to consider for the management of occupational injuries and illnesses.

Overview of Primary Care

$\overline{\text{I}}$

Position Statements

A number of organizations have published position statements related to primary care and primary health care.

A. Agency for Health Care Policy and Research: *Primary care* is an array of integrated and coordinated health services with the following characteristics:
1. Services are accessible and acceptable to the client.
2. First-contact, or front-line, services, are comprehensive in scope.
3. Services are coordinated and continuous over time.
4. Service providers are accountable for the quality and potential effects of the services.
5. Primary care services are person-centered and holistic, which means they involve all levels of prevention; that is, services are not limited to a single organ or system or to a specific disease process (Nutting, 1991).

B. World Health Organization (WHO) Alma-Ata Declaration of 1978: Primary health care by the year 2000 will have the following characteristics (Krebs, 1983; Barnes, Eribes, Juarbe, et al., 1995):
1. Primary health care will consist of essential health care, which is universally accessible to individuals and families in the community.
2. Primary health care will be acceptable to the community with their full participation, and at a cost that the community and country can afford.

TABLE 10-1

Objectives of Clinical Preventive Services

---

1. Increase years of healthy life to at least 65 years.

2. Increase to at least 50 percent the proportion of people who have received, as a minimum within the appropriate interval, all of the screening and immunization services and at least one of the counseling services appropriate for their age and gender as recommended by the U.S. Preventive Services Task Force.

3. Increase to at least 95 percent the proportion of people who have a specific source of ongoing primary care for coordination of their preventive and episodic health care.

4. Improve financing and delivery of clinical preventive services so that virtually no American has a financial barrier to receiving at a minimum, the screening, counseling, and immunization services recommended by the U.S. Preventive Services Task Force.

5. Assure that at least 90 percent of people for whom primary care services are provided directly by publicly funded programs are offered, at a minimum, the screening, counseling, and immunization services recommended by the U.S. Preventive Services Task Force.

6. Increase to at least 50 percent the proportion of primary care providers who provide their patients with the screening, counseling, and immunizations recommended by the U.S. Preventive Services Task Force.

7. Increase to at least 90 percent the proportion of people who are served by a local health department that assesses and assures access to essential clinical preventive services.

8. Increase the proportion of all degrees in the health professions and allied and associated health profession fields awarded to members of under-represented racial and ethnic minority groups.

Source: USDHHS (1991). *Healthy People 2000: National Health Promotion and Disease Prevention Objectives,* Chapter 21.

---

    3. Primary health care will serve as the nucleus of the country's health care system, and of the overall social and economic development of the community.

C. The Institute of Medicine: Primary care is the provision of integrated, accessible health care services by clinicians who are accountable for addressing a large majority of personal health care needs, developing a sustained partnership with clients, and practicing in the context of family and community (Donaldson, Yordy, & Vanselow, 1994, pg. 15).

D. Healthy People 2000 Review: 1995–1996 (United States Department of Health and Human Services [USDHHS], 1996) outlined the following:
    1. Three broad goals for the country are to:
        a. Increase the span of healthy life for Americans
        b. Reduce health disparities among Americans
        c. Achieve access to preventive services for all Americans
    2. Chapter 21 of *Healthy People 2000,* Clinical Preventive Services (USDHHS,1991; 1994a), includes eight objectives relevant to primary care delivery (see Table 10-1), in addition, preventive services for specific diseases and health-related behaviors are addressed in other chapters of *Healthy People 2000.*
    3. "Put Prevention into Practice" is a program of the Office of Disease Prevention and Health Promotion; it includes health education materials, *The Clinician's Handbook of Preventive Services,* and other resources (USDHHS, 1994).
    4. *The Guide to Clinical Preventive Services* (2nd ed.) provides research-based screening recommendations for the clinician (U.S. Prevention Services Task Force, 1996).

E. The American Association of Occupational Health Nurses and the American Nurses' Association, in support of Nursing's Agenda for Health Care Reform, published *Innovation at the Worksite: Delivery of Nurse-Managed Primary Health Care Services,* noting the added value of providing primary care at a convenient worksite location for both employees and their dependents (Burgel, 1993).

II

Primary Care: Prevention-based Services

A. Health promotion
   1. Begins with people who are basically healthy
   2. Uses strategies related to personal lifestyle—those personal choices made in a social context—that can have a powerful influence over one's health status (USDHHS, 1991; 1996)
   3. Includes the promotion of physical exercise and the reduction of the use of alcohol and tobacco

B. Health protection strategies
   1. Are related to environmental or regulatory measures that confer protection on large population groups
   2. Include food and drug safety and environmental health initiatives (USDHHS, 1991; 1996).

C. Primary prevention refers to those health promotion and health protection measures that prevent the occurrence of disease and injury.

D. Secondary prevention is the early detection and treatment of disease and injury so that progression is slowed or complications are limited.
   1. Screening is a secondary prevention measure to detect asymptomatic disease early in the disease progression; for example, mammography is a screening method that can detect breast cancer before a woman has symptoms of this disease.
   2. Screening is used as a prevention strategy when there is evidence that the morbidity or mortality of a condition will be decreased as a result of early detection and treatment.

E. Tertiary prevention is the prevention of disability through rehabilitative efforts.

III

Primary Care Skills

The provision of primary care services requires the following special skills and knowledge:

A. Expertise in physical assessment and history-taking techniques

B. Expertise in clinical decision making and the diagnosis and treatment of injury and illness

C. An ability to communicate effectively about strategies for self-care and the ability to negotiate lifestyle modification plans

D. Comfort in a role as a generalist, managing multiple health problems

E. Awareness of the connection between the physical and psychosocial aspects of illness

F. Knowing when to refer

G. Recognition of the linkage between worksite exposure and adverse health effects; and the linkage of worker health status and a safe work environment

$\overline{IV}$

Primary Care Delivery at the Worksite

A. Advantages of Primary Care Delivery at the Worksite
1. It provides for convenience for employees and dependents, with less down-time for visits to off-site health care providers.
2. It presents a greater opportunity to manage quality, outcomes, and cost of care.
3. It allows a more immediate determination of work-related etiology or aggravation of the symptom and/or disease.
4. Accommodations are made in a more expeditious manner, with greater control of compliance with the Americans with Disabilities Act (see Chapter 4).
5. Cost savings are realized by controlling duplicate administrative costs.
6. It reinforces a self-care approach to health.

B. Arrangements for Primary Care Delivery at the Worksite
1. The scope of services delivered at the worksite varies among employers, as follows:
   a. On-site services depend on the size of the workforce, the hazard profile of the company, the health benefit coverage status of the workforce, the resources of the company, and the proximity of community health services.
   b. Primary care services may extend to all employees, insured employees, dependents, and/or retirees.
   c. Personnel arrangements may include health care providers either as employees of the company or as independent contractors; contractual arrangements with a health maintenance organization for on-site providers may also be developed.
   d. Services may range from full-service, on-site with 24-hour call to triage and referral.
   e. Services may focus on either occupational or nonoccupational conditions, or both.
2. Components of primary care services include:
   a. Diagnosis and treatment of health conditions, including emergency care, minor acute care, chronic illness management, and 24-hour call
   b. Prevention-based services, including health-promotion programs and screening programs such as health surveillance
   c. Case management of occupational and nonoccupational health problems

C. Ethical and Legal Issues in Primary Care
1. Ethical principles: autonomy, non-maleficence, beneficence, distributive justice (see Chapter 4)
   a. Confidentiality of personal health information of workers and their dependents must be maintained.
   b. The primary care provider must balance the "duty to warn" against the right to privacy of the employee or dependent.
   c. Limited resources are already dedicated to occupational health and safety; if primary care is provided at the worksite, will occupational health and safety have a lower priority?

       d. Workers have a right to know about the hazards in their work settings as well as a right to be notified of an exposure or abnormal physical finding

  2. Legal issues

      a. Potential liability issues arising from primary care services provided at the worksite:

         1) Is there an employee-employer relationship between workers and on-site, employer-paid health personnel? If yes, then workers' compensation would be the only recourse for any injury that resulted from provider negligence.

         2) Is there a client-provider relationship, with the employer-paid health personnel considered an independent contractor? If yes, then a negligent provider could be sued for medical malpractice.

         3) Does the employer-paid health personnel hold dual capacity? Dual capacity recognizes the co-employee role and exercises independent judgment in the client-provider relationship.

      b. The legal use and protection of personal health information requires a review of the confidentiality of health information statutes, which vary from state to state.

      c. Legal statutes regarding the scope of practice of a registered nurse, a nurse practitioner, or a medical doctor need to be reviewed prior to developing a primary care service at a worksite.

Health Assessment of the Worker
$\overline{\text{V}}$

Health History

    A health history provides a database of both subjective and objective data that encompasses all aspects of the worker's health, including occupational experiences and work exposures.

A. Benefits of a health history

  1. Identification of problems and immediate concerns may be revealed

  2. Provides a method to explore the possible causes of a problem; prevents an assumption that a problem is related to a disease process rather than exposure (Rosenstock & Cullen, 1994)

  3. Provides update on past health concerns

B. Components of a health history (Bates, 1995; Bowers & Thompson, 1992; Rogers, 1994)

  1. Client profile: identifies demographic data, age, sex, and nationality

  2. Major concerns; chief complaint; reason for visit—illness, injury, or routine check-up

  3. Current health status and history of prior illnesses/injuries and hospitalizations

  4. Lifestyle activities and risk factors such as tobacco and alcohol use, nutritional factors, and personal safety issues (such as seat belt use)

  5. Current medications: should include both prescribed and over-the-counter (OTC) medications

  6. Allergies: food, respiratory, seasonal, or dermatitis

  7. Current status of immunizations, including those for foreign travel, if necessary

8. Family history: provides information on genetic/hereditary risk factors, chronic disease in family, and any significant family problems
9. Psychosocial history: coping mechanism, history of any problems; assesses mental capacity and ability to function
10. Socioeconomic history: income status, home, living conditions
11. Information on family, support systems, and marital status
12. History of exposures including those in workplace, in hobbies, at home, and in the community.
13. Review of systems: collects data on the process of a disease related to any of the body systems
14. Information regarding ability to perform the activities of daily living

C. Generic health history
1. Used for routine physical examinations or episodic visits
2. Provides generalized health data
3. Progressive from birth to present
4. Encompasses all aspects of worker health, occupational exposures, and lifestyle
5. Updates on each visit to health care provider

D. Occupational/environmental exposure and history (see Table 10-2)
1. Purposes:
   a. Supplements routine history relating to personal health
   b. Provides epidemiological correlation between symptoms and activities or exposures
   c. Helps to prevent misdiagnosis of occupational or environmental health problems
   d. Used for prevention of aggravation of existing injury/illness
   e. Used for teaching and counseling worker on self-care
2. Defining characteristics include:
   a. Systematic, thorough description of worker's current and prior work history and exposures
   b. Incorporates both work- and non-work-related activities
   c. Updates on periodic basis so that changes can be noted
3. Employment history consists of (Agency for Toxic Substances and Disease Registry, 1992; Burgel, 1991; Wegman, Levy, & Halperen, 1995):
   a. Demographic and biographical data
   b. Date of history
   c. Type and length of different jobs
   d. Activities leading to exposures
   e. Occurrence of illness/injury and time of development
   f. Use of personal protective equipment and type

E. Limitations of the health history
1. Reliability of source of information
2. Unknown factors relating to health, such as family history
3. Worker's knowledge or lack of knowledge about exposures
4. Worker's understanding of the health implications of certain activities
5. Incomplete information—important data not obtained
6. Too much information; hard to interpret

TABLE 10-2

Work and Exposure History

Date: _____

Name: _____   SS#

_____

Male _____ Female _____   Birth date

_____

Describe your current job._____

What is your job title?_____

Are you exposed to any of the following health hazards?

　　Dust _____　Fumes _____　Solvents _____

　　Chemicals _____　name(s)

　　Noise _____　Vibrations _____　Heat _____　Cold _____

　　Repetitive motion _____　(if yes, specify type 　　　)

　　Other types of exposures or concerns

How long in current job?_____

Describe a typical work day. _____

Is protective equipment required in your job?　Yes _____ No _____

　　(If yes, specify type)

　　Gloves _____　Goggles/Face shield _____　Hearing protection _____

　　Safety glasses _____　Mask respirator _____　Air-supplied respirator _____

　　Coveralls/apron _____　Other types (list)

Past Employment History

Job	No. of Years	Job Title	Exposures	Protective Equip. (yes/no; type)

Additional Activities/Exposures

What hobbies are you involved with? (list)_____

　　Are chemicals, metals, or other substances involved? (list)_____

　　Does anyone in your family work in a job that involves exposure? (e.g., lead or asbestos)

　　Please explain. _____

Where do you live?_____

　　Are there any factories or public dumps near your home?

　　Yes _____　No _____　Explain_____

Smoking History: Do you smoke?　Yes _____　How long? _____　No _____

　　Does anyone else in your household smoke?　Yes _____　No _____

At home, do you work with:

　　Household cleaners?　Yes _____　No _____　(type)

　　Pesticides?　Yes _____　No _____　(type)

　　Herbicides　Yes _____　No _____　(type)

Are you involved in farming activities?　Yes _____　No _____

Current Health Status

Do you consider yourself to be in good health?　Yes _____　No _____

　　If no, do you consider your health problems to be related to your work? Please explain.

　　Does anyone else in your work area have conditions similar to yours?　Yes _____　No _____

　　If yes, please explain._____

Sources: Burgel, 1991; Agency for Toxic Substances and Disease Registry, 1995; Wegman, Levy, & Halpern, 1995.

VI

The Interview

Obtaining a useful and accurate health history depends upon the skill of the interviewer to elicit the needed information from the worker.

A. The interview is a face-to-face or telephone interaction with the worker for the purpose of obtaining necessary health information.

B. Key elements for a successful interview are as follows:
1. The setting should be private, comfortable, and nonthreatening.
2. Lead into the interview process gradually; establish rapport and trust.
3. Begin with present—keep in mind the reason for the specific visit.
4. Listen to the worker; do not supply answers.
5. Clarify points of information.

C. The objectives of the health history are to:
1. Obtain accurate information about worker's health and emotional status and to gather data to assist in diagnosis.
2. Provide worker with understanding of illness.
3. Assure worker of support during course of treatment and follow-up.

D. The advantages of interview
1. Interviews can clarify ambiguous information obtained from the health history and can provide additional information to assist in problem solving and understanding of situation.
2. General, nondirective questions establish trust and help identify specific problems.
3. The interview process provides an opportunity to counsel the worker on health maintenance and preventive activities.

E. Guiding the worker through the process:
1. Consider the type of interview—voluntary or involuntary?
2. Can the worker speak freely?
3. Availability of time for the interview; is it scheduled or unscheduled?
4. Plan in advance when possible to allow both the health care provider and the worker time to prepare for the interview.
5. Accept the problem as stated, but look for underlying problems when necessary.
6. Accept the values of the worker and do not allow personal bias to influence behaviors.

F. Technique for interviewing (Bates, 1995; Bowers & Thompson, 1992; Cassidy, 1993)
1. Nondirective questions encourage the worker to talk.
2. Direct, probing questions elicit more detailed information.
3. Understanding and accepting can convey empathy.
4. Reassurance helps to relax the worker and encourage trust.
5. The interviewer should word questions to obtain as much or as little information as needed.
6. The interviewer should use words and statements that the worker can understand.
7. Be sensitive to nonverbal clues, such as body movements, eye contact, or silence.

8. Be considerate of cultural differences.
9. Be as direct as necessary to gain information.
10. End the interview when the needed information is obtained or at the end of the scheduled time.
11. Always offer to be available at a later date.

Physical Examinations of the Worker
VII

The Physical Examination

A. The purposes of the physical examination in the occupational setting
1. To identify health problems, detect disease process in presymptomatic stage, evaluate lifestyle, job requirements, and workplace exposures that may result in adverse health outcome
2. To obtain information that may be used as a foundation for direct care for the worker

B. Characteristics of the physical examination
1. Every physical examination should be accompanied by a health history.
2. Nursing assessment should be objective and nonjudgmental.
3. Ethical concerns should be considered; confidentiality should be maintained.
4. Findings should be summarized and recorded.
5. The worker should be notified regarding results.
6. Counseling and plans for follow-up should be based on findings.

C. Techniques for physical examination (Kozier, Erb, Blas, & Wilkinson, 1995):
1. *Inspection* uses the sense of sight to look at the individual and to observe for variations from the norm or from previously observed state.
2. *Palpation* uses the sense of touch to feel with hands and fingers to check temperature, moisture, texture, size, pulsation, vibrations, presence of joint swelling, nodules, masses, joint mobility, organ size and location.
3. *Percussion* may be the direct striking of a finger against skin or the indirect striking of a finger against a finger lying against an individual's skin—a technique used to determine the density, size, and location of underlying organs; sounds range from tympanic to resonant, hyperresonant, dull, or flat.
4. *Auscultation* is the process of listening directly with the ear or with a stethoscope to assess sounds produced by the various organs and tissues.

D. Equipment
The following equipment may be needed in order to conduct a physical examination: stethoscope with bell and diaphragm, balance-beam scale, oto/ophthalmoscope, sphygmomanometer, thermometer, tape measure, percussion hammer, tongue blades, glove, penlight, tuning fork, guaiac test, lubricating jelly, vaginal speculum, gown, and drape. (This list is not exhaustive; in some instances, other equipment may be needed, depending on the nature of the examination.)

E. Sequence of examination
1. The examination should be performed in a systematic manner.
   * Skin and appendages (the hands are a good place to start; their examination provides important information and helps the individual to relax)
   * Reflexes—a nonthreatening procedure
   * Head, eyes, ears, nose, mouth, and pharynx
   * Neck—thyroid and nodes

- Thorax and posterior chest
- Anterior chest—heart, lungs, carotid and aortic arteries, breasts
- Abdomen—renal and femoral arteries, liver, intestines, stomach
- Musculoskeletal—continuous throughout examination
- Neurological—continuous throughout examination
- Mental status—continuous throughout examination
- Genitalia and pap (if indicated)
- Lower extremities—peripheral vascular system of legs

2. Abnormal findings should be managed by the occupational health nurse or referred to the appropriate health care provider.

VIII

Types of Examinations

A. Baseline health examination
1. Baseline examination may be performed as part of a preplacement examination or upon the implementation of a health monitoring/surveillance program.
2. Appropriate screenings are included: for example, vital signs, height, weight, spirometry, vision, audiometry, urinalysis, and blood chemistry with complete blood count.
3. Advantages of baseline information include:
   a. Findings are used to aid the worker in seeking care or maintaining functional health status.
   b. Findings provide documentation of a current illness or injury.
   c. Information can be used for health and self-care instruction.
   d. Findings provide baseline data for future comparisons.
      - Normal changes occur in all systems throughout a lifespan
      - Changes may be associated with lifestyle, home, or workplace exposures. (See Table 10-3.)

B. Preplacement physical examination
1. Purposes of the preplacement physical following a job offer:
   a. May serve as the baseline examination
   b. Focuses on ability to perform the essential functions of the job
   c. Assures protection of the worker from known risk factors
   d. Provides information so that the worker can be placed in a job that does not compromise the worker's current health status
   e. Assesses the worker's need for accommodation
   f. Identifies any previously undiagnosed health problems
   g. Assures compliance with local, state, or other mandated programs
   h. Introduces the worker to a health care system that is focused on prevention and early detection of disease
2. Components of the preplacement examination include:
   a. Appropriate screenings, as discussed in baseline physicals
   b. The focus on systems that may be affected by job performance
   c. Complete health history
3. Preplacement examination considerations are (Bunkeen & Cooper, 1985; Kemerer & Runiere, 1990; Rogers, 1994):
   a. The examiner should have the necessary skills to perform the examination as well as the knowledge of the job requirements.

TABLE 10-3

Normal Changes of Aging

System	Changes
Integumentary	**Skin:** Decrease of the following: subcutaneous fat, sweat glands, extra-cellular water, melanin, and circulation to extremities **Hair:** thinning/loss, decreased pigment and oil **Nails:** decreased peripheral blood supply, increased keratin
Respiratory	**Decreased:** recoil—alveolar walls thicken; vital capacity and tidal volume; ciliary movement; strength of expiratory muscles; number of alveoli/larger size **Increased:** septi loss; residual air and dead space; thoracic wall rigidity
Cardiovascular	**Cardiac Function: Decreased:** force of contraction, stroke volume, cardiac volume **Cardiac Rate:** resting rate unchanged with age; exercise increases output, but to a reduced maximal rate; slowed response to stress with only slightly increased rate **Blood Vessels:** elastic fibers straighten, fragments; accumulation of collagen and calcium
Gastrointestinal	**Loss of Teeth/Dentures**—can affect nutrition **Decrease of the following:** taste buds, saliva volume and salivary amylase, tone and motility of esophagus, stomach, and intestines, gastric acid production, external intestinal sphincter reflex **Increased:** biliary stones
Genitourinary	**Renal:** polyuria—atrophy of collecting tubules **Decrease of the following**: nephrons, 40% fewer by age 85; renal plasma flow; glomerular rate; renal artery flow—by 50%
Bladder	**Decrease of the following:** muscle tone, sphincter control, capacity
Gonads	**Male**—Decreased testosterone **Female**—Decreased estrogen/progesterone
Musculoskeletal	**Muscles:** decreased mass; adipose replaces muscle cells; collagen fibers become more rigid **Bones:** decreased mass; demineralization, and protein matrix loss (greatest in post-menopausal women) **Joints:** cartilage erosion; increased calcium deposits; decreased water in cartilage

Neurologic	**Brain**
	    Decreased: number of cells, pyramidal tract functions, and blood flow and oxygen utilization
	    Increased: plaque/pigment accumulation
	Nerves: Decreased conduction velocity
	Receptors: Decreased number/function
	Cognitive: no decrease in I.Q, learning and problem solving remain

Sensory	**Taste:** Decreased number/function of taste buds **Smell:** fiber loss in olfactory bulb; cellular degeneration in parietal lobe **Touch:** Decreased receptors/less sensitive to tactile environment **Vision:** Decreased: acuity, accommodation, dark adaptation, lens clarity, and tear production **Hearing:** Decreased: acuity, pitch discrimination, and sensitivity to higher frequency **Increased:** vertigo, cerumen, and tinnitus

Sources: Kozier et al. (1995), Lewis & Collier (1987).

    b. The examiner must be provided a copy of the job analysis that specifies specific requirements, such as climbing ladders, lifting 30 pounds on continuous basis, reaching 70 inches to push button to start a machine.
    c. The physical examination should focus on the requirements/physical demands of a particular job.
    d. The physical examination is performed to match the worker to the job; for the purpose of employment, the examination is restricted to a worker's fitness for a job-related task.

C. Americans with Disabilities Act (ADA) examination:
  1. Purposes of ADA examination
    a. To remove barriers against potential workers with known disabilities (Pruitt, 1995)
    b. To assess the need for reasonable accommodation for the worker with disability
    c. To assess the condition of the worker at the time of the examination without considering the possibility that a disability could develop in the future
  2. Considerations related to ADA examination
    a. Restrictions to prevent employment must be specific to the job.
    b. The disabled worker must be able to perform the essential functions of the job.
    c. All applicants for the same job must have the same evaluation.
    d. It is the responsibility of the individual worker to notify the employer of any needed accommodation.
  3. Considerations in the placement of a worker
    • A hearing-impaired person should not be placed in a job that requires unimpaired hearing.
    • A worker should have sufficient physical stamina and strength for a job that requires continuous manual labor.
    • If a worker has an impaired sense of smell, he/she should not work in an area where normal sense of smell is needed, such as in an area where there is risk of chemical exposure.
    • A worker should have no impairment of respiratory and cardiovascular function for a job the requires wearing a respirator.
    • Jobs requiring rotating shifts should be avoided if a worker needs set hours of work (for example, a diabetic who is insulin dependent and has difficulty controlling blood glucose).

D. An interval, or periodic, examination
  1. Supplements and adds to the baseline physical
  2. Provides ongoing health status information
  3. Screening and interval examinations should have a selective approach
    a. Based on age and sex
    b. Geared toward health status and/or risk factors (American College of Physicians, 1981; Breslow & Somers, 1977; Obler & LaForce, 1989).
  4. Provides for continued assurance of compatibility with a job
  5. May result in detection and diagnosis of previously undiagnosed problems

E. A preretirement, or exit, physical
  1. Provided upon retirement or termination
  2. Extent of examination dependent on date of last physical and age of worker
  3. Based on exposure history (i.e., to noise or asbestos) or based on other mandated programs by company policy or governmental regulations

IX

Specialty Examinations

A. Fitness-for-duty evaluation
   1. Purpose: to assure that the worker is physically and mentally capable of performing job functions and to assure safety of the worker and the public (Pransky, Frumkin, & Himmelstein, 1988).
   2. Considerations in determining the worker's capacity to work
      a. Frequency and duration of continuous activity; environmental or mental stressors of job
      b. The worker's characteristics—age, fitness, skill level
      c. Ability of the worker to perform the job without risk of injury or illness to self and/or co-workers
   3. Factors that may interfere with the worker's ability
      a. Health history—presence of illness/injury or history of disabling condition, risk factors (hypertension, obesity, and so forth)
      b. Genetic makeup—strength, height, weight
      c. Behavioral patterns (e.g., a smoking habit, lack of exercise, poor nutrition)
      d. Emotional or psychological problems, such as phobias
   4. Can job be modified to facilitate the worker's successful performance of job?

B. Internal job-transfer evaluation
   1. Some considerations are similar to preplacement, such as the ability to perform the job or the need for workplace modifications.
   2. Will the transfer to a new job place the worker at increased risk for injury or aggravation of an existing problem?
   3. Does a change in the health status of the worker require transfer to a new job?
   4. Can the worker safely perform the essential tasks of the new job?

C. Return-to-work evaluation
   1. Purpose: to assess the worker's ability to resume work after time away from work; the goal is to return the worker to productive employment.
   2. The evaluation should document the worker's fitness or the need for modification in the job task or hours of work.
   3. Placement on return to work should ensure that there will be no aggravation of preexisting injury or illness.
   4. Considerations:
      • If the worker can return to the same job with no restrictions, then no further action is required.
      • If modifications are needed, what type? (reasonable accommodation? work available?)
      • Do any new requirements fit within the framework of company policies?
   5. Tools for assessment
      • Job analysis
      • Ergonomic analysis
      • Functional capacity of worker
   6. Managing the worker's return to work
      • Modified work: could include reducing the number of hours of work and changing the type of task to be performed
      • Work conditioning: occurs on the job and refers to a gradual working back into the regular job
      • Work hardening: may be job simulation, external to the workplace

TABLE 10-4

Request for Medical Evaluation

I. Supervisor's reason for bringing worker to medical attention (using the supervisor's own words):

_____

Time of arrival in Occupational Health Service—_____:_____ AM/PM

II. Objective observations by the health professional (check all that apply):

_____ Cooperative _____ Oriented to time, place, person
_____ Confused _____ Agitated _____ Inappropriate euphoria
_____ Drowsy _____ Seems unable to respond rationally to simple questions
Other: _____

Speech Pattern:
_____ Slurring _____ Inability to form words _____ Coherent speech
Other: _____

Breath:
_____ Garlicky _____ Sweet _____ Alcohol-like _____ within normal limits
Other: _____

Eyes:
_____ "Bloodshot" _____ Glassy-eyed _____ Pin-point pupils
_____ Unequal pupil size _____ PERL _____ Nystagmus
Other: _____

Finger-to-nose—Can touch nose with fingertips from outstretched position:
_____ Yes _____ No

Tandem Gait—Can walk heel to toe without stumbling or hesitating
With eyes open: _____ Yes _____ No
With eyes closed: _____ Yes _____ No

Blood Pressure: _____
Pulse: _____
Oral Temperature: _____ F

III. Working assessment as to status and casual factors (check all that apply):

_____ Deemed fit for duty
_____ Deemed medically unfit for duty, possibly due to:
_____ Opiates
_____ Alcohol
_____ Other drugs
_____ Workplace toxin
_____ Diabetic symptoms
_____ Infectious causes
_____ Cerebrovascular incident
_____ Other

IV. Recommended actions at this time (check all that apply):

_____ Worker not to be returned to duty
_____ Worker advised to seek medical care
_____ Worker not to drive (Transportation to be arranged. If worker insists on driving and you believe him/her impaired, explain that you must notify police.)
_____ A relative has been informed of the situation (no diagnosis to be stated or implied).
_____ Screening tests offered to rule out specific toxin where appropriate test is available.
_____ Alcohol (breath or blood)
_____ Other drugs (urine)
_____ Blood sugar elevation
_____ Investigation of possible work related toxic exposure to be initiated.

V. Further comments:

Health Care Provider _____ RN/MD Date _____

Employee _____ Date _____

SSN _____

Source: Pederson, M. T., Muldoon, S., & Curtis, E. C. (1993). (Used with permission.)

- Counseling: teaching preventive measures, such as proper lifting or performing stressful job requirements
- Pain management: use of effective measures such as stress management or proper use of medications while on the job
- Transfer to job with less strenuous physical demands, if available, or retrain (Pranksy, Frumkin, & Himmelstein, 1988)

D. Requested evaluations may be performed under the following circumstances (Penderson, Muldoon, & Curtes, 1993):
  1. If management is concerned about the worker's physical ability to perform the job
  2. As a result of the worker's erratic job performance
  3. If management is concerned regarding the worker's mental ability to perform the job
  4. When there are indications or suspicions of substance abuse
  5. For post-accident testing, per company policy
  6. In case of the worker's altered work behaviors

E. Nursing assessment should be objective, nonjudgmental, and based on data.

F. Ethical concerns and confidentiality should be maintained for nonrelated findings.

G. A thorough interview should be included in the evaluation (see Table 10-4).

Screening in the Occupational Setting

Health Screening

A. *Screening* is defined as "the identification of an unrecognized disease or defect by applying tests, examinations, or procedures" (Cahall & Vester, 1985).

B. Purpose and characteristics:
  1. Screenings provide a means to collect general health data to determine the general health status of the worker.
  2. Screenings are prevention oriented.
  3. Screenings are used to discriminate persons who have a disease from a population of those who do not.
  4. Screenings may be a one-time activity or may be repeated at regular intervals.

C. Criteria for health screening
  1. The disease must be one where early diagnosis and intervention has a positive affect on morbidity and mortality (for example, a sigmoidoscopy screening to detect colorectal cancer)
  2. The method of administering the test must be acceptable to both the person administering the test as well as the worker receiving the test.
  3. Efficacy: the test must be able to detect the target condition earlier than it could be detected without screening and with sufficient accuracy to avoid large number of false negative results (sensitivity) and false positive results (specificity). (See Chapter 7 for an explanation of sensitivity and specificity.)
  4. The occupational health nurse should be properly educated to perform the test, recognize abnormals, counsel, refer, and provide care for the worker.

D. Mandatory surveillance examinations

1. The term "medical surveillance" is used by the Occupational Safety and Health Administration (OSHA) in describing protocol for monitoring specific exposures; however, the processes and personnel involved in this monitoring extend beyond medicine; hence it is actually a type of "health surveillance."

2. The purpose of a surveillance examination is to:
   a. Protect the worker from exposures that may cause adverse health effects
   b. Assure the worker's ability to perform the job activity
   c. Fulfill governmental surveillance requirements, such as those outlined in the standards for asbestos and lead exposure

---

TABLE 10-5

Examples of OSHA Standards Requiring Medical Surveillance

Standard #	Substance
29 CFR 1910.1000	hazardous materials (hazmat)
29 CFR 1910.1001	asbestos
29 CFR 1910.1002	coal tar pitch volatiles
29 CFR 1910.1003	4-nitrobiphenyl
29 CFR 1910.1004	alpha naphthylamine
29 CFR 1910.1006	methyl chloromethyl ether
29 CFR 1910.1007	3,3'-dichlorobenzidine and its salts
29 CFR 1910.1008	bis-chloromethyl ether
29 CFR 1910.1009	beta-naphthylamine
29 CFR 1910.1010	benzidine
29 CFR 1910.1011	4-aminodiphenyl
29 CFR 1910.1012	ethyleneimine
29 CFR 1910.1013	beta-propiolactone
29 CFR 1910.1014	2-acetylaminofluorene
29 CFR 1910.1015	4-dimethylaminoazobenzene
29 CFR 1910.1016	n-nitrosodimethylamine
29 CFR 1910.1017	vinyl chloride
29 CFR 1910.1018	inorganic arsenic
29 CFR 1910.1025	lead
29 CFR 1910.1027	cadmium
29 CFR 1910.1028	benzene
29 CFR 1910.1029	coke oven emissions
29 CFR 1910.1043	cotton dust
29 CFR 1910.1044	1,2-dibromo-3-chloropropane
29 CFR 1910.1045	acrylonitrile
29 CFR 1910.1047	ethylene oxide
29 CFR 1910.1048	formaldehyde
29 CFR 1910.1050	4,4'-methylenedianiline

Examples of OSHA Standards That Require Medical Clearance

Standard #	Specific Activity
29 CFR 1910.134	respiratory protection
29 CFR 1910.156	fire fighters

Post Exposure Surveillance

29 CFR 1910.1030	blood borne pathogens
29 CFR 1910.95	noise exposure

Source: Occupational Safety and Health Standards for General Industry (1994).

   3. The scope of health surveillance includes:
      a. Training for both professionals and workers
      b. Interpretation of test results
      c. Quality-control actions and assurance
      d. Confidentiality of the worker's test result, to be released only on a "need to know" basis
      e. Recordkeeping and trend analysis
   4. Health surveillance is geared toward and related to a specific exposure (e.g., lead or asbestos) or an activity (e.g., fire fighters or crane operators). (See Table 10-5.)
E. Purposes of health/medical surveillance
   1. To identify a specific instance of illness or a health trend in order to prevent recurrence of new cases
   2. To focus on specific exposure and target organs
   3. To define a specific high-risk population on the basis of an exposure history known from environmental monitoring
   4. As an ongoing process, can be used to determine effectiveness of environmental control
F. Characteristics of mandated screening and surveillance examinations
   1. Systematic and performed at identified intervals whose frequency is defined by standard or incidence of exposure
   2. Uses periodic diagnostic tests for detecting or monitoring a specific agent
      a. All tests require preplacement or preassignment health evaluation.
      b. Periodic evaluation is ongoing.
      c. Evaluation is done after an accidental/emergency exposure.
      d. Some standards require medical evaluation at termination.
   3. Recognized methods of surveillance include chest x-ray, urinalysis, liver function testing, kidney function studies, complete blood work, audiometric, spirometry, or other test needed for specific indicators of organ systems status.
   4. The frequency of testing depends on the incidence of disease in a specific target population.
   5. A written opinion is required from the person who conducts the examination.

XI

Biological Monitoring

A. Purpose of monitoring:
   1. Identification of specific types of needed surveillance
   2. Early recognition of indication of exposure
   3. Evaluates the exposure level and the health risk by evaluating the internal dose of the chemical or its metabolites
   4. Tests the effectiveness of environmental controls and personal protective equipment
B. Sources of samples for biologic monitoring include: blood, urine, hair, or expired air.
C. Variables that affect the biological monitoring of individuals
   1. Route of entry
   2. Age of worker
   3. Sex of worker
   4. Body composition (fatty mass)
   5. Pregnancy and disease process
   6. Personal hygiene and habits (handwashing, smoking)

D. Factors to consider are:
1. How is the chemical absorbed?
2. Distribution of chemical
3. Biotransformation (accumulation and/or elimination) of the chemical
4. Are there metabolic interferences between industrial agents and use of alcohol, drugs or tobacco, pesticide residues, and food additives? (Rempel, 1990; Amdur, Doull, & Klaassen, 1993)

XII

Implications for Occupational Health Nursing

The occupational health nurse has the following roles in health/medical surveillance and monitoring.

A. Assurance of proper record maintenance

B. Collaboration in the development of policy for testing (who to test; selection of testing method; frequency of testing; reporting of abnormals; referral plan for abnormals)

C. Performance of test examination

D. Interpretation of test, referral, follow-up, care plans

E. Maintenance of confidentiality, record retention, and storage

F. Health education—recommending changes in personal and work habits

G. Instruction in self-care techniques for prevention and early detection

H. Counseling or referral for conditions unrelated to exposusre

Direct Care: Management of Illness and Injury
XIII

Direct Care at the Worksite

In many occupational health settings, the occupational health nurse is the primary provider of health care to the worker population. The occupational health nurse assumes the responsibility of providing health management of all occupational and many nonoccupational health problems.

A. The occupational health nurse may assume the roles of:
1. Direct care provider
2. Urgent care provider
3. Health emergency manager

B. Guidelines for direct care are provided by:
1. State Nurse Practice Act, Pharmacy Act, and Medical Practice Acts
2. American Association Occupational Health Nurses (AAOHN) Standards of Practice (Appendix A)
3. AAOHN Code of Ethics (Appendix B)
4. Qualifications and abilities of the occupational health nurse
5. Employer requirements: policies and procedures
6. Nurse/physician relationship: protocols and guidelines for practice
7. Geographic location of industry in relation to an emergency medical service
8. Clinical practice guidelines; sources are:
    - *Clinician's Handbook of Preventive Services: Put Prevention into Practice* (1994) Department of Health and Human Services
    - Community agencies (e.g., American Cancer Society, American Diabetes Association, American Heart Association)

- National Institute of Health
- Professional groups, such as American Colleges of Obstetricians and Gynecologists, American College of Physicians, American Academy of Ophthalmology

C. Characteristics of direct care in occupational health nursing
1. Direct care may be provided for both occupational and nonoccupational health problems.
   a. Occupational problems include conditions the which are work related or aggravated by work.
   b. If nonoccupational, the condition is usually
      - Emergent
      - A self-limiting illness, such as a respiratory infection
      - A chronic illness that is responding well to a recognized treatment plan
      - An acute illness that calls for a quick referral to an outside care provider
2. On-site treatment allows workers to stay on the job, decreasing their time away from work.
3. Direct care is a multidisciplinary approach the which includes other health care providers (e.g., physicians, industrial hygienists, safety personnel, and other adjunct health care providers).
4. Direct care includes primary prevention services, such as the provision of adult immunizations (Table 10-6).

D. Over-the-counter medications (OTC), also known as nonprescription medications, are often provided as part of an organized occupational health service (AAOHN, 1995).
1. Advantages of over-the-counter (OTC) medications are:
   a. Allow for prompt treatment of a worker's injury or illness
   b. Result in less lost work time
   c. Save the employer money through increased productivity
2. OTC medications may be used by the general public only "in the presence of adequate packaging and appropriate instructions" (AAOHN, 1995).
3. Administration of OTCs by the occupational health nurse requires:
   - Knowledge of state laws, including the nurse practice act and the pharmacy act
   - Knowledge of company policies
   - Knowledge of licensure requirements of staff
4. Considerations for the occupational health nurse when administering OTCs in the occupational setting (AAOHN, 1995):
   a. Evaluate the appropriateness for their use in the occupational setting; for example, consider whether they may cause drowsiness, which could lead to injury on the job.
   b. Be knowledgeable about the medication, including its action and its possible side effects.
   c. Consider its possible interaction with a prescription medication.
   d. Be prepared for adverse reactions.
   e. Consider the impact of the medication on an existing illness.
5. Options related to OTC medication use (AAOHN, 1995):
   a. Eliminate the dispensation of OTC medications entirely.
   b. Provide a vending machine for OTC medications.
   c. Develop a self-administered medication system for employees.
   d. Develop procedures and guidelines for the dispensation of OTC medications.

TABLE 10-6

Adult Immunizations—General Recommendations

Vaccine	Population	Frequency
Tetanus & Diphtheria (Td)	Everyone	Initial series (usually in childhood)
		Adult series if needed
		Td booster every 10 years
Hepatitis B	Health care workers	Initial series of 3 doses—first dose, followed by second at one month; third dose 6 months after first dose
	Sexually active people	
	High-risk groups	
Hepatitis A	Travelers	Primary dose, then booster 6–12 months after primary dose
	Military personnel	
	High-risk sexual group	
	Substance abusers	
	Institutional workers	
Measles, Mumps, Rubella (MMR)	Born after 1956	1 Dose
	Lack proof of immunity	
Influenza	Health care workers	Annually
	Over age 65	
	High-risk groups	
Pneumococcal	High-risk groups	Initial—one dose
	Over age 65	If given at younger age, reimmunize at age 65 if more than 6 years since initial dose

Travelers to high-risk countries should contact health care provider and/or CDC for specific needed immunizations.

Package inserts for vaccine will advise of dosage, contraindications, side effects, and reporting requirements. VAERS, 1-800-822-7967.

Sources: *Guide for adult immunization,* (3rd ed.) (1994), American College of Physicians Task Force; Smith Kline Beecham (1995); Havrix Hepatitis A, Inactivated (Monograph).

Direct Care for Four Categories of Illness and Injury

The following sections briefly describes *emergent, urgent, acute* and *chronic* conditions that may be seen in the occupational setting. For more detailed information, refer to appropriate texts and references.

XIV

Emergent Injury/Illness

A. *Shock* can present as: anxiety, confusion, dizziness, stupor, tachycardia, weak pulse, cool moist skin, poor capillary refill, sweating, and pallor.

  1. Common types of shock include:
     a. Hypovolemia: blood volume loss can occur in multiple trauma, crushing injuries, amputations, broken/fractured bones, heat exhaustion
     b. Anaphylaxis, which can result from food/drug allergies, insect bites, or chemicals in the workplace; its symptoms are described in Table 10-7.
  2. General treatment of shock
     a. Regardless of etiology, treat as an emergency.
     b. Advanced life support (ALS) should be notified immediately.
     c. Emergency measures should be applied while awaiting ALS (Hoole, Pickard, Ouimette, Lohr, & Greenberg, 1995; Ho & Sanders, 1990; Ganong, 1995).

B. Burns
  1. Types of burns (Hau, 1994):
     a. Thermal: extent of burn depends on temperature and exposure.
     b. Electrical: alternating current follows the path of least resistance; an electrical burn has an entrance and an exit wound.
     c. Chemical burns are of two types:
        • Acid: damage is immediately apparent.
        • Alkali: hours can pass before damage is apparent.
     d. The recognized universal treatment for chemical exposure is to irrigate with water, except for lime in which case the affected part should be brushed first.
  2. Classification of burns:
     a. First degree: mixed partial thickness of skin; redness
     b. Second degree: epidermis involved; blistering
     c. Third degree: involves all layers of skin; severe tissue damage

C. *Seizure* is an involuntary muscle contraction associated with loss of consciousness, incontinence (Hoole, Pickard, Ouimette, Lohr & Greenberg, 1995).
  1. Etiology includes: epilepsy, drugs and/or alcohol, hypoglycemia, brain lesions, eclampsia, meningitis, acute overwhelming infection, heat exposure, hypoxia related to chemical exposure

---

TABLE 10-7

Clinical Manifestations of Anaphylaxis

System	Signs/Symptoms
Respiratory	nasal congestion, nasal itching, sneezing, nasal mucosal edema, rhinitis, rhinorrhea, dyspnea, hoarseness, throat tightness, stridor, cough, wheezing, chest tightness, cyanosis
Circulatory	lightheadedness, generalized weakness, syncope, chest pain, ECG changes (tachycardia)
Skin	urticaria, erythema, hives, flushing, pruritus, periorbital edema, non-pitting edema
GI	nausea, vomiting, abdominal cramping
CNS	apprehension, headache, confusion, anxiety secondary to cerebral hypoxia, sense of impending doom

Sources: Hoole, Pickard, Ouimette, Lohr, & Greenberg, 1995; Ho & Sanders, 1990; Ganong, 1995.

2. Signs of seizure include: sudden onset, vaso-vagal response, loss of consciousness, absence of respirations, tonic/clonic muscle movements, eyeballs rolled upward, contorted expression—neck hyperextended, postictal phase (drowsiness, disorientation).
3. Treatment of seizure (follow specific clinic directives)
   a. Prevent self-injury—keep in lying position.
   b. Observe (DO NOT TREAT) during active seizure.
   c. Maintain patent airway.

D. Head injury (Hau, 1994, p. 89–90)
1. Mild injury involves no signs or symptoms of brain or skull injury.
2. Severe injury may involve: loss of consciousness (LOC), headache, skull fracture/depressed skull fracture, concussion, unequal pupils, fluid (cerebrospinal) from nose or ears, speech/memory deficit.
3. Head injury may result in a concussion, subdural/epidural hematoma, cerebral edema, and associated cervical spine injury.
4. Standard treatment includes (Hau, 1994, p. 90): universal precaution, 30-degree head elevation if no cervical injury, monitor vital signs, initiate emergency medical services, keep employee calm, prepare for seizures and vomiting.
5. Other procedures may include:
   a. Oral suctioning as necessary (vomiting; avoid nasal suctioning)
   b. Covering open head wound with sterile gauze, avoiding pressure on injury site
   c. Providing airway support
   d. Electrolyte replacement

XV

Urgent/Minor Acute Injury

A. Eye injuries resulting from exposure (Rogers, Randolph, & Mastroianni, 1996)
1. Injuries may result from exposure to chemical, physical, or biological agents.
   a. Acid burns cause damage rapidly but are generally less serious than alkaline burns.
   b. Alkaline burns (especially particulate burns such as lime) are more serious than acid burns because even after removal of the agent, tiny particles lodged in the skin may continue to burn, causing progressive damage.
   c. Detergents cause water loss in eye tissues.
   d. UV radiation burns, such as those from a welder arc, may not show symptoms for 6–12 hours after exposure.
2. Symptoms include: burning pain, blurred vision, tearing, decreased visual acuity, exudates, erythema, edema of eyes and surrounding tissue.
3. Universal treatment for eye injury: immediately irrigate eyes with copious amounts of water or normal saline. Other activities include:
   a. Determine the chemical etiology—examine Material Safety Data Sheets.
   b. Remove contact with the offending agent.
   c. Continue flushing with tepid water for 15–20 minutes; use the Morgan lens (per protocol) and ensure that the eyelids are irrigated externally.
   d. Check the worker's visual acuity with a hand-held vision screener (Jaeger Card).
   e. Refer to an ophthalmologist for: persistent pain, chemical involvement, and/or decreased post-treatment visual acuity.

BOX 10-1

Sample Protocol for Nursing Diagnosis of Corneal Abrasion

1. Sterile fluorescein strip is touched to the internal lower lid (fluorescein will spread across the eye).
2. Have patient blink several times.
3. Examine the eye under light.
4. Defects/abrasions in the conjunctival layer will stain bright green.
5. Refer to an appropriate provider for antibiotic treatment.
6. Severe corneal abrasions can lead to corneal erosion if not properly treated within 24 hours post-injury.

B. Eye injuries resulting from trauma to the eye
   1. Types of eye injuries
      a. Corneal abrasion (foreign bodies become embedded in the conjunctiva under the upper eyelid). Invert the lid to facilitate inspection and removal of the irritant (see Box 10-1).
      b. Direct penetration or perforation of eye
      c. Eye injury that results from head trauma
   2. Collecting data about eye injury
      a. A rapid yet thorough injury history must be obtained.
         • What was the worker doing?
         • Did the incident involve head trauma?
         • Were chemicals involved?
         • Was the worker wearing safety glasses?
      b. Symptoms of minor injury include: irritation, tearing, red sclera/conjunctiva, corneal irritation, periorbital edema, photophobia.
      c. Symptoms of major injury include:
         • Diminished vision, sudden loss of vision (may indicate detached retina), and/or hemorrhage
         • Papilledema (redness, congestion, blurred margins of disc when viewed with an ophthalmoscope)
         • Blood in the anterior chamber (gravity settles blood to the bottom of the iris) may indicate spontaneous hemorrhage, scleral rupture, major intraocular hemorrhage.
   3. Treatments for eye trauma (see Box 10-2 for eye tray equipment)
      a. Universal treatment for eye injury: flushing alone may remove the foreign body from the eye.
      b. Never remove an impaled object (may require surgical repair—urgent).
      c. If the lid cannot close because of the object; stabilize the object and place a wet dressing next to the cornea, between the lids; provide a bulky dressing to encompass the impaled object.
      d. Patch the uninjured eye also to prevent bilateral sympathetic movement.
      e. Transport to an emergency department with an ophthalmologist or staff.

C. Diabetic emergencies: hypoglycemia or hyperglycemia (abnormally low or high serum glucose)
   1. Signs/symptoms include: tremors/weakness, light-headedness, diaphoresis, anxiety, confusion, cool/pale skin, nausea/vomiting, decreased level of consciousness, rapid/bounding pulse.
   2. Actions required: stabilize, monitor, and refer.

BOX 10-2

Eye Tray (Equipment and Supplies)

Most worksite eye injuries can be evaluated and treated with a simple setup that includes the following:

1. Hand-held flashlight with fresh batteries
2. Opthalmoscope
3. Visual activity chart (Snellen or Jaegar)

4. Sterile, 6-inch, cotton-tipped applicators
5. Sterile isotonic saline—(2) 1000-ml bags
6. Morgan lens
7. Sterile fluorescein papers
8. Ultraviolet lamp
9. Properacaine 0.5% or tetracaine 0.5% ophthalmic solution
10. Eye patches and eye-patch holders with wraparound head bandage

---

D. Hypertensive crisis (Ganong, 1995; Rogers, Randolph, & Mastroianni, 1996)
  1. The crisis is characterized by blood pressure reading of 200/110 or higher.
  2. Etiology may include untreated hypertension or chemical exposure.
  3. The employee may present with headache, angina, peripheral edema, dyspnea, orthopnea, nausea/vomiting, jugular venous distention, periorbital edema, flushed face, red sclera.
  4. Treatment: stabilize, monitor, and refer.

E. Fractures are the result of a break or crack in the bone continuity.
  1. Types of fractures:
     a. Closed fracture: skin intact with no opening wound to the surface
     b. Open fracture: open wound, protruding bone, and damage to soft tissue
  2. Symptoms of fracture include: a snap or popping sensation at the time of injury, deformity and pain at the site of the fracture, swelling, discoloration, tenderness, shortening of the injured limb, decreased range of motion or function of the limb.
  3. Actions required: assess the type of fracture, stabilize, and arrange or coordinate transport to an appropriate care facility, for example, an emergency room or a free-standing emergency clinic.

XVI

Acute Injuries and Illnesses

A. Lumbosacral strain (LSS)
  1. Etiology of LSS
     a. LSS arises from strain of the ligaments and musculature of the lumbosacral area (Hoole, Pickard, Ouimette, Lohr, & Greenberg, 1995, p. 258).
     b. Strain does not involve vertebrae, articular cartilage, or nerve roots: 80% of the population will experience back pain at some point in their adult life (Hoole et al., 1995).
     c. LSS is generally related to a specific event or series of repetitive movements that precipitated the pain.
  2. Symptoms include mild to severe pain across the lumbosacral area that is worsened by sudden movement.
  3. Treatment protocol for LSS
     a. Apply ice to affected area, replacing ice every 20 minutes.

b. Administer over-the-counter antiinflammatory medications per established directives.

c. Provide written work modification, following established directives and company policies.

B. Other acute injuries (Rogers, Randolph, & Mastroianni, 1996)

1. These include lacerations, abrasions, and/or contusions.
2. Treatment is based on type and extent of injury.
   a. A Tetanus booster of .5 ml intramuscularly may be required if immunization is not up to date. (Assess for primary series.)
   b. If the wound is open, clean it with normal saline or Betadine solution.
   c. Refer the employee for wound closure as appropriate.

XVII

Chronic Injury/Illness

A. A work-related musculoskeletal disorder (WRMSD) refers to an injury or illness that cannot be attributed to one specific event and of which symptoms occur over a period of time.

1. WRMSD includes the following diagnostic terms: overuse syndrome, cumulative trauma disorders, myalgia, thoracic outlet syndrome, rotator cuff tears, epicondylitis, tenosynovitis (deQuervain's, ganglion cysts, trigger finger, and carpal tunnel syndrome) (Putz-Anderson, 1988).
2. Without adequate recovery, micro-traumas result in pain, discomfort, numbness, reduced strength, and inhibited dexterity (Cherniack, 1994).
3. Ergonomic stressors include repetition, force, extreme or static postures, vibration, and static loading.

B. Management of work-related musculoskeletal disorder

1. Assessment includes:
   a. History and physical examination
   b. Evaluation of pain type (Controlling Cumulative Trauma Disorders, 1994)
      • Type I: pain that lasts for more than one day after an activity
      • Type II: pain during activity that does not restrict performance
      • Type III: pain during activity that restricts performance
      • Type IV: pain that is chronic and occurs even at rest
   c. Evaluation of worksite and work design.
2. *Conservative treatment* is recommended for WRMSD of upper extremities; this may include:
   a. Resting and/or immobilization of affected body part during acute phase
   b. Specific job restrictions
   c. Modification of work area to fit the person
   d. Ice massage to affected part to relieve symptoms
   e. Therapeutic muscle massage
   f. Antiinflammatory drugs
   g. Work conditioning and/or work hardening after acute phase
3. A *functional capacity evaluation* may be conducted to determine the worker's physical ability to perform the job task.

C. Chronic pain syndrome (see Table 10-8)

1. Manifestations of chronic pain syndrome
   a. Excessive (beyond "normal") reaction to pain
   b. Intense response to relatively minor injuries
   c. Prolonged subjective perception of pain

TABLE 10-8

8 Characteristics Related to Chronic Pain Syndrome

Duration	• generally prolonged pain of 6 months' duration • chronic pain characteristics can appear within first 2 weeks
Dramatization	• unusual, exaggerated, verbal and nonverbal expressions of pain • theatrical behavior • indignant if validity of pain is questioned
Diagnostic dilemma	• extensive history of evaluations by multiple health care providers • repeated diagnostic studies • clinical impressions tend to be vague
Duration of drug use	• willing recipient of multiple drugs • substance abuse and dependence may be noted (alcohol, tobacco)
Dependence	• becomes dependent on physician, spouse, and family • makes excessive demands for medical care
Depression	• coping mechanisms are impaired • exhibits unhappiness, despair, anxiety, irritability, hostility, insomnia • low self-esteem
Disuse	• self-imposed limitations in activity • development of generalized deconditioning
Dysfunction	• social withdrawal and isolation further contributes to patient's sense of disability

Source: Menzel, N. N. (1994). *Workers' compensation management from A to Z: A "How to" guide with forms.* OEM Press. Used with permission.

2. Diagnostic considerations
    a. Differentiate from symptom exaggeration/magnification or malingering.
    b. Responses to chronic pain are usually not a conscious process.
    c. Ongoing health intervention may be counterproductive.
3. Treatment considerations
    a. Oftentimes, less health intervention is more effective.
    b. A psychological evaluation may be required.
    c. Remain objective (caring and professional) with employee despite open hostility.
    d. Increased out-of-work time leads to decreased chance of recovery.

Strategies for Direct Care

The primary goal when providing occupational health services is to prevent injury or illness and, when a disability has occurred, to assist the worker throughout the process so that he/she may successfully return to work.

XVIII

Case Management

Case management is "a process of coordinating an individual client's health care services in order to achieve optimal, quality care delivered in a cost-effective manner" (AAOHN, 1994).

A. The case manager coordinates services with appropriate health care professionals.

B. The case manager monitors the economic aspects of treatment.

C. Assessment, planning, and implementation of the worker's care and progress toward returning to work is part of the process.

D. The case manager provides evaluation and follow-up of the worker's progress. (More details on case management can be found in Chapter 12.)

XIX
Work Conditioning

Work conditioning is working internally within the workplace to return the worker to work and provide gradual conditioning in the process.

A. Considerations for implementing work conditioning include:
1. Has the worker reached a point in the rehabilitation process of maximum improvement without the need for further intervention?
2. Is the worker a proper candidate for work conditioning through modification of job task or limitation of time at work?
3. Can the worker return to the job task for a full day?
4. What are the worker's limitations and disability?
5. Will performing the job task do harm to the worker?
6. What are company and departmental policies? Is there work available?

B. Options in performance of the job
1. The worker performs the regular job task for part of a scheduled shift.
2. The worker performs the job following modification of a certain job task.

C. The goal of work conditioning is a gradual return to full-time work with minimal disruptions for the worker and the employer.

D. Work conditioning is mutually beneficial for both the worker and employer since it saves money for the company and provides income to the worker.

XX
Work Hardening

Work hardening comprises activities designed to facilitate easing the worker back to work.

A. Characteristics of work hardening
1. Takes place externally (away from the workplace)
2. Simulates the particular job task and functions of the worker
3. Evaluates the workers capacity and tolerance for the job
4. Gradually increases activities in order to increase physical conditioning of worker
5. Matches work abilities to job demands
6. Generally lasts from 3 to 6 weeks, depending on the needs of the worker

B. Benefits of work hardening
1. Provides conditioning of employee to rebuild tolerance, physical strength, and stamina
2. Keeps the worker oriented to work and provides a contact with the work environment
3. Provides a routine for the worker and simulates an 8-hour workday

4. Can assist in elevating the worker's self-esteem
5. Through performance of simulated work activities, may reduce fears of reinjury in the workplace
6. Results in early return to work, which is economical and beneficial for both the worker and the employer
7. Can provide objective and measurable data for assessing the worker's progress

C. Roles of the occupational health nurse in work hardening include:
1. In cases where the occupational health nurse is the case manager, there may be an external case manager; the occupational health nurse acts as the liaison between the external case manager and management.
2. The occupational health nurse coordinates and identifies appropriate referral sources.
3. The occupational health nurse provides follow-up on a regular basis to assess a worker's progress.
4. The occupational health nurse provides education and counseling and teaches the worker self-care techniques to aid in a quick recovery (Lepping, 1990).

BIBLIOGRAPHY

Agency for Toxic Substances and Disease Registry. (1992). Taking an exposure history. *Case studies in environmental medicine.* Atlanta: U.S. Department of Health and Human Services, National Institute for Occupational Safety and Health.

Amdur, M. O., Doull, J., & Klaassen, C. D. (Eds.). (1993). *Cassarette and Doull's toxicology: The basic science of poisons.* (4th ed.) New York: Macmillan Publishing Company.

American Association of Occupational Health Nurses (1994). Position statement: The certified occupational health nurse as case manager. *AAOHN Journal, 42*(4).

American Association of Occupational Health Nurses (1995). Advisory: *Over-the-counter medications.* Author.

American College of Physicians (1994). *Guide for adult immunization* (3rd ed.), Philadelphia: Author.

American College of Physicians. (1981). Periodic health examinations: A guide for designing individualized preventive health care in the asymptomatic patient. *Annals of Internal Medicine. 95,* 729–723.

Barnes, D., Eribes, C., Juarbe, T., Nelson, M., Proctor, S., Sawyer, L., Shaul, M., & Meleis, A. (1995). Primary health care and primary care: A confusion of philosophies. *Nursing Outlook, 43*(1), 7–16.

Bates, B. (1995). *A guide to physical examination and history taking* (6th ed.). Philadelphia: J. B. Lippincott Company.

Bowers, A. C., & Thompson, J. M. (1992). *Clinical manual of health assessment* (4th ed.). St. Louis, MO: Mosby Year Book, Inc.

Breslow, L., & Somers, A. R. (1977). The lifetime health-monitoring program. *New England Journal of Medicine. 29*(11), 601–608.

Burkeen, O. E., & Cooper, G. (1985). Pre-placement health assessment: The occupational health nurses role. *AAOHN Update Series, 1*(15) 2–7.

Burgel, B. J. (1991). Occupational health history. In L. N. Ray & L. K. Glazner, *Clinical guidelines for occupational health nurses* (2nd ed.). CAOHN. Tucson, AZ: Sundance Press.

Burgel, B. J. (1993). *Innovation at the worksite: Delivery of nurse-managed primary health care services.* Washington, DC: American Nurses' Publishing, Inc.

Cahall, J. B., & Vester, J. C. (1985). The principles and process of screening. *AAOHN Update Series, 1*(20) 1–7.

Cassidy, C. A. (1993). Taking the employee's history of the present problem. *AAOHN Update Series, 5*(7) 2–8.

Cherniack, M. (1994). Upper extremity disorders. In L. Rosenstock & M. Cullen, (Eds.) *Textbook of Clinical and environmental medicine.* Philadelphia: W. B. Saunders Co.

Controlling cumulative trauma disorders: Practical ergonomics and medical intervention. A seminar for nurses. Sept. 1994. Greensboro, NC: Health & Hygiene, Inc.

Donaldson, M., Yordy, K., & Vanselow, N. (Eds.). (1994). *Defining primary care: An interim report.* Washington, DC: National Academy Press.

Ganong, W. F. (1995). *Review of medical physiology* (17th ed.). Norwalk, Conn.: Appleton & Lange.

Hau, M. (1994). *In control—site specific occupational health and safety series—While help is on the way.* Chicago: Health Products Marketing, Inc.

Ho, M. T., & Sanders, C. E. (Eds.). (1990). *Current emergency diagnosis and treatment.* (3rd ed.) Englewood Cliffs, NJ: Prentice-Hall.

Hoole, A. J., Pichard., C. G. Jr., Quimette, R. M., Lohr, J. A., & Greenberg, R. A. (1995). *Patient guidelines for nurse practitioners.* (4th ed.). Philadelphia: J. P. Lippincott Company.

Kemerer, S., & Raniere, T. M. (1990). Cost effective job placement physical examination: A decision making framework. *AAOHN Journal, 38*(5), 236–242.

Kozier, B., Erb, G., Blais, K., & Wilkinson, J. M. (1995). *Fundamentals of nursing: Concepts, process and practice.* (4th ed.) Reading, MA: Addison-Wesley Publishing Company, Inc..

Krebs, D. (1983). Nursing in primary health care. *International Nursing Review, 30*(5), 141–145.

Lepping, V. (1990). Work hardening: A valuable resource for the occupational health nurse. *AAOHN Journal. 38*(7), 313–317.

Lewis, S. M., & Collier, I. C. (1987). *Medical-surgical nursing: Assessment and management of clinical problems* (4th ed.). New York: McGraw-Hill Book Co.

Menzel, N. N. (1994). *Workers' compensation management from A to Z: A "How to" guide with forms.* Beverly, MA: OEM Press.

Nutting, P. A. (Ed.) (1991). A research agenda for primary care: Summary report of a conference. Pub. AHCPR 91-08. Washington, DC: USDHHS.

Obler, S. K., & LaForce, F. M., (1989). The periodic physical examination in asymptomatic adults. *Annals of Internal Medicine. 110*(3) 214–226.

Occupational safety and health standards for general industry, (29CFR, Part 1910) with Amendments as of September 1, 1994, Promulgated by the Occupational Safety and Health Administration, United States Department of Labor.

Pederson, M. T., Muldoon, S., & Curtes, E.C., (1993). Request for medical evaluation. *AAOHN Journal. 41*(5) 241–244.

Pransky, G. S., Frumkin, H., & Himmelstein, J. S. (1988). Decision making in worker fitness and risk evaluation. In J. S. Himmelstein & G. S. Pransky (Eds.) *Occupational medicine: State of the art review, 3*(2) 179–191.

Pruitt, R. H. (1995). Pre-placement evaluation: Thriving within the A.D.A. guidelines. *AAOHN Journal. 43*(3) 124–130.

Putz-Anderson, V. (1988). *Cumulative trauma disorders: A manual for musculoskeletal diseases of the upper limbs.* Cincinnati: Taylor & Francis Bristol, Inc.

Rempel, D. (1990). Medical surveillance in the workplace overview. *Occupational Medicine. State of Art Review. 5*(3) 435–438.

Rogers, B. (1994). *Occupational health nursing: Concepts and practice.* Philadelphia: W. B. Saunders Co.

Rogers, B., Randolph, S. A., & Mastroianni, K. (1996). *Occupational health nursing guidelines for primary clinical conditions.* (2nd ed.) Beverly, MA: OEM Press.

Rosenstock, L. & Cullen, M. (1994). *Textbook of clinical occupational and environmental medicine.* Philadelphia: W. B. Saunders Co.

Smith-Kline Beecham (1995). *Havrix hepatitis. A vaccine inactivated* (Monograph). Philadelphia: Author.

U.S. Department of Health and Human Services. (1991). *Healthy People 2000: National Health Promotion and Disease Prevention Objectives.* DHHS Pub. No. (PHS) 91-50212. Washington, DC: U.S. Government Printing Office.

U.S. Department of Health and Human Services. (1994). *The Clinician's Handbook of Preventive Services.* Washington, DC: International Medical Publishing, Inc.

U.S. Department of Health and Human Services. (1996). *Healthy People 2000 Review 1995–1996..* DHHS Pub. No. (PHS) 96-1256. Washington, DC: U.S. Government Printing Office.

U.S. Preventive Service Task Force (1989). *Guide to clinical preventive services: An assessment of the effectiveness of 169 interventions.* Baltimore: Williams & Wilkins.

Wegman, D. H., Levy, B. S., & Halperen, W. E. (1995). Recognizing occupational disease, In B. H. Levy & D. H. Wegman (eds). *Recognizing and Preventing Work-related Disease,* (3rd. ed.), Boston: Little, Brown and Company.

CHAPTER

11

Health Promotion and Adult Education

MAJOR TOPICS

- *Health promotion*
- *Health behavior change models*
- *Levels of prevention*
- *Adult education*
- *Effective presentations*

Health promotion and adult education are vital parts of occupational health practice today and for the future. The basic principles of adult education provide tools that can be applied to health education and to health promotion in the workplace. By helping individuals assess their health needs and by developing strategies to meet organizational needs, the occupational health nurse can help create an environment that values and supports healthy workers.

Introduction to Health Promotion

I

What Is Health Promotion?

"Health promotion is the science and art of helping people change their lifestyle to move towards a state of optimal health" (O'Donnell, 1989).

A. The health promotion movement began with the 19th-century epidemiological revolution.
1. 19th century: The focus was on hygiene, sanitation, housing, and working conditions (Rogers, 1994).
2. 20th century: The emphasis was on disease prevention and health (Rogers, 1994).
3. Early 1980s: Less than 5% of employers had health promotion programs (O'Donnell & Harris, 1994).
4. Late 1980s and 1990s: 80% of employers with 50 or more employees have some form of health promotion programs (O'Donnell & Harris, 1994).

B. Health promotion focuses on the promotion of optimal health through:
1. Prevention of illness/injury
2. Presentation of health education programs
3. Promotion of personal responsibility for one's health
4. Development of strategies for behavioral change

C. Health promotion activities are conducted by and draw upon the expertise of health professionals from many fields.
1. Examples of fields are nursing, health education, medicine, psychology, nutrition, occupational and physical therapy, safety, and ergonomics.
2. Occupational health nurses are often responsible for developing health promotion programs in work settings.

D. The rationale for health promotion includes:
1. The costs of treating preventable illness and injury increase the cost of health care.
2. Health promotion has the potential to improve the quality of life.

E. When incorporating health promotion in the workplace, one must consider:
1. The consistency of the program with the organizational mission and goals
2. The costs and benefits of the program
3. Benefits for the workers, which include:
    a. Demonstration of management's proactive position
    b. Workers' improved sense of well-being
    c. Possible reduction in overall health care costs
4. Benefits for employers, which include:
    a. Improvement in workers' performance and productivity
    b. Reduction in benefit costs
    c. Lowered operating costs
    d. Enhanced company image
    e. Improved workplace quality

F. Three levels of health promotion are:
1. *Awareness* programs that increase the level of interest in a health-related topic and may include newsletters, flyers, posters, seminars, and health fairs (O'Donnell & Harris, 1994)
2. *Lifestyle* or *behavior change* programs that are designed to help individuals adopt health related behaviors, such as regular exercise, good nutrition, stress management, and smoking cessation (Selleck, Sirles, and Newman, 1989)
3. *Creating environments* that support and encourage healthy lifestyles (O'Donnell & Harris, 1994)

II

National Health Promotion Objectives

A. *Healthy People 2000: National Health Promotion and Disease Prevention Objectives* (U.S. Department of Health and Human Services, 1991) describes the national objectives related to major chronic illness, injuries, and infectious diseases; its major emphasis is health promotion and disease prevention.

B. There are 15 objectives that address increased training and education for occupational health and safety personnel, improved surveillance activities, and increased research in occupational health and safety. See Table 11-1, which provides the segmentation of the priority areas, including health promotion, protection, preventive services, surveillance, and data systems.

III

Health Behavior Change Models

As occupational health nurses work with clients to assist them in changing their lifestyle behaviors, it is critical to have an understanding of the theories regarding behavior change. With this knowledge, the nurse will be in a better position to help clients overcome their barriers and move toward successful outcomes.

TABLE 11-1
Healthy People 2000: Priority Areas

Health Promotion
1. Physical Activity and Fitness
2. Nutrition
3. Tobacco
4. Alcohol and Other Drugs
5. Family Planning
6. Mental Health and Mental Disorders
7. Violent and Abusive Behavior
8. Educational and Community-Based Programs

Health Protection
9. Unintentional Injuries
10. Occupational Safety and Health
11. Environmental Health
12. Food and Drug Safety
13. Oral Health

Preventive Services
14. Maternal and Infant Health
15. Heart Disease and Stroke
16. Cancer
17. Diabetes and Chronic Disabling Conditions

18. HIV Infection
19. Sexually Transmitted Diseases
20. Immunization and Infectious Diseases
21. Clinical Preventive Services

Surveillance and Data Systems
22. Surveillance and Data Systems

Age-Related Objectives
Children
Adolescents and Young Adults
Adults
Older Adults

Special Population Objectives
People with Low Income
Blacks
Hispanics
Asians and Pacific Islanders
American Indians and Native Alaskans
People with Disabilities

Source: USDHHS Healthy People 2000: (1991). Washington, D.C. DHHS Publication No. 91-50212, 7.

A. The *Health Belief Model* was developed by Godfrey Hochbaum, Stephen Kegeles, Howard Leventhal, and Irwin Rosenstock in the 1950s (Rosenstock, 1990).
1. Major components of the model:
   a. *Perceived susceptibility* is an individual's subjective estimation of his or her own personal risk of developing a specific health problem.
   b. *Perceived severity* refers to an individual's own personal judgment of how serious a health condition may be; perceived susceptibility and perceived severity are often combined into *perceived threat*.
   c. *Perceived benefits* are an individual's estimation of how effective a health recommendation may be in removing the threat.
   d. *Perceived barriers* are an individual's estimation of the obstacles to the performance of a health-related behavior.
2. The likelihood of an action being taken is driven by the positive difference between the perceived barriers and the perceived benefits (O'Donnell & Harris, 1994).

B. There are several *social learning theories* that are built around the concept that people's thoughts have a strong effect on their behavior and that their behavior affects their thoughts (O'Donnell & Harris, 1994); two examples are:
1. *The Locus of Control Theory:*
   a. An individual's belief (outcome expectation) that their own behavior determines reinforcements (outcomes) is called *internal locus of control.*
   b. An individual's belief that reinforcements are controlled by others is called *external locus of control.*
   c. Theoretically, "internals" are more likely to take control of their health and to engage in health promotion activities than are "externals."
2. *The Self-Efficacy Theory* (Bandura, 1986) assesses the individual's "belief that he/she can achieve a desired outcome."

C. The *Health Promotion Model* by Pender (1996) incorporated social learning theory and the Health Belief Model. Concepts from Pender's model include:
1. Health promotion is directed at increasing the level of well-being and self-actualization of an individual or group.
2. Health promoting behaviors are viewed as proactive rather than reactive.

D. The *Theory of Reasoned Action* (Ajzen & Fishbein, 1975) proposes that behavioral intentions are the result of one's attitude and subjective norms.
1. Attitudes are determined by beliefs regarding the consequences of a behavior and one's positive or negative evaluation of those consequences.
2. Subjective norms refer to a person's beliefs or perceptions about what others think he or she should do.
3. Intentions are the immediate determinant of behavior.

E. The *Theory of Planned Behavior* (Ajzen, 1988) builds on the *Theory of Reasoned Action*; the element added to the Theory of Reasoned Action is the belief that one has the resources to perform the behavior.

F. The *Theory of Social Behavior* (Triandis, 1980) states that the probability of an act occurring in a specific situation is equal to the sum of the person's habit and intention.

G. The *Protection Motivation Theory* (Prentice-Dunn & Rogers, 1986) combines features of the Health Belief Model with self-efficacy theory and other social psychological constructs such as fear, arousal, appraisal, and coping.

H. The *Health Action Process Approach* (Schwarzer, 1992) states that health behavior change takes place over time.

I. The *Model of Health Promotion Behavior* (O'Donnell, 1989) refers to the assumption that self-efficacy beliefs play a central role regarding health beliefs and behavior.

J. The *Transtheoretical Model of Behavior Change,* also known as the *Stages of Change Model,* describes the process of behavioral change as occurring in a series of five stages: precontemplation, contemplation, preparation, action, and maintenance (Prochaska & DiClemente, 1983).

IV

Levels of Prevention

Three levels of prevention that are a part of comprehensive health promotion programs (Leavell and Clark, 1965) are the following:

A. *Primary prevention* is aimed at eliminating or reducing the risk of disease through specific actions; examples include immunizations, stress management, smoking avoidance, risk factor appraisal, seat belt use, worksite walk-throughs, and personal protective equipment use.

B. *Secondary prevention* is directed at early case-finding and diagnosis of individuals with disease in order to institute prompt interventions; examples include screening programs, health surveillance, monitoring health/illness trend data, and preplacement/periodic exams.

C. *Tertiary prevention* is directed at rehabilitating and restoring individuals to their maximum health potential; examples include disability case management, early return to work, chronic illness monitoring, and substance abuse rehabilitation.

$\overline{\textbf{V}}$

Framework for a Health Promotion Program

(See Figure 11-1. See Chapter 8 for more details regarding the various components described in the following section.)

A. Health promotion program planning
1. Include management in early stages of planning.
   a. Management must be convinced of the value of health promotion and wellness.
      1) Provide management with an estimate of cost savings (including indirect cost savings such as reduced absenteeism, increased productivity) that will be realized as a result of the program.
      2) Use supportive background, including case histories of successful programs, to generate management support.
   b. Management should be kept informed of all program activities and invited to participate in planning as appropriate.

FIGURE 11-1 *Guiding Framework for Workplace Health Promotion Programs*

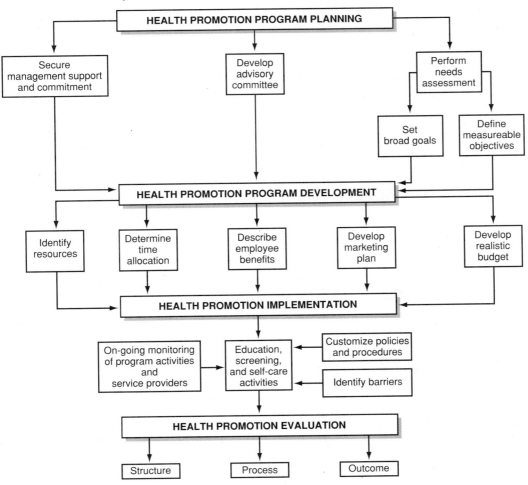

Source: Adapted from Rogers (1994). Original work used with permission.

  2. Advisory committees that are representative of the employee populations should be formed; representatives should include management, line supervisors, union members, benefits manager, as well as members of the employee population.

    a. The advisory committee provides assistance and advice throughout all stages of the program, from planning to evaluation.

    b. Workers' involvement and support of programs at this level are critical to a program's success.

  3. In order to develop appropriate goals and objectives to guide program implementation and evaluation, a well-planned needs assessment must be conducted.

    a. A needs assessment may be used to collect information about the interests and health status of employees through written surveys, interviews, focus groups, or a combination of these methods.

    b. Workers' compensation data, insurance data, absenteeism reports, and other data that reflect health care costs within an organization are an important component of the needs assessment.

    c. A health risk appraisal is an efficient and relatively inexpensive tool that can identify a specific employee's health behavior and risks. (See Box 11-1.)

B. Health promotion program development

  1. Resources must be identified when developing a health promotion program.

    a. Personnel includes the individuals who will implement the program.

BOX 11-1

Health Risk Appraisal

- A Health Risk Appraisal (HRA) is a health education tool that is used to compare an individual's health-related behaviors and characteristics with those of the general population by comparing statistics and epidemiological data. An HRA estimates an individual's life expectancy based on current risk behaviors, and it calculates the amount of risk that could be eliminated by making appropriate behavioral changes.

- A Health Risk Appraisal is easy to administer, is confidential, provides information specific to the individual, and is easy to interpret. It includes a section that recommends corrective action, and it provides positive feedback for results that demonstrate healthy behaviors.

- A Health Risk Appraisal is used to assess nutrition/weight-management needs, fitness, stress levels, drug and alcohol problems, smoking behaviors, safety behaviors, and cancer signs and risks.

- The benefits of a Health Risk Appraisal include the following:

  □ It provides the health care counselor with a rational teaching aid that can be used as a point of focus during discussions about health and behavior.

  □ It relies on a self-administered questionnaire, simple physiologic measurements, and computer-assisted calculations.

  □ It can be used with large groups because it is efficient and relatively inexpensive.

  □ It is science-based; it uses precise data based on appropriate studies.

1) Programs may be implemented by personnel from health services within the organization, or they may be outsourced to outside businesses.
2) Programs may require personnel with special skills and knowledge, such as an exercise physiologist to lead an exercise program.
3) Personnel from various community agencies, such as the American Cancer Society or the American Red Cross, offer services or programs that can be provided to worksites.

   b. Audiovisual equipment may be essential, as well as other equipment specific to the program (i.e., screening supplies, exercise devices).

   c. Paper, pencils, computer products, and other incidental supplies should be readily available.

   d. The availability of facilities and space appropriate for the purposes of the activity should be determined.

2. Determine the time required to develop the program and the time needed for workers to use the program; negotiate with the company for program versus company time.

3. Investigate the existing and potential benefits of the program.

   a. Existing benefits may include insurance incentives for employees who participate in certain activities.

   b. Potential benefits might be negotiated with management; for example, a "wellness" day could be traded for a certain number of sick days.

4. Marketing strategies will be most successful if the employees affected by the program participate in the program.

5. A successful program will depend on the inclusion of a realistic and a feasible budget; if costs exceed available resources, the occupational health nurse will be required to either submit a revised budget to management or to adjust the programs to accommodate the available funds.

C. Health promotion program implementation

1. The primary strategy used in health promotion programs is education; screening and self-care activities are also important elements of a program. (*Note:* Referral and follow-up procedures must always be included as part of a screening program.)

2. Once a program is implemented, it is continually monitored in order to assess time frames, costs, and management interest and support; adjustments are made as needed.

3. The advantages and disadvantages of the health service providers (in-house or outsourced) should be constantly monitored (see Chapter 8 for a description of advantages and disadvantages); if it is determined that disadvantages outweigh the advantages, the providers of services may need to be replaced.

4. Existing policies and procedures that affect the provision of health promotion services should be customized to meet the needs of the organization.

5. Barriers to program implementation must be identified and considered in future planning.

D. Health promotion program evaluation using *structure, process,* and *outcome.* (For more detailed information regarding structure, process, and outcome, see Chapter 8.)

1. Examples of the structural elements to be considered in the evaluation include:

   a. The qualifications and adequacy of the staff involved in all phases of the program

   b. The appropriateness of the equipment and supplies used to carry out the program

    c. The demographics of workers who participated in the program

    d. The appropriateness of the facilities

    e. The match of the program with the mission and goals of the organization

    f. Management's commitment to wellness and support of the program

2. Examples of process elements to be considered in an evaluation include:

    a. The specific activities that characterize the program (i.e., if a diabetic screening program is in place, are the protocols and procedures state-of-the-art and appropriate for this employee population?)

    b. Evidence of collaboration and support among the various personnel involved in the program

    c. A monitoring system in place that is adequate to detect changes when needed

    d. Documentation and recordkeeping that meet any legal requirements as well as serve as an effective means of maintaining the communication needs of the company

3. Examples of outcome elements to be considered in an evaluation include:

    a. Injury, illness, and absenteeism records

    b. Surveys that evaluate knowledge about self-care (i.e., American Cancer Society screening guidelines) and attitudes about health (i.e., reflected in an expressed desire to participate in healthy behaviors)

    c. Epidemiological data that reflect behavioral choices related to health (i.e., decreased smoking rates)

    d. Observations of health activities (i.e., increased use of company exercise equipment)

4. The costs and benefits are a critical outcome measure that may determine whether a company will continue to support a program. (Chapter 8 describes steps in conducting cost-effectiveness/cost-benefit analyses.)

VI

Lifestyle and Health Promotion

Modifiable lifestyles have been identified as being a major cause of premature deaths in the United States.

A. *Addiction behaviors* are characterized by the following: compulsion, loss of control, and continued involvement despite adverse consequences.

    1. Tobacco use accounts for 30% of all cancer deaths and is a major risk factor for cardiovascular disease; smoking is one form of addictive behavior. (See Table 11-2.)

    2. Alcohol is the most misused drug.

        a. When combined with other drugs, it can dangerously potentiate the effects of both.

        b. One out of every four families in the United States suffers from an alcohol or drug-related problem; family members may "adapt" by becoming codependents or "enablers" (see Table 11-3).

    3. Drug misuse includes misuse or abuse of caffeine, alcohol, nicotine, cocaine, marijuana, designer drugs (drugs that are manufactured in an illegal laboratory and mimic a controlled substance), and prescription drugs.

B. *Stress* is a contributing risk factor to cardiovascular disease and more than half of the visits to health care professionals are for stress-related disorders.

TABLE 11-2

The Fagerstrom Test for Nicotine Dependence

Questions		Points
1. How soon after you wake in the morning do you smoke your first cigarette?	within 5 min.	3
	6–30 min.	2
	31–60 min.	1
	After 60 min.	0
2. Do you find it difficult to refrain from smoking in places where it is forbidden, e.g., church, library, cinema?	Yes	1
	No	0
3. Which cigarettes would you most hate to give up?	First one in the A.M.	1
	All others	0
4. How many cigarettes do you smoke per day?	10 or fewer	0
	11–20	1
	21–30	2
	31 or more	3
5. Do you smoke more frequently during the first hours after waking than during the rest of the day?	Yes	1
	No	0
6. Do you smoke even if you are so ill that you are in bed most of the day?	Yes	1
	No	0

Score: 1–6 = Low to moderate dependence
7–11 = High dependence

Source: Flynn, T. J., & Manley, M. W. April, (1990)

C. *Diet* is associated with 6 of the top 10 causes of death: heart disease, stroke, ather-osclerosis, non-insulin-dependent diabetes, cancer, and chronic liver disease.
  1. Eating foods low in fat and high in fiber reduces the risk of heart disease and cancer.
  2. Low-fat, high-fiber diets also help to control body weight, which is a growing concern, according to the U.S. Public Health Service, since approximately 34% of Americans are overweight (USDHHS, 1995).
  3. A mind-body philosophy suggests that the body's appetite can be managed by being aware of the hunger level both before and after eating and by accepting and liking oneself.

TABLE 11-3

Alcohol and Other Drug Validation Question Set (CAGE Questionnaire)

C Have you ever felt the need to *cut down* on your drinking?

A Have you ever felt *annoyed* by criticism of your drinking?

G Have you ever felt *guilty* about drinking?

E Have you ever used an *eye*-opener or taken a drink the first thing in the morning to steady your nerves or get rid of a hangover?

A positive response to two or more questions creates a high degree of suspicion regarding alcohol dependency.

TABLE 11-4
Safe Driving Tips

- Do not drink alcohol and drive:
  - ☐ Use a designated driver
  - ☐ Use a taxicab
- Use seatbelts consistently
- Use infant/child car seats correctly and consistently

TABLE 11-5
Modes of Transmission for HIV/AIDS

- Homosexual transmission
- Heterosexual transmission
- Transfusion transmission
- Needle sharing among intravenous drug users
- Mother-to-child transmission
- Accidental needle-sticks

D. Regular physical activity helps prevent coronary heart disease, high blood pressure, non-insulin-dependent diabetes mellitus, cancer, osteoporosis, obesity, mental health problems and low back problems.
  1. Physiologic evidence demonstrates that physical activity improves many biologic measures associated with health and physiological functioning (USDHHS, 1995).
  2. People even in their 90s can increase their strength and flexibility through exercise.

E. Cancer awareness
  1. Skin cancer is the most common type of cancer; lung cancer, however, causes the most deaths.
  2. Breast cancer is the most common cancer among women in the United States, occurring in 1 out of every 9; some studies suggest it may be affected by a high-fat diet and excessive alcohol consumption.
  3. The risk for uterine cancer increases with age (over 45) and with obesity.
  4. The main type of cancer seen in men over 60 years of age is prostate cancer.

F. Alcohol-related traffic accidents are the leading cause of death and spinal cord injuries in young Americans.
  1. In 1987, approximately one-half of the deaths in the United States were alcohol-related.
  2. In 1988, auto death rates improved, with an estimated 1,500 lives saved due to a 45% nationwide rate of seatbelt use. (See Table 11-4 for safe driving tips.)
  3. Safety also includes preventing falls, fires, and traffic accidents, both on and off the job.

G. The World Health Organization (WHO) recognizes the human immunodeficiency virus (HIV) infection as a worldwide epidemic, for which prevention is the only control; currently there is no cure (see Table 11-5).

H. The occupational setting is an ideal location for the development of health promotion programs.
  1. Health promotion programs are an essential part of a comprehensive health and safety program in the occupational setting.
  2. The timing and type of program will be based on the needs of the worker populations (see Table 11-6).

VII

Employee Assistance Programs (EAP)

A. An *employee assistance program* is a work-based program designed to provide support services to employees and, in some cases, employees' families who have personal issues that may affect their well-being and their ability to perform their jobs.

TABLE 11-6

Program Development in the Occupational Setting

Health Promotion Activity	Type of Program	When Program Is Appropriate
A. Addictive Behaviors:		

1. **Tobacco Use**	Smoking Cessation
	Nicotine Gum/Patches
	Individual Behavioral
	   Modification
		Smoker wants to quit:
		   Assess dependency for
		   appropriate program and
		   support. (See Table 11-2.)

2. **Alcohol and/or Drug Misuse**	Awareness
	Referral
	Employee Assistance
	Community
		Job performance degenerates
		Absentee pattern appears
		   (See Cage Questionnaire in
		   Table 11-3.)

B. Stress Reduction	Biofeedback Time Management Visual Imagery Exercise Humor	Company experiences changes (i.e., downsizing) Increased client visits Increased EAP utilization

C. Nutrition	General Nutrition
	Weight Management
	Low Fat/Low Cholesterol
	Cooking Demonstrations
	Nutrition Tables Interpretation
		Elevated cholesterol level
		HRA results are out of the
		   norm
		Reports of high blood
		   pressure
		Concern about weight

D. Fitness	Recreational
	Flexibility
	Strengthening
	Aerobic
		Anytime: everyone benefits
		   from exercise and activity.
		   (Recommended level assessed
		   at preplacement physical)

E. Cancer Awareness		
1. **Breast**	Cancer Awareness Breast Self-Exam Instruction Clinical Breast Exams Mammography	When worker population includes female workers who are age 20 and older
2. **Uterine**	Annual Pap Smears	
3. **Prostate** 4. **Testicular**	PSA with Digital Exam Testicular Self-Exam Instruction Clinical Testicular Exams	When worker population includes male workers who are age 20 and older
5. **Skin** 6. **Colon**	Skin Cancer Awareness Fecal Occult Blood Test Sigmoidoscopy	Anytime: All workers can benefit from this knowledge.
F. Safety	Safety Awareness/Education Driving Safety Fire Awareness Safety Carbon Monoxide Safety	Anytime: Entire worker population can benefit from this information.
G. HIV/AIDS	HIV/AIDS Awareness World AIDS Day Recognition	Anytime: All workers, particularly those at high risk can benefit from these activities. (See Table 11-5.)

1. EAPs were originally designed to deal with alcohol and substance abuse problems.
2. EAPs now address an array of problems, including family, legal, financial, interpersonal, and organizational issues (Travers & McDougall, 1995).

B. Standards for programs and professionals providing EAP services are developed by:
1. The Employee Assistance Professional Association
2. The Employee Assistance Society of North America

C. Objectives of an EAP include:
1. To effectively and efficiently provide services for ameliorating the mental health problems as well as alcoholism and other drug-related problems of the workforce
2. To identify employees with job performance problems and to respond to those seeking assistance by directing them toward the best assistance possible and providing continuing support and guidance throughout the problem-solving period
3. To serve as a resource for management and labor in intervening with employees whose personal problems affect their job performance

D. The core technology of EAPs include (Gilbert, 1994):
1. Identification of employees' behavioral problems, based on job performance
2. Provision of expert consultation to employers and managers
3. Availability and appropriate use of constructive confrontation
4. Creation and maintenance of linkages between the work organization and community resources
5. Evaluation of success in employee assistance utilization, primarily on the basis of job performance

E. Criteria for successful programs are as follows:
1. Confidentiality
2. Accessibility of voluntary self-referral with an on-site or off-site counselor
3. Ability of supervisors to identify and refer employees with problems

F. Models for EAPs include:
1. Internal programs
   a. Staffed by employees of the sponsoring agency
   b. Standard is one staff member for each 2,000 employees
   c. Advantage: familiarity with the culture of the organization
   d. Disadvantage: employee concerns about confidentiality
2. External programs
   a. Contracted by the organization
   b. Services provided by a variety of treatment centers, private companies, and other organizations
   c. Advantage: more accessible to small and medium-sized companies
   d. Disadvantage: may not provide convenient access for employees
3. Combination of internal and external programs

G. The nature of services varies among organizations (Travers & McDougall, 1995). Some organizations may:
1. Offer assessment, short-term counseling, diagnostic and referral services
2. Be available during nonbusiness hours and for crisis counseling 7 days a week, 24 hours a day
3. Assist in the development of a company's mental health policies

4. Provide employee orientation, supervisory training, and union representation
5. Offer group education programs, such as stress management, conflict resolution, parenting
6. Occasionally offer prepaid alcohol and drug rehabilitation services

H. The role of the occupational health nurse in providing employee assistance services will depend on the nature of services within the organization and on the nurse's knowledge base and educational preparation.
1. Occupational health nurses should be able to detect and recognize signs of potential psychological or emotional distress among employees; these employees should be referred as appropriate.
2. Counseling services related to lifestyle and health behaviors, personal issues, and work-related problems may be provided as part of routine care in the occupational setting; the provision of formal counseling sessions usually requires advanced preparation and credentialing in an appropriate field, such as clinical psychology.
3. Occupational health nurses should work with management to ensure that confidential and appropriate employee health services are part of a comprehensive occupational safety and health program.
4. Occupational health nurses may provide crisis intervention to employees, who are then referred to counselors in an employee assistance program.
5. Occupational health nurses may serve as liaison between the management of the company and the employee assistance program.
6. Occupational health nurses may participate in the development of the program from the assessment to the evaluation.

Introduction to Adult Education
VIII

Adult Education

A. Characteristics of adult education
1. *Adult education* is the purposeful exploration by adults of a field of knowledge, attainment of skills, or a collective reflection upon common experiences.
   a. Explorations take place in group settings.
   b. Explorations are influenced by the participants' collection of experiences, skills, and knowledge.
   c. Experiences, skills, and knowledge influence how new ideas are received, how new skills are acquired, and how experiences of others are interpreted.
2. Settings for programs include continuing education, training, networks, self-directed learning, and community activity (Brookfield, 1991).
3. The principles of adult education are vital to occupational health nurses because they provide adult populations with preventive health information and assist them to modify their lifestyle behaviors.
4. Participants of adult education are likely to have a variety of learning styles that affect their ability to acquire and retain information.
   a. Using multiple methods of presenting information will maximize the effectiveness of health education programs.
   b. Teaching styles should be adjusted to accommodate the needs of the learner; for example, older workers may require written material with large print and a setting that facilitates their ability to hear the speaker.

B. The central principles of effective adult education
   1. Participation is voluntary, with adults engaging in learning of their own volition.
   2. Facilitation is characterized by a respect among participants for each other's self worth.
   3. Facilitators and learners are engaged in a cooperative group process involving a continuous renegotiation of activities and priorities.
   4. Learners and facilitators are involved in a continual process of activity, reflection on activity, collaborative analysis of the activity, new activity, reflection, and so on.
   5. Facilitation inspires adults to appreciate that values, beliefs, behaviors, and ideologies are culturally transmitted and to critically reflect on aspects of their professional, personal, and political lives.
   6. The aim of facilitation is the nurturing of self-directed, empowered, and proactive adults (Brookfield, 1991).

C. *Self directed learning* is the process in which individuals take the initiative in designing learning experiences, diagnosing needs, locating resources, and evaluating learning for themselves (Knowles, 1975).
   1. *Contracts* written by students are the chief mechanism used to enhance self-direction and allow students to diagnose their learning needs, to plan activities, and to identify and select relevant resources.
   2. Techniques for self-directed learning involve the development of problem-solving skills to enhance students' ability to respond to typical problems and challenges.
   3. Self-directed learners rely heavily on peer learning groups for support, information exchange, stimulus of new ideas, and locating relevant resources.
   4. More time is required for extended exploration of curricular concerns, diagnosis and exploration of *felt needs* (of learners), and *prescribed needs* (by educators) and negotiation of an agreed-upon learning plan.
   5. Learners take control of their learning by becoming invested and grounded in their own concerns and circumstances (Brookfield, 1991).

D. Models for teaching adults
   1. Facilitators assist adults to meet educational needs that adults perceive and express as meaningful and important.
   2. Resource people assist adults to locate individuals and material resources to complete the learning efforts the students have defined (Brookfield, 1991).

E. Teaching involves presenting alternatives, questioning givens, and scrutinizing the self.
   1. Characteristics of effective teaching include:
      a. The ability to set an emotional atmosphere conducive to learning
      b. The ability to use learners' experiences as educational resources
      c. The provision of evaluative information to students
      d. The ability to encourage collaboration and participation
   2. The best teaching methods for self-directed learning include:
      a. Leading discussions that present intellectual challenges in a non-threatening setting
      b. Forming peer learning groups to experiment with ideas
      c. Encouraging the expression of opinions and alternative interpretations
      d. Providing lectures, demonstrations, independent study, and programmed computer learning

F. Adult educational programs are series of learning experiences designed to achieve, in a limited period of time, certain specific instructional objectives (Brookfield, 1991); overall planning includes:

1. Identifying the gaps between the learner's current and desired proficiencies
2. Assessing learning needs by the use of questionnaires, conducting individual interviews, observation of participants, or consulting with experts
3. Using behavioral objectives to state the intended outcome or proficiency level the learner should obtain as a result of participating in the educational experience. (See Table 11-7.)

TABLE 11-7

American Association of Occupational Health Nurses, Inc.
Behavioral Objectives

A behavioral objective states what the learner will be able to do on completion of a continuing education activity. A behavioral objective identifies the terminal behavior or outcome of the program.

Objectives are critical to continuing education activity development because they: 1) reflect input from learners relative to educational needs; 2) determine the selection of content and teaching methods; and 3) provide a guide to the evaluation phase.

Be sure that all written objectives:
• use verbs that describe an ACTION that can be OBSERVED
• are measurable within the teaching time frame
• consist of only one action verb per objective
• describe the learner outcome, not the instructor's process or approach
• are appropriate for the designated teaching method(s)

Behavioral Terms to Use			
apply*	define	distinguish	relate
analyze*	demonstrate*	explain	repeat
choose	describe	identify	revise*
compare	design*	list	select
compile*	develop*	outline	state
conduct*	differentiate	name	summarize
critique*	discuss	recall	synthesize*

*Use these action verbs with teaching methods that involve participants beyond a lecture/discussion approach, e.g., return skills demonstration, written/group exercises, etc.

Avoid using words that describe mental responses that cannot be measured, or terms that are broad, vague, difficult to measure, and permit a variety of interpretation.

Nonbehavioral Terms to Avoid		
appreciate	enjoy	perceive
be acquainted with	gain a working knowledge of	recognize
be aware of	grasp the significance of	remember
be familiar with	have knowledge of	sympathize with
comprehend	increased interest in	think
develop an appreciation of	know	understand
develop conceptual thinking	learn	

Source: Printed with permission of the American Association of Occupational Health Nurses

4. Developing a plan that considers the objectives, outcomes, characteristics of the learner, size of the group, available times, equipment, facilities, and budget
5. Evaluating the program in terms of attainment of behaviors
   - *Summative* evaluations are used to justify the program and focus on the program's worth and impact on the outcomes (a cost-benefit analysis, for example).
   - *Formative* evaluations focus on the procedures in the programs and are used for decision making to make improvements in the program (standardized tests and inventories, for example).

IX

Philosophies of Adult Education

Adult educators' philosophies and systems of beliefs develop from values, principles, and experience.

A. Personal values will affect adult educators' approaches to program development.

B. Adult educators should develop and employ a working philosophy of adult education:
   1. To provide a point of reference upon which to base activities
   2. To help avoid pitfalls in strategy development

C. Recognized philosophies that can guide the adult educator include (see Table 11-8):
   - Liberalism: Knowledge is transmitted from expert to novice.
   - Humanism: Knowledge is acquired voluntarily based on individual needs and is self-directed, experimental, self-evaluated, and facilitative.
   - Progressivism: Knowledge is accumulated experimentally by use of one's senses and interaction with the world.
   - Behaviorism: Knowledge is provided by use of scientific method and through programmed learning.
   - Radicalism: Knowledge is gained through dialogue, dialectical process of reflection and action, problem posing, and critical thinking.
   - Deconstruction: Knowledge is achieved through linguistic-literary analysis, by constructing individual reality, using dialectical process of reflection and action, problem posing, and critical thinking

D. Eclectic approaches can be developed either by selecting certain elements of identified theories or by adopting one particular theory and building on it.

E. It is advantageous for adult educators to utilize some philosophical or systematic approach in their practice (Ward, 1993; Zinn, 1990).

F. Some concerns in adult education are the objectives of the program, needs of participants, curriculum, program content, analysis of the teaching/learning process, and the relationship of the education to the community in which the education takes place.

X

Motivating Adults to Learn

Motivation is the concept that explains why people behave as they do.

A. Adults and motivation
   1. When adults are motivated to learn, they work harder, learn more, have a sense of enjoyment and achievement, and want to continue to learn (Wlodkowski, 1993).
   2. Motivation is not controlled by teachers but can be stimulated, influenced, and effected by them.

text continues on page 251

TABLE 11-8

Adult Education Philosophies: Comparative Analysis and Summary Evaluation (CASE) of Philosophies

Philosophies

Analytical Components	Liberalism	Humanism	Progressivism	Behaviorism	Radicalism	Deconstruction
Origins	Circa, 4th Century B.C... Ancient Greeks, rise of Republic-Democratic state, classic ideals, Judeo-Christian, and western origins	16th Century Western origins (Greco-Roman) and Eastern influences (Buddhism and Confucianism), 18th century enlightenment and existentialism of 20th century	16th century European rationalist, empirical and scientific thought, 19th Century pragmatism/romanticism, and the industrial revolution	18th Century Darwinism, scientific realism, positivism, rise of empiricism, and 20th Century school of American psychology	Anarchists of 1800's, the Freudian left, Marxists, Socialists, Christianity, liberation theology, radical feminism, labor movement, and existentialism	Radical-analytic concepts initiated in France—gained increased notice in U.S. (intellectual circles) in 1970s, 1980s and 1990s
Purposes	To enlighten the citizenry, to pursue absolute truth, to attain wisdom, to foster development of individual as good virtuous being, and to support a democratic society	To enhance personal growth, self-fulfillment and development of the whole person, and to achieve individual autonomy	To develop individual abilities and social consciousness, to foster a practical understanding of the world, and to maintain the democratic state while promoting social reform	To control overt behavior of the organism and to scientifically condition individuals to operate within their environment	To develop the process by which revolutionary personal, political, social, and economic changes are brought about	To construct reality in terms of the individual acting within a specific socio-political climate, and to construct and critically approach reality
Instructional Strategies	Knowledge is transmitted from expert to novice: Socratic method (discussion and dialogue-problem posing and response) lecture and classical readings	Knowledge is acquired voluntarily based on individual needs; and is self-directed, experimental, self-evaluated and facilitative	Knowledge is accumulated experimentally by use of one's senses and interaction with world, experience, by scientific methods, and by problem solving techniques	Knowledge is provided by use of scientific method, and through programmed learning: using strict sequence of stimulus and response to reinforce desired behaviors and to extinguish the undesirable	Knowledge is gained through dialogue, dialectical process of reflection and action, problem posing, and critical thinking	Knowledge is achieved through linguistic literary analysis, by constructing individual reality, using dialectical process of reflection and action, problem posing and critical thinking
Teacher/Learner Relationship	Vertical: Pedagogical (pedantic)	More horizontal than vertical: A collaborative facilitative process	More horizontal than vertical: a reciprocal process	Vertical: Teacher controlled and directed	Horizontal: Teacher-Learner equality	Vertical: Learner focused
Relationship Between Individual, Society and State	Education is to produce an informed citizenry supportive of the democratic state	Education is to develop self-actualized citizenry who will indirectly support democratic state	Education is to focus on individual-social development which will generally support the democratic state and will directly influence social changes.	Education is to be used to control the environment so as to direct the behavior of individuals within society thereby supporting the current controlling systems in authority	Education is to produce socially and politically aware individuals who are capable of bringing about social and political change in existing governing systems	Education is concerned with the development of the individual's critical thinking and with the exposure of oppression, and in turn, political action to bring about changes in existing governing/ruling systems.

(continued)

TABLE 11-8

Adult Education Philosophies: Comparative Analysis and Summary Evaluation (CASE) of Philosophies (continued)

Philosophies

Analytical Components	Liberalism	Humanism	Progressivism	Behaviorism	Radicalism	Deconstruction
Relationship to Political and Economic Systems	Highly subject to political climate and economic conditions, i.e. in last century and a half, government has supported need of productive workhorse rather then enlightened populace	Political/economic climate does not substantially affect humanistic programs inasmuch as most are individual and small group matters vs. large social-political movements	Political/economic climate may have substantial effect on support of social reforms which may have an effect and be affected by politics	Politics and economics play a significant role in the design of the state, which, in turn, directly affects overt behavior	Highly affected and may significantly affect politics and economy which are critical elements in social change	Political and economic forms are tool of critical analysis which may, in turn, affect political and economic forms
Representative Proponents and Movements	Socrates, Plato, Augustine, Thomas Aquinas, Thomas Jefferson, Everett Dean Martin, and Jacques Maritain Franklin's Junto, founding of early American Universities, lyceums, Chautauqua, university extension programs, Great Books Program, and Elderhostel	Maslow, Rogers, May, Tough, McKenzie, and Brookfield Human potential seminars, encounter-type groups, training groups (T-groups) Knowles' andragogy, counseling, self-directed learning projects	John Dewey, Eduard Lindeman, Benne, Bergevin and Jane Addams Settlement houses in urban areas for Immigrants; land grant universities, Cooperative Extension Service, citizenship education and community development, community colleges, adult basic education, and vocational education	J. B. Watson, E. L. Thorndike, and B. F. Skinner Binary computer programs and skills, programmed learning, competency based education, and behavior modification	Ivan Illich, John Ohlinger, Paulo Freire, Gramsci, Habermas, and Mezirow Horton's Highlander Folk School, Freire's literacy training used in Third World countries, and popular education	Jacques Derrida, Paul de Man, J. Harris Miller, Barbara Johnson, Stanley Fish, Annabel Patterson and Jane Tompkins Cultural diversity and pluralism
Criticisms	Anti-vocational stance, often considered elitist, oppressive, and ethnocentric	Normlessness, lack of standards for learning process, no accountability, and exaggerated emphasis on learner's needs	Experiential learning alone may be inadequate, anti-intellectualism and indefinite role of teacher	Big Brothers Image; Individual has no control over external forces, individual is a pawn; discounts higher cognitive processes, reductionistic, and dehumanizing, discounts faith, emotion, and beliefs	Belief that revolutionary approach is only method to change society; challenges all aspects of culture and its structures, polarizes relationships between oppressors and the oppressed	All western values are intrinsically oppressive; only political action can free people from dominant ideology or hegemony, oppressive unyielding—totally negates absolutes: all is relative, and anti-liberal stance
Contributions	Significant influence in mainstream adult education; instrumental in development of early American universities numerous adult education programs and other institutions	Strong emphasis on individual learner and self development, instrumental in providing adult education with a more humane face; and strong force in adult education	Significant role in social movement and reforms fostered integration of immigrants into society focused attention on experiential learning and scientific methodology	Developments in programmed learning, contract learning, behavior modification programs, accountability; competency-based education, extensive use in continuing professional education and in training and development	Significant role in raising critical consciousness and producing social change	Emphasis on critical examination of language, recognition of various cultural groups, and acknowledgment of diversity

Synopsis developed from Dr. Nancy E. Hagan, "Philosophy and Adult Education" by Robert M. Ward

B. Instructors who are able to motivate
  1. Are experts who know beneficial information, can explain it well, and are prepared to convey their knowledge through instruction
  2. Use motivation to arouse behavior, give direction or purpose to behavior, cause behavior to persist, and influence the learner to choose a particular behavior
  3. Have a realistic understanding of the needs and expectations of adults that influence their motivation to learn
  4. Teach in a manner that expresses care for the learner and knowledge of the subject, together with the intent to encourage similar feelings in the learner
  5. Present instructional material in a logical and orderly manner thus providing clarity to difficult and new information (Wlodkowski, 1993).

C. Motivating factors are defined as follows:
  1. An *attitude* is a combination of concepts, information, and emotions that result in a predisposition to respond favorably or unfavorably to particular people, groups, ideas, events, and objectives.
       a. Attitudes may be acquired through experience, direct instruction, or identification of role behavior.
       b. Attitudes can be modified by a new experience.
  2. A *need* is a condition experienced by the individual as an internal (*intrinsic*) or external (*extrinsic*) force that leads the person to move in the direction of a goal; identifying and addressing the learner's needs will enhance motivation.
  3. *Stimulation* is any change in perception or experience with the environment that makes people active; it sustains adult learning behavior; attention, interest, and involvement are goals for learner participation.
  4. An *affect* is the emotional experience of feeling, concerns, and passions that influence behaviors; when appropriate, the instructor should relate content and instructional procedures to learner concerns.
  5. *Competence* and *self-confidence* are motivating forces in learning; consistent feedback to learners regarding their mastery, progress, and responsibility will enhance their learning.
  6. *Reinforcement* is a positive or negative response to an individual's behavior that affects the probability of the behavior's recurrence (Wlodkowski, 1993).

XI

Teaching Methods and Techniques
(See Table 11-9.)

A. Learning contract: a formal agreement written by learner detailing conditions of learning, including timelines and written evaluation

B. Lecture: a planned oral discourse on a particular subject by a qualified person

C. Discussion: an exchange of ideas between teacher and learner about subjects and issues

D. Mentorship: an informal role in which the teaching function is primarily a means to advancement and secondarily a contribution to the learner

E. Case study: an in-depth study of a representative problem or situation

F. Demonstration: a presentation showing how something works and the procedures followed when using it

G. Simulation: a method of obtaining skills, competence, or knowledge by participating in activities similar to a real life activity of interest

text continues on page 256

TABLE 11-9
Teaching Methods and Techniques

	Definition	Purpose	Specifics	Advantages	Limitations
Learning Contracts	Formal agreement written by learner detailing what will be learned, how learning will be accomplished, timeline, and written evaluation	Individualizes the learning process	Components include objectives, resources and strategies, target dates for completion, evidence of accomplishment and evaluation strategies	Flexible; learners control the process; preferred methods.	Uncomfortable for learners and teacher if not used before; learners question quality of learning; teacher placed at risk for excess time pressures
Lecture	A planned oral discourse on a particular subject by a highly qualified individual	Cognitive transfer of information from teacher; framework for learning activities; identifies, explains, and clarifies different concepts, problems or ideas; challenges beliefs, attitudes, and behaviors; and stimulates the audience to further inquiry	Preparation includes preplanning, organization, compliance with time constraints, handouts and practice	Precise and orderly format; popular; useful when no handouts; use for large groups; forum for one on one and enhances listening	Audience is exposed to one view; biased information may be given; discourages learners from the teaching, learning interaction; not able to determine impact on audience; speaker not know audience level of knowledge or experience; evaluated on entertainment value rather than content
Discussion	Allows learners and teacher to talk about subjects and issues	Allows cognitive and affective exploration of issues	Prepare by setting discussion themes; providing resource materials; evoking consensual rules; personalizing discussion topics; and attending to group composition	Most favored, inclusive, and participatory	May uncover emotional issues which may need to be dealt with before further learning can take place
Mentorship	Designates an informal role in which the teaching function is recognized primarily as a means to personal and institutional advancement and only secondarily as contribution to the overall well-being of the protégé	Promotes the development of the learner	Role of the mentor involves being supportive, challenging, and visionary	Promotes critical thinking; develops personal power and independence; provides a role model	Provides an environment where power may be misused, emotional dependence fostered and favoritism practiced. Hero worship, values conflicts and feelings of abandonment may be experienced
Case Study	An in-depth study of a problem or situation	Presents real life examples for study	Types include: case reports, analysis, and discussion. Design the study by focusing on the problem; developing supporting materials; reviewing; and field testing the case	Causes critical thinking;-develops decision making; problem solving skills; and is participatory	Long preparation time; requires a facilitator to think on the spot

(continued)

252

TABLE 11-9

Teaching Methods and Techniques (continued)

	Definition	Purpose	Specifics	Advantages	Limitations
Demonstration	Presents how something works and the procedures followed in using it	Arouses interest and motivation; directs attention; supports verbal explanation; enables economical use of time and resources; and provides step by step guidelines in performing tasks or improving skills	Types include: instructional, participant volunteers, and full participation Roles Teachers must be technically expert; able to analyze process and break into small steps; and have all materials ready for use Learner must practice each step; communicate problems and practice deficiencies	Illustrates point to enable learners to comprehend complex and difficult materials in a short time; reduces gaps between the learner and practice; and provides variety to facilitate different learning styles	Discourages some learners; difficult to isolate tasks, skills, and procedures into step-by-step manuals; time consuming; uses only small groups; and limited individualized feedback
Simulation	A technique that enables learners to obtain skills, competence, or knowledge by becoming involved in activities that are similar to those in real life	An attempt to address real problems under real life conditions and discuss them; develops complex cognitive skills such as decision making, evaluating, and synthesizing; impacts the learners' values, beliefs and attitudes; induces empathy; sharpens interpersonal communication skills; and help learners unlearn negative attitudes or behaviors	Types include: role play, case study, and critical incident Steps are experience, sharing, processing, generalizing, and application Roles Facilitator should explain the purpose; give short, clear, and understandable instructions; provide relevant, real life situations; involve problem solving appropriate to the level of the learner; have adequate interaction with learners; and give appropriate feedback. Learners should participate in all activities; develop an attitude of sharing and support; have open feedback with facilitators, and apply knowledge, skills or attitudes to personal life situations	An opportunity to apply teaming to a new situation; participatory; no consequences of wrong decisions; immediate feedback; generates new ideas and changed attitudes; and is cost effective	Negative learning may occur if situation too complex; teacher must be proficient; expensive to design and conduct; and time consuming

(continued)

TABLE 11-9

Teaching Methods and Techniques (continued)

	Definition	Purpose	Specifics	Advantages	Limitations
Forum	An open discussion carried on by one or more resource persons and an entire group	Clarifies or explores information from a lecture or panel presentation; promotes audience participation by contributing ideas and opinions; stimulate discussions; and identifies community needs and interests for further programming	Participants are moderator, resource person, and audience	Informal; interactive; audience access to clarify points with speaker	Time issues may arise; audience intimidated if large group; need large facility; and need experienced moderator to handle large groups
Panel	A small group of three to six people who sit around a table in the presence of an audience and have a purposeful conversation on a topic in which they have specialized knowledge	Addresses several points of view; stimulates interest; identifies and clarifies problems and issues; and promotes a variety of informative opinions	Participants are moderator, panel members, and audience	Opportunity to hear a variety of opinions or points of views from knowledgeable speakers; informal, unrehearsed, and spontaneous results	Skilled moderator needed to direct panelists and avoid chaos; knowledgeable speakers needed
Symposium	A series of presentations given by two to five persons of notable authority on different aspects of the same themes or closely related themes	Different perspectives; helps people understand how related parts of a topic contribute to the whole topic and stimulates new thoughts and ideas on a topic	Participants are chairperson, speakers, and audience	Brings together knowledgeable speakers and audience benefits from hearing different points of view	Formal process; decreases audience participation; and may be repetitious
Computer Enhanced Education	Uses computers as an enhancement to the teacher-learner transaction	Vehicle for instruction; drill and practice; simulation and games; dialogues and programming; resources; and tools.	Develops group and individual learning opportunities; critically evaluates the needs of the learner; provides opportunities for problem solving; gives current feedback; and visual and graphic aide	Provides individually tailored programs; flexible information in a variety of sensory modems; and interactive with immediate feedback	Limited by appropriateness of software
Distance Education	Describes all teaching-learning arrangements in which the learner and teacher are normally separated by space and or by time; so that the communication between them is through print, writing, electronic media, or other interactive telecommunication	Provides access to learning for more people	Process includes study guides, interaction instruction, student support, and evaluation	Permits learning integrated with work and family life; learner controls study process; encourages reflective thinking; allows for large populations; and provides individualized learning	Learner must be able to read, write and possibly use computers; be motivated to continue to learn; have good support, feedback and follow-up processes

(continued)

TABLE 11-9
Teaching Methods and Techniques (continued)

	Definition	Purpose	Specifics	Advantages	Limitations
Nominal Group Technique	Group technique is a predesignated pattern for human instruction that offers a better potential for progress toward goals than instructed random behavior Group process is the factors which are concerned with how people learn together (the way) as contrasted to what they learn (the content)	Uses an instructional or problem solving method to facilitate learning, to meet the goals of the participants learners, and to generate, explore and communicate ideas	Develop the technique by formulating questions; generating ideas; developing a round robin listing; discussing ideas; voting on individual ideas; and tabulating the vote	Restricts the influence of the group leader; reduces the influences of dominant group members; efficient use of time	Must have well formed questions; not consensus model, group leader is limited to the role of facilitator, and limits emergence of a leader by restricting the decision making process
Brainstorming	A technic for the stimulation of creative thinking for the development of new ideas				

Adapted from Adult Learning Methods, Michael W. Galbraith (editor) (1990)

H. Forum: an open discussion with one or more resource person(s) and an entire group

I. Panel: a small group of 3 to 6 persons who have a purposeful discussion of a topic about which they have specialized knowledge; discussion is in presence of an audience

J. Symposium: a series of presentations by 2 to 5 persons of notable authority on different aspects of the same or closely related themes

K. Computer-enhanced education: use of computers as an enhancement to teacher-learner interaction

L. Distance education: communication between teacher and learner occurs through print, writing, telephone, or electronic media

M. Nominal group technique: a type of group process that emphasizes the *way* people learn as contrasted to *what* they learn

N. Brainstorming: a sharing of free-flowing ideas that is intended to stimulate creative thinking and the development of new ideas

XII

Effective Presentations

Presentations involve the preparation and delivery of critical subject matter in a logical and condensed form, leading to effective communication (Morrisey & Sechrest, 1987).

A. Elements of a presentation
   1. The goal of any presentation is effective communication, which means getting the message across in a manner that accomplishes the stated objectives.
   2. Audience needs must be identified in order to reach the goals; audience needs are the determining factor in the selection of appropriate resource materials.
   3. Meaningful content is supported by presentation aids, presentation techniques, and logistical details.

B. Types of presentations
   1. *Persuasive* or *selling* presentations pique the interest of potential participants, convince management of program approval, or sell existing customers on making changes.
   2. *Explanatory* presentations make new information available or refresh an audience's understanding of a given topic by providing a general familiarization overview or description of new development.
   3. *Instructional* presentations teach how to use something, such as a new procedure or piece of equipment.
   4. An *oral report* brings the audience up to date on a subject they already know something about, by providing details suited to the needs and interest of the audience.

C. Preparing the presentation
   1. Establish written behavioral objectives, stating specific expected results and measurable accomplishments. (See Table 11-7.)
   2. Audience analysis includes:
      a. Identification of the objectives for the audience
      b. Development of an overall approach to achieve objectives
      c. Description of the social and demographic characteristics of the audience
      d. Selection of appropriate information and techniques

3. Prepare a preliminary plan consisting of no more than five main ideas or concepts, and discuss it with the officials who are planning the event.
   a. The plan is a guide for the presenter, keeping ideas channeled, focusing on points to be emphasized, and preventing the omission of information.
   b. Know the audience: If possible, determine the number of participants, where they work, what type of work they do, and their attitudes toward the subject.
   c. Make modifications as necessary prior to the presentation.
4. Select resource information to determine the purpose of the presentation material to be covered and the level of detail needed to meet the audience's needs.
   Questions to be answered:
   • What is the purpose of this presentation?
   • What do the participants expect and need from this presentation?
   • What should be covered? What should be eliminated?
   • What amount of detail is necessary?
   • Will members of the audience have limitations that require adjustments? (e.g., physical disabilities, language limitations, illiteracy, or other barriers to learning)
   • What can be withheld from the presentation but offered as a resource?
5. Organize the materials into the introduction, body, and conclusion of the presentation.
   a. The introduction should include:
      • A direct statement concerning the subject of the presentation and its importance
      • Some audience interest linked to the subject
      • Examples leading directly to the subject
      • Strong quotations related to the subject
      • Important statistics that emphasize a point
      • Strong or anecdotal information illustrating the subject
   b. The body of the presentation should consider:
      • Visual illustrations as important aids to support the content
      • Reiteration, statistics, comparisons, analogies, and expert testimony to present the main ideas
   c. The conclusion should consist of:
      • A summary of the main ideas
      • A review of the purpose of the presentation
      • An appeal for audience action
6. Practice the presentation aloud to yourself; or videotape or audiotape the practice session; or give a pilot presentation.
7. Evaluation
   a. Evaluation is a critical component in assessing the effectiveness and efficiency of a program intervention in achieving a predetermined objective.
   b. Evaluations cannot be accomplished without taking into account people and their environments.
   c. By using the planning process data, measurable objectives, and program participants, a meaningful evaluation can be undertaken (Morrisey & Sechrest, 1987).
D. Development and utilization of audiovisuals
   1. People retain about 30% of what they hear; about 20% of what they see; and about 50% of what they both hear and see; visual aids are used in a presentation to facilitate learning.

TABLE 11-10

Specific Media Tools

	Definition	Advantages	Disadvantages
Overhead Projector	An electric device designed to project transparent materials as large as 10 by 10 inches and as small as 2 by 2 inches.	The projected image is visible in a lighted room and transparencies are made inexpensively	Teachers must be able to talk and use transparencies simultaneously; and machines require electric outlet and bulb.
Slides	A small piece of film on which a single pictorial graphic image has been placed for still projection	Convenient to use, easy to obtain in high quality, relatively inexpensive, easy to use with no more than 5 to 6 lines per slide, and can be made from anything that is drawn, painted, written, typewritten, printed or photographed.	Slides must be viewed in a darkened room; each presentation requires filing, storage and organizing slides
Video	Motion on tape shown on a television monitor with sound	Provides a common stimulus for students, with specific examples which achieve identification and involvement of the viewer with characters and situations presented	Expensive; not all information being presented may be consistent with what is being presented; must be shown in a darkened room and equipment often fails
Flip Charts	A series of bound sheets of paper or posterboard that can be flipped over, one at a time, to show a series of thoughts, pictures, outline points, questions, cartoons or symbols	Portable, economical and versatile; can be prepared ahead of time and used repeatedly.	Not useful with large audiences; do not store easily; and good handwriting skills are needed to develop
Handouts	Printed or duplicated material given to learners, such as outlines, job descriptions, bulletins, cartoons, charts, and problems	Allows learners to receive the same information and to be able to review or reference after presentation	A supplement not substitute for presentation and may distract from the main point, or confuse the learner
Audio Recorder	Recorded sound on a magnetic tape	Flexible timing and interruption of instruction; inexpensive, reusable and easy to use; and tape is useful in large and small groups	Poorly prepared or used materials may distract or discourage learners
Chalkboard	A board whose writing surface is specially treated for use with chalk	Minimal cost; allows for spontaneity; audience involvement; and on the spot revisions	Not a permanent record with limited use in a large group
Models	Scaled representation, which may be equal in size, smaller or larger than original	A model shows clearly and quickly "how" and "why" something works and permits close up observation, investigation, and analysis	Commercial models are costly to purchase; require large storage space, special atmospheric conditions or extreme care in handling

Adapted from *Effective Business and Technical Presentations*, G. L. Morrisey and T. L. Sechrest

2. Characteristics of effective visual aids are as follows:
      a. They each represent one key concept.
      b. They are appropriate to the audience.
      c. Text is restricted to a maximum of 6 words per line and 10 lines per visual, consisting of short phrases and key words rather than complete sentences.
      d. They use color or contrast to highlight important points.
      e. They represent facts accurately.
      f. They should be checked for spelling and accuracy; they can be unconvincing if inaccurate or misspelled.
   3. To maintain quality, the presentation should contain no more than one visual for every two minutes of presentation time; the presentation, not the visuals, should be the center of attention.
   4. Guidelines for using media include: visibility or audibility, ease of operation, and accessibility.
      a. Consider room size, number of people, any distracting noises, seating arrangement, visual obstacles, and lighting.
      b. Organize the equipment before the presentation; arrange presentation components in sequence, and designate someone to help with lighting, if needed.
      c. Select aids based on availability, cost, and convenience.
   5. Specific tools used in teaching include: overhead projector, slides, video, flip charts, handouts, audio recorder, chalkboards, and models. (See Table 11-10 for advantages and disadvantages of each.)
   6. Aids to further understanding (*Note:* When using any of the aids listed in this section, it is important to consider that all nonoriginal material may be subject to copyright.)
      a. The purpose of a *chart* is to direct thinking; clarify points; summarize; show trends, relationships, and comparisons. There are numerous types of charts (see Table 11-11).

TABLE 11-11

Types of Charts

- *Highlight charts* present a direct copy or emphasize a point.
- *Time sequence charts* show relationships over a period of time.
- *Organizational charts* indicate the relationships among individuals, departments, and jobs.
- *Cause-and-effect charts* illustrate causal relationships.
- *Flow charts* show the relation of parts to the finished whole or to the direction of movement of a process (e.g., PERT [Program Evaluation and Review Technique] charts).
- *Inventory charts* show a picture of an object with its parts labeled off to the side.
- *Dissection charts* present enlarged, transparent, or cut-away views of an object.
- *Diagrammatic* or *schematic charts* provide a simple portrayal of a complex subject by means of symbols.
- *Multibar graphs* represent comparable data using horizontal or vertical bars.
- *Divided-bar graphs* show the relation of parts to the whole by using a single bar divided into parts by lines.
- *Line graphs* display information using a horizontal scale and a vertical scale.
- *Pie graphs* show relations of parts to the whole, like a divided-bar graph.
- *Pictographs* represent comparable quantities in a given time by use of symbols such as a stack of coins representing comparable costs

Source: Morrisey & Sechrest, (1987).

b. *Illustrations, diagrams,* and *maps* clarify points, emphasize trends, get attention, or show relationships or differences.

c. *Exhibits* show finished products, demonstrate the results of good and bad practices, attract attention, arouse and hold interest, and adequately illustrate an idea.

d. *Manuals, pamphlets, outlines,* and *bulletins* provide standard information and guidelines as well as reference and background material.

e. *Cartoons, posters,* and *signs* attract attention, arouse interest and often promote critical thinking.

f. *Photographs* and *illustrations* from textbooks or magazines tie the discussion to actual situations and people, illustrate the immediate relevance of a topic, or show local activities.

g. *Examples* and *stories* relieve tension, fix an idea, get attention, illustrate a point, clarify a situation, or break away from a delicate subject.

h. *Field trips* present a subject in its natural setting, stimulate interest, blend theory with practical application, and provide additional material for study (Morrisey & Sechrest, 1987).

E. Logistics: preparing for a presentation

1. Invite the audience to the presentation by letter, memo, phone call, formal announcement, electronic mail, or word of mouth.

2. Room set-up options depend on the size and shape of the meeting room, size and nature of the audience, type of presentation, delivery method, and kind of participation wanted from the audience; options include the following:

a. *Auditorium* style is used for large groups when there is no need for the audience to write or consult reference materials and when audience participation is limited to a question-and-answer period; generally, no tables or writing areas are available for participants.

b. *Classroom* style is useful for relatively formal situations where participants need to write or actively use reference materials; then, tables or desks are provided.

c. *Horseshoe,* or U-shaped, style is useful when eye contact with the audience and relatively informal discussions are desirable and participants may write or use materials easily; this is most desirable for small groups.

d. *Buzz* style is useful when small-group discussions are conducted as part of the presentation; these discussions can be held easily at small tables distributed around in the room.

e. *Chevron* or *herringbone* style is useful for group discussions, creating a more formal climate than buzz style and a less formal climate than classroom style; rectangular tables are preferred.

f. *T-shape, hollow square,* and *conference* styles are useful if no instructor or audiovisual aids are used (Hau & Hau, 1994).

3. Equipment that may be needed includes a table for projection equipment, extension cords, spare bulbs, flip chart, and markers.

4. Always check equipment, room temperature, and lighting; put slides, transparencies, and handouts in order; hide displays that should be out of sight before presentation; number transparencies or slides in order in case they become mixed up.

5. Coordinate arrangements at the presentation site by giving clear instructions regarding the specific needs; arrange for shipping materials in advance; arrive early to prepare the room; and always know how to operate equipment personally.

6. Announce "housekeeping" details before the presentation begins: rules regarding smoking, eating, or drinking; restroom locations; time and location of breaks; and registration requirements (Morrisey & Sechrest, 1987).

F. Deliver the presentation
1. Effective communication is a two-way process, involving both the speaker and the listener, that leads to some form of action or response.
2. In the communication process, the listener is the more important of the two members.
3. Platform techniques such as eye contact with the audience, appropriate dress, confidence, and relaxed hand movements are important behaviors to exhibit.
   a. Gestures can be effective if they are properly synchronized with certain words or phrases and are not overused.
   b. Body movements are effective in releasing some of the speakers' tension, drawing attention back to the speaker from the visual aid, and changing the pace of the presentation.
   c. Facial expressions should be lively, varied, and appropriate to the mood of the audience.
   d. Concentrate on reducing distracting mannerisms such as lip licking, nose patting, ear tugging, stretching, or playing with pens, rubber bands, or paper clips.
4. Develop good voice quality: a natural, conversational pitch and inflection; a level of volume that can be heard by all; a rate and tempo that varies enough to maintain the audience's interest; and deliberate pauses, used as needed.
   a. "Uh" results when the thought process interrupts the speech process and is eliminated with increased familiarity with the subject.
   b. Trailing sentences or loss of voice at the end of sentences lose the audience.
   c. Faulty pronunciation and poor enunciation can be corrected by checking the dictionary for correct pronunciations and by adopting a manner of speaking that is clear, precise, and easy to listen to.
5. Tools facilitate the delivery of a speaker's message.
   a. A *lectern* provides a surface on which notes may be placed; provides an out-of-sight storage space for aids and handouts; gives a resting place for hands; establishes a type of relationship with the audience.
      • Remaining behind the lectern establishes a formal relation with the audience.
      • Moving to the side or front of the lectern removes the barriers and is less formal.
   b. The *pointer* draws attention to specific items on a visual aid and should be put down when not in use.
   c. The *podium* or *lavaliere microphones* should be used in practice until the presenter is speaking comfortably in a natural voice and with equipment at the proper height or on the lapel close to the mouth.
6. Learning to deal with audiences' questions is a vital skill for presenters.
   a. Conducting question-and-answer sessions involves accepting the question as a compliment from the participant, being prepared for possible questions, paraphrasing the question to ensure that everyone understands it, making the question relevant to the discussion, and trying to give a correct answer.
   b. Dealing with some difficult situations requires experience.
      • Arguments should be postponed until after the session, since they limit the participation of the rest of the audience.

- "Curves" or "loaded" questions may be intended to put the speaker on the spot, so end the discussion quickly and move on.
- Long-winded questioners should be handled by picking out a word or an idea that is being expressed and show its relationship to the presentation; or as a last resort only, cut the questioner off in the interest of time.
- The audience grows tired very quickly of a questioner who takes over to make a speech; the presenter should take control of the situation by asking the questioner to ask the question and then move on.
- A question may come up for which the speaker has no answer; in that case, the speaker should admit it and ask the group if they have an answer (Morrisey & Sechrest, 1987).

G. Always finish the presentation or program by evaluating the process and content.
1. Allow participants to rate the instructor.
2. Participants should evaluate whether the program addressed the stated goals and objectives as well as their own personal objectives.
3. Participants should be evaluated to determine the knowledge they gained during the presentation; this could be done using a pre-test, post-test format.

BIBLIOGRAPHY

Anspaugh, D. J., Hamrick, M. K., & Rosato, F. D. (1994). *Wellness concepts and applications* (5th ed.). St. Louis: Mosby-Year Book, Inc.

Ajzen, I. (1988). *Attitudes, personality, and behavior.* Milton Keynes: Open University Press.

Bandura, A. (1986). *Social foundations of thought and action: A social cognitive theory.* Englewood Cliffs, NJ: Prentice-Hall.

Brookfield, S. D. (1991). *Understanding and facilitating adult learning.* San Francisco: Jossey-Bass, Inc.

Chopra, D. (1994). *Perfect Weight.* New York: Harmony Books.

Elias, J. L., & Merriam, S. (1994). *Philosophical foundation of adult education* (Rev. ed.). Malabar, FL: Krieger Publishing Company.

Flynn, T. J., & Manley, M. W. (1990, April). *How to help your patients stop smoking.* American Cancer Society/National Cancer Institute. (NIHP No. 90-3064).

Galbraith, M. W. (Ed.). (1990) *Adult learning methods.* Malabar, FL: Krieger Publishing Company.

Gilbert, B. (1994). Employee assistance programs: History and program description. *AAOHN Journal, 42*(10), 488–493.

Green, L., & Krueter, M. (1991). *Health promotion planning: An educational and environmental approach.* Mountain View, CA: Mayfield Publishing Company.

Gustafson, M. B., & Corcoran, S. A. (1978). *Teachers' Desk Reference.* Oradell, NJ: Medical Economics Company.

Hau, M. L., & Hau, K. A. (1994). *In control . . . So now you're a trainer.* Chicago: Health Products Marketing, Inc.

Hoff, R. (1988). *I can see you naked.* Kansas City: Andrews and McMeel.

Knowles, M. S. (1975). *Self-directed learning: A guide for learners and teachers.* New York: Cambridge Books.

Leavell, H., & Clark, E. (1965). *Preventive medicine for the doctor in the community.* New York: McGraw Hill.

Morrisey, G. L., & Sechrest, T. L. (1987). *Effective business and technical presentations* (3rd ed.). Reading, MA: Addison-Wesley Publishing Co., Inc.

O'Donnell, M. D. (1989). Definition of health promotion: Part III: Expanding the definition. *American Journal of Health Promotion, 3*(3), 5.

O'Donnell, M. D., & Harris, J. (1994). *Health promotion in the workplace* (2nd ed.). New York: Delmar Publishers, Inc.

Ozmon, H., & Craver, S. (1990). *Philosophical foundations of education* (4th ed.). Columbus, OH: Merrill Publishing Company.

Pender, N. (1996). *Health promotion in nursing practice* (3rd ed.). Stamford, CT: Appleton & Lange.

Prentice-Dunn, S., & Rogers, R. W. (1986). Protection motivation theory and preventive health: Beyond the health belief model. *Health education research: Theory and practice 1*, (3) 153–161.

Prochaska, J. O., & DiClemente, C. C. (1983). Stages and processes of self-change of smoking: Towards an integrative model of change. *Journal of Consulting and Clinical Psychology 51*(3), 390–395.

Rogers, B. (1994). *Occupational health nursing concepts and practice*. Philadelphia: W.B. Saunders Company.

Rosenstock, I. M. (1990). The health belief model: Explaining health behavior through expectancies. In *Health behavior and health education: Theory, research, and practice*. San Francisco: Jossey-Bass.

Schwanzer, R. (1992). Adaptation and maintenance of health behaviors: A critical review of theoretical approaches. In Schwanzer, R. (Ed.), *Self-efficacy: Thought control of action*. New York: Hemisphere.

Selleck, C., Sirles, A., & Newman, K. (1989). Health promotion at the workplace. *AAOHN Journal, 37*(10), 412–422.

Travers, P. H., & McDougall, C. (1995). Guidelines for an occupational health & safelty service. Atlanta: AAOHN Publications.

Triandis, H.C. (1980). Values, attitudes, and interpersonal behavior. In M. N. Page (Ed.), Nebraska Symposium on Motivation, 1979. Lincoln, NE: University of Nebraska Press.

United States Department of Health and Human Services (1991). *Healthy people 2000: National health promotion and disease prevention objectives* (DHHS Publication No. 91-50212, pp. 94–110). Washington, DC: U.S. Government Printing Office.

United States Department of Health and Human Services (1995). *Healthy people 2000: Midcourse review and 1995 revisions* (Stock No. 017-001-00-56-5). Washington, DC: U.S. Government Printing Office.

Wachs, J., & Parker-Conrad, J. (1990). Occupational health nursing in 1990 and the coming decade. *Applied Occupational and Environmental Hygiene, 5*(4), 200–203.

Ward, R. M. (1993). Adult education philosophies. Developed from Hagan, N. E., Philosophy and adult education. Unpublished data.

Wlodkowski, R. J. (1993). *Enhancing adult motivation to learn*. San Francisco: Jossey-Bass, Inc.

Woolf, S. H. (1996). What not to do and why. In S. H. Woolf, S. Jonas, & R. S. Lawrence (Eds.). *Health promotion and disease prevention in clinical practice* (Rev. ed.) (pp. 448–463). Baltimore, MD: Williams & Wilkins.

Woolf, S.H., & Lawrence, R.S. (1996). The physical examination: Where to look for preclinical disease. In S. H. Woolf, S. Jonas, & R. S. Lawrence (Eds.). *Health promotion and disease prevention in clinical practice* (pp. 49–84). Baltimore, MD: Williams & Wilkins.

Zinn, L. M. (1990). Identifying your philosophical orientation. In M. W. Galbraith (Ed.), *Adult learning methods* (pp. 59–78). Malabar, FL: Krieger Publishing Company.

12

Examples of Occupational Health and Safety Programs

MAJOR TOPICS

- *International travel health and safety program*
- *Case management program*
- *Hearing conservation program*
- *Hazard communication program*
- *Drug and alcohol testing program*
- *Emergency preparedness/disaster plan*

This chapter describes selected samples of occupational health and safety programs that can be used as models in a variety of work settings. The basic template can be applied to most any kind of worksite program. Some of the programs are mandated by law (Hearing Conservation, Hazard Communication, Drug and Alcohol Testing); others may be of interest to specific industries or businesses (International Travel Health and Safety, Emergency Preparedness/Disaster Plan). The section on Case Management describes a program useful to all occupational health nurses who manage worker illnesses and injuries (work-related and non-work-related) as well as return-to-work programs.

International Travel Health and Safety Program

As the world economy becomes more global, an increasing number of companies are conducting a portion of their business in foreign countries. As a result, the international business traveler may be exposed to illnesses or threats to personal safety during travel to foreign countries. The travel health and safety program described in this section provides guidelines that can be used by the occupational health nurse to reduce the risk to the personal health and safety of the traveler.

I

The Purposes of the Program

The purposes of a travel health and safety program are to prepare workers for travel, provide recommendations, assure fitness for work, prevent illness, provide appropriate vaccinations, and ensure, to the greatest extent possible, the personal safety of the travelers.

II

Employer's Responsibilities

The responsibilities of management to traveling employees include:

A. Develop travel policies and procedures, including emergency evacuation or escape protocols.

B. Provide travel health and safety information appropriate to the traveler's destination.

C. Request security information from destination hotels or other accommodations (deadbolts and view holes on doors, fire safety, 24-hour security, safety-deposit boxes, etc.).

D. Provide the resources for medications, supplies, vaccinations, and counseling necessary for the traveler's health and safety.

E. Identify resources at the traveler's destination for health or safety emergencies.

III

Traveler's Responsibilities

The responsibilities of the traveler include the following:

A. Maintain a current passport and obtain visa and other necessary documents.

B. Ensure that adequate time is available for administration of vaccines prior to departure, usually 4 to 6 weeks.

C. Prepare a travel itinerary and leave a copy with family and office staff.

D. Confirm travel arrangements (tickets, hotel accommodations, car rental, etc.)

E. Review and follow all safety procedures recommended in the travel policy and procedure manual.

F. Prepare a list of phone numbers where the traveler can be contacted and names of people whom the traveler can contact in case of an emergency.

IV

Nurse's Responsibilities

The responsibilities of the occupational health nurse include the following:

A. Obtain a health history.
1. Determine significant illnesses, injuries, or current health problems.
2. Identify health risks that may prohibit travel, such as diabetes, pregnancy, or heart disease.
3. List any scars or permanent identifying marks on the body in case identity of the traveler needs to be confirmed.
4. Review any health problems encountered during previous travel or as a result of previous travel.
5. List all current medication (prescription and nonprescription).
6. Review current health and dental status and provide appropriate interventions or referrals.
7. List all allergies (to medication, food, plants, insects, vaccines, and others).

B. Determine and provide for appropriate immunizations.
1. Elicit current status of immunizations.
2. Determine which vaccines are required or recommended for the traveler's destination.
3. Provide appropriate vaccines or resources to obtain those vaccines.
4. Report adverse vaccine reactions to the local health authorities.

C. Conduct a physical examination and, if appropriate, determine any health risk prior to travel assignment.

D. Conduct testing for the human immunovirus (HIV) if required for entry, identify blood type, and perform chest x-ray if traveler will be living abroad.

E. Review special considerations for the traveler, such as pregnancy or recent surgery.

F. Refer the worker for treatment of travel-related problems and follow up on recommendations.

V

Health and Safety Education for Travel

A. Issues related to the safety of the traveler

1. Since business travelers usually travel alone, discuss personal safety, such as avoiding drawing attention to oneself as a "business traveler"; advise traveling in casual attire and being alert to surrounding activities.

2. Provide current information on the political and social climate of the traveler's destination, such as risk of terrorism, kidnapping, theft, and crime. (See Table 12-1 for list of resources.)

3. Encourage using travelers' checks or bank cards instead of carrying large sums of currency.

4. Discuss methods to reduce risk of theft of important documents and personal property.

5. Review the travelers itinerary, including:
   a. The length of stay at each destination
   b. The type of work to be performed (office versus field work)
   c. Specific hazards associated with the work to be done
   d. Type of accommodations (housing, utilities, services)

B. Business travel and stress: Business travel differs from tourism because individuals traveling for business reasons are under higher stress due to job performance requirements, tight schedules, sudden departures, separation from family and home, and increased fear of kidnapping and terrorism.

1. Considerations for short-term assignments
   a. Discuss living accommodations and schedules.
   b. Assist the traveler in understanding the culture of the destination country and how to dress appropriately.
   c. Provide the traveler with resources for health care or emergency situations.

2. Considerations for long-term assignments
   a. Discuss stress, loneliness, job demands, living in hotels, and traveling alone.
   b. Offer training and country-specific culture programs to those preparing to work abroad.
   c. Provide a copy of the appropriate evacuation procedure and be clear about instructions.
   d. Identify resources for health or psychological concerns for the traveler (e.g., an employee assistance counselor, if available, or insurance for health care).
   e. If family is to be living abroad with the traveler, provide information on housing accommodations, the lifestyle and culture of the destination country, and schooling options for dependents.

TABLE 12-1

International Travel Safety and Health Program Resources

The Travel Medicine Advisor Update
American Health Consultants
P.O. Box 740056, Atlanta, GA 30374
Phone: (404) 262-7436; FAX: (404) 262-7837

World Status Map: Official Advisories for International Travelers
Box 466, Merrifield, VA 22116

American Society of Tropical Medicine and Hygiene
60 Revere Drive, Suite 500, Northbrook, IL 60062
Phone: (708) 480-9592; FAX: (708) 480-9282

Centers for Disease Control and Prevention, Atlanta, GA 30333
* CDC Hot Line (recorded messages 24 hours a day) (404) 332-4559
* International Travel, 1994 (Publication)
   Purchase from: U.S. Government Printing Office,
   Washington DC 20402
   Phone: (202) 783-3238

Travel Medicine Software
International Travel Safety and Health Program
TRAVAX. Travel Health Information Services
Phone: (608) 831-2331; FAX: (414) 774-4060

The Immunization Alert
International Health Database
93 Timber Drive, Storrs, CT 06266
Phone: (800) 584-1999

Travel Care, c/o Care Ware, Inc.
9555 Poole Street, La Jolla, CA 92037
Phone: (619) 455-1484; FAX: (619) 455-5429

C. Issues related to the health of the traveler
  1. In many countries, illnesses such as "traveler's diarrhea" can be caused by food or water contaminated with bacteria, viruses, or parasites; high-risk foods to avoid include:
     a. Undercooked meat, poultry, or seafood, which may contain harmful organisms
     b. Raw fruits or vegetables, which may contain harmful bacteria if not thoroughly washed with a chlorine solution
     c. Tap water (including ice made from tap water), which may be unchlorinated and be contaminated with fecal material
     d. Unpasteurized dairy products, which may contain such organisms as the salmonella bacteria
  2. Prevention of illness may be further enhanced by the following recommendations:
     a. Give hepatitis A vaccine (for high endemic areas).
     b. Drink bottled water, or purify water through boiling for at least ten minutes, or use water-purification tablets as recommended.
     c. Follow the basic principles for safe handling of foods.
     d. Follow the basic principles of good hygienic practices.

TABLE 12-2

Traveler's Medical Kit Recommendations

Essential Items

An adequate supply of medications for health conditions specific to the traveler

Additional prescriptions (with generic name) as determined by physician

Copies of medical and eyeglasses prescriptions

Nonprescription Items:

Analgesic (aspirin, acetaminophen, ibuprofen)

Antibiotic skin ointment (Bacitracin, Betadine, Mycitracin)

Antiseptic (providone iodine)

Anticonstipation (many brands of laxatives are available)

Antidiarrheal (lopermide [Immodium AD, bismuth subsalicylate [Pepto Bismol])

Anti-motion sickness (meclizine [Bonine], dimenhydrinate [Dramamine])

Antihistamines (diphenhydramine [Benadryl])

Adhesive bandages (Band-Aids, Curad)

Antacids (Tums, Rolaids, Maalox)

Oral rehydrating salts (available at sporting goods stores)

Disposable thermometers (Fever Scan)

Water purification tablets

Prescription Items

Altitude sickness prophylactics (acetazolamide [Diamox])

Antibiotics (oral doxycycline, ciprofloxacin, or erythromycin)

Antimalarials (mefloquine, choloquine, or doxycycline)

Sleeping medications (Halcion, Restoril)

Additional Medical Supplies

Disposable syringes and needles

Latex gloves

Skin closures (Steri-Strips)

Suture removal kit

---

3. Management of traveler's illnesses may include:
   a. Oral rehydrating fluids (electrolyte solutions) for diarrhea
   b. Prophylactic antibiotics to prevent certain bacteria-caused illnesses
   c. Good hygienic practices to avoid reinfection (e.g., proper disposal of contaminated items, thorough hand washing)
4. Assemble an appropriate medical emergency kit (see Table 12-2).

VI

Control of Prevalent Communicable Diseases

A. Malaria is a febrile illness caused by the blood parasite plasmodium, of which there are four species (p. falciparum is the species with the greatest potential to kill and is the most important to prevent [Health Hints for the Tropics, 1993]).
   1. Symptoms may include fever, chills, muscle aches, headache, and occasionally, vomiting, diarrhea, and coughing.
   2. Risks
      a. In some areas, mosquito activity is high and malaria occurs.
      b. Mosquito activity is highest at night, especially just after dusk.
      c. The highest rate of mosquito activity occurs in Africa, where mosquitoes carry the malaria parasite.
      d. The risk increases during rainy and hot seasons.
   3. Prevention
      a. Use antimosquito measures, such as repellents (permethrin), long-sleeved clothing, long pants, and mosquito netting.
      b. Sleep in screened or air-conditioned rooms if possible.
   4. Control
      a. There is currently no vaccine against malaria available.
      b. Antimalarial medications (chemoprophylaxis) include mefloquine, doxycyline, and chloroquine.

5. Treatment
   a. Medications such as Fansidar (sulphadoxine-pyrimethamine) and Halfan (halofantrine) may be taken as self-treatment if fever and/or flu-like symptoms occur.
   b. Self-treatment is only a temporary measure, and prompt health evaluation is imperative.

B. Sexually transmitted diseases (STDs): Individuals traveling abroad may be at risk for contracting STDs if they engage in sex while abroad; thus, the health care provider must include education specific to STDs.
   1. Individuals assigned to long-term assignments abroad are more likely to engage in casual sex than short-term travelers.
   2. Discuss the possibility of casual sex abroad, and emphasize abstinence.
   3. Encourage the use of condoms and other safe sex practices.
   4. Warn about the effects of alcohol and drugs, which may contribute to careless sexual behavior.
   5. Discuss cultural attitudes concerning prostitution in the traveler's destination country.

C. Selected physiological health hazards: see Table 12-3.

TABLE 12-3

Selected Physiological Health Hazards

Jet Lag: Jet lag is the disruption of the traveler's sleep-wake cycle. It usually occurs when traveling over two or more time zones.

Symptoms	Prevention
Insomnia	Adjust sleep schedule.
Fatigue	Drink extra fluids (preferably water).
Poor concentration	Reduce coffee and alcohol consumption.
Irritability	Exposure to light may help in resetting circadian rhythm.
Headache	
Myalgia	

Altitude Sickness: Altitude sickness is a cluster of symptoms caused by lack of oxygen. The symptoms may include headache, shortness of breath, lightheadedness, fatigue, insomnia, loss of appetite, and nausea. It can be life threatening.

Risk Factors	Prevention	Treatment
Ascent over 6000 feet	High carbohydrate diet	Descent and rest
Rapid ascent without acclimation	Extra fluid intake	Aspirin or acetaminophen
Obesity	Reduce strenuous activity	
Strenuous activity at high altitudes	Slow, gradual ascent	Diamox
Use of sleeping pills or sedatives	Acetazolamide (250 mg every 8 hours for 3–5 days before ascent)	
Previous history of altitude sickness		

VII

Post-Travel Evaluation

This type of evaluation is usually not necessary for short-term travelers.

A. Provide immediate evaluation for signs or symptoms of illness.

B. Perform the following post-travel assessment:
1. History and physical examination to include:
   a. Urinalysis
   b. Stool for ova and parasites if returning from high-risk area
   c. Tuberculosis skin test
2. Post-travel debriefing
   a. Discussion of problems encountered during travel/stay
   b. Recommendations for future travelers

Case Management Program

Case management is a critical function of the occupational health nursing role; it not only examines the quality and cost of health care, but helps to ensure that services are delivered in a timely fashion. Case management services may be provided from the onset of an injury or illness to the worker's return to work or an optional alternative. The occupational health nurse needs excellent communication and negotiation skills to administer a successful case management program.

VIII

The Purpose of the Program

The purpose of a *case management program* is to provide quality care 1) by the appropriate provider, 2) in the appropriate setting, and 3) at an appropriate cost.

A. *Case management* is a process of coordinating an individual client's health care services to achieve optimal, quality care delivered in a cost-effective manner (AAOHN, 1994).

B. Case management can be focused solely on high-cost, catastrophic cases, which have multiple providers and fragmented care; or it can be viewed as an early intervention approach whose purpose is to monitor the quality of care and outcomes of every case.

C. Case management can be limited to work-related injury or illness cases, or it may include non-work-related injury and illness for workers and their dependents.

D. Case management is designed to prevent fragmented care and delayed recovery, and to facilitate employee's return to appropriate modified duty or full duty.

E. The primary goal of case management is to rationalize the care provided with a clear measurement of health outcomes; this may or may not result in cost savings.

IX

Levels/Models of Case Management

A. The key benefits of *on-site case management* include full knowledge of the workers, their dependents, the work process, supervisors, and community providers.

B. *Telephone case management* enables the case manager to link appropriate health care resources to a worker or dependent at a distant location.

C. *Off-site case management* services may be provided by the workers' compensation insurance carrier or purchased from an outside case management vendor.

X

Case Management and the Occupational Health Nurse

A. Comprehensive case management is ideally provided by occupational health nurses; because of the emphasis on return to pre-injury function, occupational health nurses are well positioned to support an appropriate return-to-work plan as a case management goal (AAOHN, 1994; ABOHN, 1994).

B. Case management can include many different service roles, such as advocate, planner, consultant, diagnostician, and/or counselor.

XI

Functions and Process of Case Management

The following case management functions, as originally outlined by Weils & Karl (1985), mirror the steps of the nursing process.

A. Client identification and outreach (determination of eligibility for services)

B. Individual assessment and diagnosis (determination of the level of functioning and the service needs of the client)

C. Service planning and resource identification with clients who are members of the service network

D. Linking the client to the needed service

E. Service implementation and coordination (service assessment and trouble shooting)

F. Monitoring the process of service delivery

G. Advocacy for clients in the service network

H. Evaluation of service delivery and case management

XII

Structural Elements of Case Management

The following structural elements are all client focused, and they interrelate in a dynamic way to reach anticipated case management outcomes (Weil & Karls, 1985; Burgel, 1991).

A. *Service effectiveness* refers to choosing the appropriate provider and the appropriate diagnostic and therapeutic interventions for the level of injury/illness; alternative services (e.g., home care) may need to be negotiated for maximum effectiveness.

B. *Service efficiency* refers to timely interventions during the acute phase of injury/illness.

C. *Service integration* aims to avoid multiple providers and reduce fragmentation of care; excellent communication skills are needed for this structural element of case management.

D. *Cost effectiveness* considers the cost of services when choosing the provider, setting, or intervention for the level of injury/illness.

XIII

Establishment of a Case Management Program

A. Assessment
1. Gather benefit-utilization data for non-work-related health problems for both workers and dependents, specifically for:
   a. High-cost cases
   b. Repeat hospitalization
   c. Extension of hospitalization
   d. Selected diagnosis (for example: spinal cord injuries, premature births, all cancer cases, all organ transplants, all psychiatric diagnoses)
   e. Geographic coverage of workers and dependents
   f. Numerous providers involved in a case
2. Collect workers' compensation data by geographic region, department, and job class on:
   a. Numbers and costs of first-aid, medical-only and lost-time cases, and the range of diagnoses
   b. The type of permanent disability award and vocational rehabilitation costs
   c. High-reserve cases
   d. Workers' compensation experience rating
   e. Litigation costs
   f. Referral data on number and type of specialty referral, wait time before seeing specialist, length of physical therapy prescription, and so forth
   g. Selected diagnoses, such as soft tissue injury, upper-extremity musculo-skeletal disorders, low back pain, all stress claims
3. Review health-benefit coverage for workers and dependents for:
   a. Preexisting condition exclusions
   b. Mental health benefits (inpatient, outpatient, partial stays)
   c. Home-care coverage
   d. Preauthorization procedures
   e. Second opinion requirements
   f. Out-of-pocket costs
   g. Prescription coverage
   h. Percentage of workers and dependents not covered by an employee-sponsored health plan
4. Review medical leave-of-absence policies and communication/linkage between human resources and the occupational health service.
5. Assess modified-duty program success:
   a. Number of successful return-to-work programs
   b. Supervisor satisfaction
   c. Number of reinjury cases
   d. Overall cost of accommodations

B. Data analyses and/or diagnoses
1. Determine regional and programmatic "hot spots," where outcomes and costs have not been well monitored.
2. Conduct a brief, retrospective, cost-effectiveness analysis to determine if case management could have made a positive impact on a sample of interest.
   a. Select two or three high-cost, lost-time cases.
   b. Detail health costs and temporary/permanent disability costs.

     c. Determine key outcome criteria/benchmarks, based on the natural history of the injury/illness and on published clinical pathways; for example, a benchmark for an acute low back sprain would be ordering an MRI only if there is a presence of low back pain limitation for more than four weeks, together with physical examination evidence of nerve root dysfunction (U.S. Department of Health and Human Services, 1994).

     d. Determine if case management could have made a positive impact on case outcomes and costs (see Examples of Case Management Outcomes in Table 12-4).

  3. Document a range of anticipated cost savings based on those cases most suitable for case management.

  4. If a positive impact of case management can be demonstrated, then proceed with formal planning for a pilot project; examples of positive impacts might include:

     a. Cost saving can cover the program expenses.

     b. Less invasive diagnostic procedures are ordered.

     c. An improved quality of life results.

C. Planning

  1. Identify one or two sites to pilot a case management program; selection of sites is determined by the following:

     a. Size of the worker population, number of dependents, and pattern of injury/illness statistics

     b. Opportunity to demonstrate a positive impact within a 6- to 12-month period

     c. Management and union support

     d. Strong occupational health nursing interest and commitment

     e. Strong commitment to primary prevention of work-related hazards

  2. Develop a policy statement with program goals, objectives, and timetable.

  3. Determine the resources (telephone, computer, fax, modem, car, computer software for database management, and the staff necesary for the appropriate level of the case management program).

  4. Detail a marketing plan for workers and dependents, including communication with human resources, union, workers' compensation carrier and administrator, community referrals, and so forth.

  5. Consider establishing a planning task force to assure the successful "buy-in" by workers and dependents.

  6. Establish evaluation criteria.

D. Implementation

  1. Initiate a trigger system to notify the occupational health services of those cases to be included in the case management pilot.

  2. Link the client to the needed services, using appropriate communication skills to share the rationale for treatment choices.

  3. Throughout the case management process, utilize primary, secondary, and tertiary prevention-based nursing interventions to prevent delayed recovery. (See Table 12-5.)

  4. Document time, nature of contact, and anticipated outcome in a database management computer system, together with estimated cost savings. Focus on a realistic return-to-work date.

E. Evaluation

  1. Establish periodic quality checks to determine if:

     a. The notification system is capturing all the cases that meet the case management criteria.

TABLE 12-4

Examples of Case Management Outcomes

Case Study	Case Management Impact
Case One: A magnetic resonance imaging test (MRI) was inappropriately ordered for low back pain, with three weeks off work and no prescribed physical therapy for the worker.	**Intervention:** Question the MRI order based on physical findings and history presented; investigate opportunity for modified duty with employer; identify physical therapy referral that emphasizes home exercise program. **Anticipated Outcomes:** Worker will have less deconditioning and less opportunity for a prolonged disability. Worker will engage in a self-care approach for back pain management. **Savings:** By denying the MRI and negotiating a modified duty assignment, savings include $1,500 for the MRI and approximately $1,200 in temporary disability costs (*Note:* Figures are examples and may vary by location or agency). **Costs:** If six sessions of physical therapy are ordered, this would add approximately $600 to the cost of the case. Case manager time is billed in units of 15 minutes, with the case initially billed at 3 units (45 minutes), specifically for telephone contact to the employer, the health care provider, the physical therapist and the injured worker. Indirect costs include the costs to the employer of having the worker on modified duty (if not fully productive).
Case Two: A 21-day inpatient substance abuse treatment program is prescribed for the spouse of a worker.	**Interventions:** Contact employee assistance program (EAP) and health care benefits coordinators for information on both inpatient and outpatient substance abuse treatment facilities; discuss options with psychological care provider, the client, and the client's family. **Anticipated Outcomes:** Outpatient rather than inpatient care allows for active family involvement with the treatment; a family systems approach to substance abuse treatment is the most effective. **Savings:** Authorizing a 14-day outpatient program saves $7,000 in costs. **Costs:** Case manager time to analyze the outcome data of the outpatient program, in addition to initial phone contact with the EAP and health care benefits coordinators, the psychological care provider, and the family, is billed at 7 units (105 minutes). Indirect costs for the family include travel time to and from the treatment facility and involvement in the family group sessions, which are required in the outpatient program.
Case Three: A worker who has end-stage acquired immune deficiency syndrome (AIDS) is admitted to the hospital for supportive care.	**Intervention:** Investigate benefit delivery to negotiate coverage for home care and/or hospice; communicate with health care provider to determine ability for client to stay in home; assess social support resources. **Anticipated Outcomes:** Use of the home for care delivery provides a better quality of life, decreased nosocomial infection rate, and may maximize limited benefit dollars. **Savings:** Depending upon length of treatment, savings would be the number of inpatient hospital days minus the costs associated with home health support. **Costs:** Home health support, in addition to case manager time over the course of the client illness, including home visits, would be anticipated costs. Indirect costs include the stress of caring for a terminally ill family member in the home.

TABLE 12-5

Nursing Interventions to Prevent Delayed Recovery

Primary Prevention Intervention Strategies

- Share the philosophy that return to work is part of the healing process; recommend modified duty.
- Jointly set a definitive date for return to work.
- Acknowledge fears/losses associated with injury/illness.
- Use work-hardening/sports medicine approach.
- Use employee assistance program.
- Educate about the limits of the workers' compensation or disability systems.

Secondary Prevention Intervention Strategies

- Identify "red flags" (for example: continued subjective complaints with no objective findings; a mortgage disability payment plan).
- View conflict as okay, and as additional data.
- Avoid extensive referrals for persistent symptoms.
- Assess whether further data are needed: violence and suicide assessment, other psychiatric symptoms indicative of underlying depression.
- Ask: "Am I doing this worker a favor by advocating more time off?"
- Help the individual acquire a healthy outlook, despite impairments.

Tertiary Prevention Intervention Strategies

- Determine permanent and stationary status as early as possible.
- Initiate rehabilitation plan in timely fashion.
- Decrease expectations of 100% recovery; help individual tolerate discomfort.
- Continue to assess the worker for underlying depression, and focus on whether the primary problem is physiological or psychological.
- Chronic pain referrals may be of value.
- Support the self-esteem of the individual.
- Gain collegial support in dealing with difficult patient situations.

---

    b. Case managers are entering appropriate data into the database management program.

    c. Services have been delivered within the anticipated time frame, with limited wait time, if referred.

    d. There is documentation of steady improvement in the worker's condition, and an active plan for return to work in a modified capacity.

    e. The permanence of the worker's recovery is determined within six months of entering the case management system, unless there are contributing variables.

    f. Analysis of the injury, if work related, has been completed, with a goal to prevent a similar incident in the future.

  2. Assessment of "customer" satisfaction to include:

    a. Satisfaction of the client and family with care coordination and communication

    b. Satisfaction of case managers with the implementation of the case management program, including the integration of any suggestions to improve the program

    c. Satisfaction of key providers and management at the referral sites, in working collaboratively with the case manager to improve outcomes of care

    d. Satisfaction of supervisors with the implementation of the modified-duty component of the case management program

   e. Satisfaction of union leadership with a fair and equitable utilization of benefits for workers and their dependents
3. Cost outcomes
   a. Evaluate direct cost saving concurrently by placing a cost value on every intervention, if possible; for example, if the nursing intervention results in saving the costs of an MRI, the direct cost saving is $1500 minus the cost of the 20-minute phone call by the case manager (see Table 12-4 for case examples).
   b. Evaluate direct cost savings retrospectively by evaluating several individual cases:
      1) From data for a particular worksite, select several cases from the case management pilot project and match them to cases that were not case managed; try to control for types of work demands and severity of worker's conditions.
      2) Evaluate frequency and costs of office visits, types and costs of diagnostic interventions, number and costs of prescriptions, number of inpatient days, and mean length of stay.
      3) Compare temporary disability payments.
      4) Determine the date of injury and the date of permanent and stationary status, as well as the amount and percent of any permanent disability award.
      5) Detail any vocational rehabilitation costs.
      6) List legal costs (health evaluations, sub rosa, attorney representation).
      7) Outline other direct cost savings in insurance premiums.
   b. Evaluate indirect cost savings:
      1) If the worker successfully returned to either modified or regular work, evaluate job performance markers, number of absent days, visits to on-site health services, visits to employee assistance providers, and other appropriate industry-specific productivity data.
      2) If the worker did not return to work, evaluate date of termination and continued costs in the social security/disability system once workers' compensation benefits are depleted.
   c. Detail expenses of the case management program, including a percentage of overhead costs and the number of hours of case management time.
   d. Determine if savings were realized with these several cases.
   e. Repeat the cost analysis for a group of claims with similar diagnoses and/or from a specific department/site/region.
4. Communicate "added value" (quality and outcomes) of case management program to management, union, human resources, and case management staff.

Hearing Conservation Program (HCP)

The passage of the Hearing Conservation Amendment to the Occupational Safety and Health Act in 1983 provided the thrust toward the development of hearing conservation programs in industry. Hearing conservation programs can be conducted either within the worksite or contracted to a certified audiology testing service. It is recommended, and in some cases required by law, that individuals performing as audiometric technicians become certified through the Council for Accreditation in Occupational Hearing Conservation. The program outlined can serve as a guide to developing a hearing conservation program. It is advised that the program coordinator review and follow requirements established by OSHA or by states with OSHA-approved state plans.

XIV

Noise-Induced Hearing Loss

Noise-induced hearing loss due to occupational exposure has been a compensable occupational disease since the 1950s.

A. 5.5 million American workers are exposed to noise levels of 85 decibels (dB) and above (U.S. Department of Labor, 1992).

B. 9 million American workers are exposed above these levels when all noisy jobs, including military, mining, construction, and transportation, are included in the data.

C. Estimates suggest that 1 million workers in the manufacturing industry alone have sustained job-related hearing loss (Suter, 1993).

XV

Purposes of the Program

The purposes of a *hearing conservation program* (HCP) are to:

A. Prevent the hearing loss of workers

B. Identify the progression of hearing loss so that preventive measures can be taken

C. Identify temporary hearing loss before it becomes permanent

D. Comply with federal regulations or OSHA-approved state plans (OSHA Noise Standard CFR 1910.95). See Table 12-6.
  1. OSHA regulations limit worksite noise exposure to 90 dBA time-weighted average (TWA) over an 8-hour work shift. Hearing conservation programs (HCPs) and hearing protection devices (HPDs) are mandatory, as are engineering controls.

TABLE 12-6

Developing Hearing Conservation Program:
Suggested Policies Based on Time-Weighted Average Ranges

TWA in dB(A)	Workers Included in the HCP	HPD Utilization	HPD Selection Options
84 or below	no	voluntary	free choice
85–89	yes	optional*	free choice
90–94	yes	required	free choice
95–99	yes	required	limited choice
100 or above	yes	required	very limited choice

*Use of a hearing protective device (HPD) will be required:
1. For any worker who shows a significant hearing change,
2. For all workers if audiometric database analysis results or group hearing trends indicate inadequate protection.

Source: Reprinted with permission from Royster, J. D., & Royster, L. H. (1990). Copyright Lewis Publishers, an imprint of CRC Press, Boca Raton, Florida.

2. HCPs are mandatory in an environment where the daily noise level equals or exceeds 85 dBA over an 8-hour, time-weighted average; appropriate HPDs are to be provided.

E. The rationale and the benefits of a worksite HCP include:
1. Better labor-management relations
2. Decreased likelihood of antisocial behaviors resulting from annoyance
3. Greater job satisfaction, increased productivity, and better quality of life, resulting from reducing noise in the workplace
4. Reduced accident rates, illnesses, and lost work time
5. Reduced risk of workers' compensation claims

XVI

Management's Role

Management has the following responsibilities:

A. Develop an HCP policy to include disciplinary action for noncompliance.

B. Identify program personnel and their responsibilities for the HCP.
1. Provide a qualified physician, an otolaryngologist, or an audiologist to supervise the program.
2. Identify the program coordinator and other personnel responsible for the program components who are enthusiastic and committed to the HCP.

C. Provide personnel, space, supplies, and funding for the program.

D. Provide all elements of the program to workers free of charge.

E. Make a good-faith effort to eliminate or reduce sources of noise and to reevaluate the noise level when there are changes in exposure.

F. Post appropriate warning signs and ear-protection requirements at entrances to areas with noise levels exceeding 85 dBA.

G. Conduct periodic evaluations to assure the quality and effectiveness of the program.

XVII

The Role of the Hearing Conservation Coordinator

The responsibilities of the hearing conservation coordinator may include the following:

A. Perform an otoscopic examination and audiometric testing (may want to seek in-service training from an occupational audiologist).

B. Coordinate the testing schedules and follow-up procedures.

C. Keep accurate, clear, and complete testing and counseling records.

D. Select, fit, and supervise the wearing of appropriate hearing-protection devices.

E. Act as liaison between workers and other members of the team.

F. Take a health or aural history on each worker participating in the program.

G. Educate and train workers on how to protect themselves from hearing loss.

H. Refer workers to appropriate sources for further testing or medical treatment when indicated.

XVIII

The Role of the Workers

A. Each worker is responsible for complying with the program by wearing appropriate hearing protection.

B. It is the responsibility of workers, especially supervisors, to encourage co-workers to wear HPDs.

C. Workers should immediately report changes in noise levels on the work floor to their supervisors, safety personnel, or other responsible individuals.

XIX

Program Requirements

A successful program requires:

A. The support, cooperation, and participation of all levels of management

B. Support of workers, since they are the most knowledgeable about the work environment

C. Cooperation of union leaders, where applicable, and/or the person responsible for worksite safety

D. Review of the OSHA standard (29 CFR 1910.95 or from an OSHA-approved state plan, where applicable)

XX

Program Goals

A. Prevent noise-induced hearing loss by reducing worker exposure to harmful noise.

B. Reduce workers' compensation costs.

C. Reduce accidents among workers.

D. Comply with state and federal regulations.

E. Improve worker efficiency and job performance.

F. Prevent loss of trained and experienced personnel.

G. Reduce cost of operating the hearing conservation program.

XXI

Noise Assessment and Control

A. If reliable information indicates noise exposure in the worksite, conduct noise measurements (to be performed by an acoustical engineer, an industrial hygienist, an occupational audiologist, or a professional proficient in noise-level measurement); include all continuous, intermittent, and impulse noise within an 80-dB(A) to 130-dB(A) range taken during a typical work situation.

1. Use only sound-level meters or noise dosimeters that meet the American National Standards Institute (ANSI) specifications (Type II instruments).

2. Use a sampling strategy that will pick up all continuous, intermittent, and impulse sound levels from 80 to 130 dBA, and include all those sound levels in the total noise measurement.

3. Permit workers and/or their representatives to observe monitoring.

4. Notify workers of noise exposure at or above an 8-hour TWA of 85 dBA.

B. Purpose and use of sound-survey results
   1. Identification of areas of the worksite where hazardous noise levels exist
   2. Identification of workers to be included in the HCP
   3. Classification of workers' noise exposures in order to define HPD policies and prioritization of areas for noise-control efforts
   4. Identification of safety hazards in terms of interference with speech communication and warning-signal detection
   5. Evaluation of noise source for noise-control purposes
   6. Documentation of noise levels for legal purposes

C. Noise-control measures
   1. Engineering controls are the most effective long-term solution and may include any of the following:
      a. Eliminate the source of noise.
      b. Redesign the process to be quieter.
      c. Isolate machinery to prevent vibrations and noise from radiating.
      d. Build enclosure around noisy machinery.
      e. Use absorptive material on walls and ceilings.
      f. Erect a barrier or noise-reducing curtain around the noisy area.
      g. Enclose the receiver in a sound-treated booth.
      h. Add a muffler to noisy tools.
      i. Keep machinery well balanced, oiled, and in good repair.
   2. Recommendations related to work practices that will decrease the risk of noise hazards should be developed.
   3. Administrative controls are implemented when engineering and work-practice controls are not feasible.
      a. Rotate workers to less noisy areas.
      b. Perform high-noise tasks when fewer workers are present.
   4. Personal protective equipment is provided when engineering and administrative control are not feasible.
      a. Provide appropriate HPDs (ear plugs, muffs, helmets).
      b. Provide a selection of appropriate styles and types at no cost to workers.

XXII

Worker Training and Education

A. Conduct the program initially for new hires and annually for workers who are included in the HCP.

B. Describe the characteristics of sound (complex combination of pure tones found in the environment that result in a vibratory disturbance in the pressure of fluid in the ear and capable of being detected by the organs of hearing).

C. Explain where noise is found.
   1. Cite occupational, recreational, and environmental sources, including cumulative effects from multiple sources. (See Table 12-7.)
   2. Provide examples of different types of noise from actual locations at the worksite (where most noise exposure occurs).

D. Describe effects of noise (in addition to hearing loss).
   1. Physical problems include effects on the cardiovascular and gastrointestinal systems, headache, stress, and fatigue.
   2. Psychological problems include annoyance, feeling of isolation among workers, masking of warning shouts and signals, and interference with speech communication.

TABLE 12-7

Some Commonly Encountered Noise Levels

Source	dB(A) Level	Effect
Jet plane	140	Acoustic trauma—may cause permanent damage to the delicate hair cells of the cochlea
Gunshot blast (impulse)	140 (pain threshold)	
Automobile horn	120	
Rock band	110	Noise-induced hearing loss: Long exposure to noise over 90 dB(A) may eventually cause permanent hearing loss.
Chain saw	110	
Car racing	110	
Motorcycle	100	
Subway	90	
Average factory	80–90	
Noisy restaurant	80	Usually will not cause permanent hearing loss
Busy traffic	75	
Conversational speech	65	
Average home	50	
Quiet office	40	
Soft whisper	30	

Source: Adapted from EPA (1978), *Protective noise levels,* EPA550/9-70-100, Environmental Protection Agency, Washington DC: Royster, J. D., & Royster, L. H. (1990).

E. Provide overview of signs and symptoms of hearing loss.
1. Tinnitus (ringing in the ear) is a sign of an overtaxed auditory system.
2. Awareness of hearing loss usually does not occur until loss is significant.
3. Perception that others are "mumbling" is often a sign of hearing loss.
4. Occupational hearing loss is usually bilateral; hearing loss in only one ear may be caused by pathological processes other than occupational exposures or acoustic trauma to that ear.

F. Explain anatomy and physiology of outer, middle, and inner ear; a diagram or model of the parts of the ear will be helpful. (See Figure 12-1.)
1. Outer ear: collects sound waves and funnels them into the ear canal.
2. Middle ear: sound impinges on ear drum and is transmitted mechanically to the bones of the middle ear (hammer, anvil, and stirrup) and transmitted to the fluid-filled cochlea in the inner ear. The hammer, anvil, and stirrup are also known as the malleus, incus, and stapes, respectively.
3. Inner ear: transmits sound waves through hair cells in the cochlea that send electrical impulses to the auditory nerve, which transmits the signals to the brain, where the sound is interpreted.

G. Explain types of hearing loss.
1. Acoustic trauma:
a. Results from a single exposure such as a loud, explosive blast or a blow to the head
b. May rupture the eardrum and damage the middle and inner ear

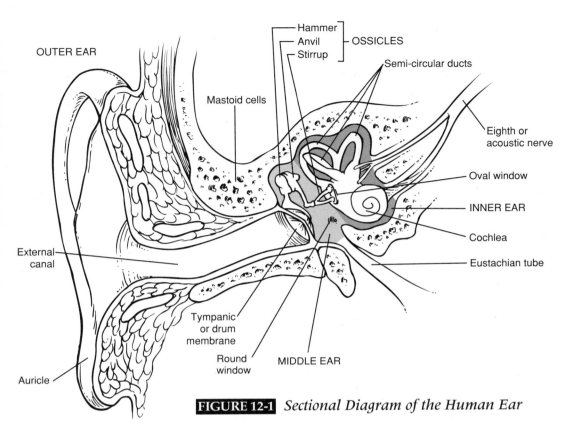

FIGURE 12-1 *Sectional Diagram of the Human Ear*

2. Sensorineural:
   a. Results in changes in the receptive cells; occurs from long-term exposure to noise
   b. Is usually bilateral
   c. Is not usually apparent until hearing loss is severe
   d. Can be caused by trauma, use of certain ototoxic drugs, aging, diseases, heredity
   e. Is usually irreversible, its severity depending on the intensity, frequency, and duration of noise exposure
3. Conductive:
   a. Occurs from obstruction of sound through the outer and inner ear
   b. May be caused by wax buildup, presence of a foreign body, ruptured eardrum, infection, otosclerosis, or injury
   c. May be (in most instances) reversed or stabilized by appropriate treatment or surgery

H. Provide *hearing-protective devices* (HPDs) at no cost, or more expensive devices at minimal cost, for workers to use when engaged in noisy activities outside the worksite. Types include:
1. Ear plugs (aural inserts): formable or molded, made of soft material (many types and styles are available).
   a. Advantages: they are small, inexpensive, easy to use, comfortable, can be worn for long periods of time.
   b. Disadvantages: they need to be kept clean, may become contaminated with dirt and grime, may cause allergic reaction in some individuals, may produce wax buildup, are difficult to monitor at a distance.

    2. Ear muffs (circumaurals): plastic-foam-filled cuffs that fit snugly against the head and are attached to an adjustable headband.
        a. Advantages: they are easy to fit and easy to monitor from a distance.
        b. Disadvantages: they are expensive, large and bulky, may be difficult to use with hard hats or respiratory equipment, and may become loose with head movement.
    3. Canal caps (semiaurals): ear-plug-like tips connected by a lightweight headband.
        a. Advantages: they are suitable for short-duration and off-and-on wearing.
        b. Disadvantages: they are uncomfortable if worn for long periods of time, and they are not suitable for areas where the noise level is high.
    4. Custom fitted ear plugs: molded to ear, solid or filtered, that allow speech to enter but reduce harmful noise.
        a. Advantages: they are suitable for very small or hard-to-fit ear canals; they can be filtered for special needs.
        b. Disadvantages: the material may shrink; the fit may change if worker gains or loses weight.

I. The *noise reduction rating* (NRR): Hearing-protective devices by law must contain a number that reflects the amount of noise that will be reduced by their use. The formula that is used in the workplace is to subtract the NRR number from the dB level of noise exposure.
    1. NRR is conducted in laboratories with selected subjects and may not reflect real work situations; a good rule of thumb is to derate the NRR by 50% (e.g., 30 dB NRR = 15 dB in the real workplace) (Sandra MacLean, Certified Industrial Audiologist, 1995, personal communication).
    2. OSHA indicates a dB(C) scale is used in NRR and needs to be corrected to dB(A) by subtracting 7 from the NRR [noise level in dB(A) – [NRR – 7] = estimated exposure in dB(A)].

J. Evaluate workers' perceptions and motivations related to the use of hearing-protective devices.
    1. Identify barriers to compliance with recommendations.
    2. Develop strategies to address concerns of workers related to the use of HPDs.

K. Fitting of HPDs
    1. Offer severals style and varying sizes.
    2. Evaluate workers to determine the types of hearing protection best suited to each worker's anatomy and job situation.
    3. Instruct workers on proper placement, limitations, and care of HPDs.
    4. Follow the manufacturers' directions.

XXIII

Audiometric Testing

A. Purpose and procedure
    1. Testing is performed to determine baseline hearing and to monitor effects of noise exposure.
    2. The test is implemented under the direction and supervision of an audiologist, an otolaryngologist, or a qualified physician.
    3. Both the test environment and the audiometer must meet criteria set by the American National Standards Institute (ANSI).
    4. The test must be performed by a licensed or certified audiologist, otolaryngologist, or physician; or by a technician who is certified by the Council for

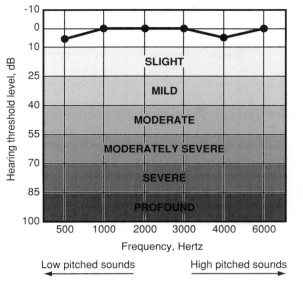

FIGURE 12-2 *Normal Audiogram and Degrees of Hearing Loss*

Source: Reprinted with permission from Royster & Royster, (1990).

Accreditation in Occupational Hearing Conservation (CAOHC), 611 E. Wells St., Milwaukee, WI 53202, (414)276-5338; or by, as OSHA states, "someone who has demonstrated competence."

   a. A worker's baseline audiogram is performed: at least 14 hours after noise exposure; or with hearing protection; or at the time of hire; or for job placement; or when a worker is transferred from a non-noisy to a noisy worksite. It is used as a reference against which future audiograms are compared.

   b. An annual (or periodic) audiogram may be performed well into the work shift to provide information on effectiveness of noise control measures; it must be taken within one year of the baseline test.

   c. An exit, or termination, audiogram is performed when worksite noise exposure ceases; it is not an OSHA requirement, but it may be important in determining the extent of employer liability for workers' compensation determination.

B. Duties of the audiometric technician may include:

   1. Calibrating the audiometer at least daily by testing the same individual with stable hearing

   2. Taking a health history and noise-exposure history

   3. Performing a visual and otoscopic examination of the ears

   4. Explaining the purpose of the test

   5. Administering a pure-tone audiometric test

   6. Providing immediate feedback and counseling

C. Audiometric evaluation

   1. Normal hearing, in general, falls within hearing threshold levels between 0 and 25 dB; it may vary slightly from left to right ear and may be age dependent. See Figure 12-2.

   2. A *standard threshold shift* (STS) (also referred to as *significant threshold shift*) is an average shift in either ear of 10 dB or more at 2000, 3000, and 4000 Hertz compared to baseline audiogram.

    a. An STS may require referral to an audiologist, an otolaryngologist, or a qualified physician.

    b. Depending upon program supervisor protocol, an exposed worker whose test reveals an STS may be retested within 30 days of the annual test before referral.

    c. Workers must be notified in writing within 21 days of determination of the STS.

  3. A *temporary threshold shift* (TTS) occurs shortly after exposure and improves gradually if the noise has not been too loud or the exposure too long. The greatest recovery takes place in 1 to 24 hours if the worker is removed from exposure. Adequacy of the HPD should be checked.

  4. A *permanent threshold shift* (PTS) occurs when hearing loss persists after removal from exposure; it is associated with damage to the delicate sensory hair cells in the inner ear. If there is no improvement within one week, the loss is usually permanent.

D. Criteria for referral to audiologist, otolaryngologist, or a qualified physician:

  1. When an infection in the ear is suspected

  2. When hearing loss is unilateral

  3. When the worker complains of pain in the ear

  4. When an STS is evident

  5. Other criteria, as determined by a supervising audiologist or physician

XXIV

Recordkeeping

A. Audiometric test records must include: name and job classification of the worker, date of the test, the examiner's name, date of the last audiometer calibration, and the worker's most recent noise exposure assessment. It is also advisable to document any worker counseling.

B. Records (noise survey forms, audiograms, exposure histories) must be kept for the duration of employment (plus thirty years is often suggested).

C. Records of noise-exposure measurements should be retained for at least two years, preferably longer.

D. Background-noise measurements of the room where work is performed should be recorded and maintained.

E. Audiometric and noise-exposure records should be accessible upon request to workers, former workers, worker-designated representatives, and others as required by law.

F. If the employer ceases to do business, all records must be transferred to the successor employer and kept in accordance with the law.

XXV

Program Evaluation

A. Assess the completeness and quality of the program components.

B. Compare annual audiograms to baseline for individuals and groups to determine the success of control measures; identify areas where further controls are needed.

C. Develop a checklist specific to the work environment to ensure that all components of the program are being followed and are in compliance with the appropriate standards.

Hazard Communication (HAZCOM) Program

The *hazard communication standard* (HCS) was promulgated by OSHA in 1983 as a means of reducing risks related to chemical exposure in the American workforce. The following *hazard communication (HazCom) program* is provided as a guide to assist in compliance with this standard. Some of the suggested elements may not be required but are included as recommendations to ensure a successful program. It is important that each program coordinator review the standards applicable to his or her jurisdiction. No single written program will work for all worksites; thus, programs should be tailored to comply with the law and to protect workers against exposures specific to their work settings.

XXVI

The Purposes of the Program

The purposes of a *hazard communication program* are as follows:

A. Ensure that the hazards of all chemicals produced or imported into the worksite are evaluated and that information concerning these hazards is transmitted to both employers and workers.

B. Prevent illness, injury, or death from exposure to hazardous chemicals and substances in the worksite.

C. Comply with OSHA's Hazard Communication Standard (HCS) 29 CFR 1910.12.

XXVII

Management's Role

Management's responsibilities for policy and program development include the following components:

A. Providing workers with a company policy statement, which should include:
  1. A statement that indicates that Company X is committed to protecting the health and safety of its workers
  2. A statement indicating that all workers will be informed of known hazardous substances that can cause illness, injury, or death
  3. A statement that all workers will be trained at time of hire, when they move to an area with new hazards, and when a new hazard is introduced into the worksite
  4. The identification of individuals (or their job titles) who will be responsible for implementation and continuation of the HazCom program

B. A written program (OSHA looks for this first) that includes:
  1. A list of hazardous chemicals present in the worksite
  2. The proper labeling of all containers of chemicals in the worksite
  3. The preparation of material safety data sheets (MSDS, ANSI Z400.1)
  4. The implementation of worker training programs about hazards of chemicals and measures that can be taken to protect workers from dangerous exposures

XXVIII

Description of the Program

A. The goals and objectives of the program are the following:
  1. Identify and assess all chemical substances in the workplace that may pose physical or health hazards to workers.

2. Communicate to all workers the presence of potentially hazardous substances in the worksite through training and provision of accessible MSDSs, which must be kept current.
3. Train all workers in the safe handling of potentially hazardous substances.
4. Properly label all chemical containers with warning notices as well as handling and disposal procedures of hazardous substances. Covered under the OSH Act are all known hazardous chemicals or chemical compounds that are not covered under other federal acts.

B. Definitions:
1. A *chemical* is defined as any element, chemical compound, or mixture of elements and/or compounds.
2. A *hazardous chemical* is defined as any chemical that is a health hazard or a physical hazard.
   a. *Health hazards* include chemicals that are known carcinogens, toxic or highly toxic agents, reproductive toxins, irritants, corrosives, sensitizers, hepatotoxins, neurotoxins, agents that act on the hematopoietic system, and agents that damage the lungs, eyes, skin, or mucous membranes.
   b. A *physical hazard* is any chemical for which there is scientifically valid evidence that it is a combustible liquid, compressed gas, explosive, flammable, an organic peroxide, pyrophoric, unstable (reactive), or water reactive.

XXIX

Elements of the Program

A. Responsibilities of a program coordinator are as follows:
1. Keep accurate inventory of all hazardous chemicals and substances used in the worksite. (It may be helpful to work with the purchasing department to identify the chemicals that have been purchased or ordered.)
2. Obtain MSDS sheets from manufacturers or suppliers of all chemicals used in the worksite.
3. Provide training programs for workers when any hazardous chemical is used in the worksite and when any new physical or health hazard is introduced into the worksite.
4. Ensure that all chemicals are properly labeled and stored.

B. Elements of worker training programs
1. The program is communicated to all current and new workers.
2. The standard is summarized during the training program.
3. The location of the written program is communicated and readily accessible to all workers.
4. The location of the list of hazardous chemical products and the master list and location of MSDSs must be communicated and accessible to all workers.
5. The program provides mechanisms for understanding its components; for example, the worker should understand:
   • How to read and understand MSDSs
   • The labeling of hazardous chemicals and products
   • The health and safety hazards of the chemicals used in the worksite
   • The safe handling and disposal of hazardous chemicals
   • The signs and symptoms of overexposure (nausea, vomiting, headache, dizziness, burn, rash, etc.)
   • Emergency procedures for exposure events
   • Methods and observations that may be used to detect the presence or release of hazardous chemicals

- The controls that are in place to protect workers, such as personal protective equipment
- Where workers can obtain more information about hazardous chemicals

C. Training for contract workers must:
1. Inform all nonemployee workers of the location of the MSDSs
2. Provide workers with personal protective equipment
3. Inform workers of the chemical hazards in their work area
4. Explain the labeling system of hazardous chemicals used by the company
5. Emphasize emergency procedures in the event of exposure

D. Training for nonroutine hazardous tasks must:
1. Provide training for the specific hazardous chemical(s) to which the workers will be exposed
2. Provide workers with personal protective equipment appropriate for the hazardous chemical(s)

XXX
Material Safety Data Sheets

Material safety data sheets (MSDSs) require the following:

A. All items on the MSDS must be completed, leaving no blank spaces.

B. All chemicals must be identified with both their generic and their common names.

C. Each chemical's characteristics must be described (e.g., liquid, vapor, solid, flammable, explosive, etc.).

D. A list of all chemicals' characteristics that make them hazardous to health must be included (e.g., carcinogenic, corrosive, highly toxic, irritant).

E. The primary routes of entry into the body—absorption, inhalation, ingestion, and injection—should be identified for each chemical.

F. Permissible exposure limits (PEL) set by the Occupational Safety and Health Administration (OSHA), and threshold limit values (TLV) set by the American Congress of Governmental Industrial Hygienists (ACGIH) must be provided.

G. Information on the chemical's listing on a hazardous chemical registry, such as the Annual Report of Carcinogens, must be included, if applicable.

H. The precautions for safe handling must be clearly described, along with the type of personal protective equipment that is recommended.

I. Measures to control exposure to the chemical, such as engineering, work practices, administrative, or personal protective equipment, must be identified.

J. Emergency and first-aid procedures if an exposure occurs must be described.

K. Date the MSDS was prepared and the name, address, and phone number of the manufacturer or other responsible party must be included.

L. The MSDS must be printed in the English language (and may, in addition, be printed in other languages).

XXXI
Trade Secrets

A. A *trade secret* is any confidential formula, pattern, process, device, information, or compilation of information that is used in an employer's business and that gives the employer an opportunity to obtain an advantage over competitors who do not know or use it.

B. A manufacturer may withhold the identity of a certain chemical when knowledge of that chemical by other manufacturers could give the latter a competitive advantage, except in the following situations:
1. A treating physician or occupational health nurse determines that a medical emergency exists and the identity of that chemical is necessary for emergency first-aid treatment.
2. In a nonemergency situation when the name of the chemical is requested in writing by a health professional (e.g., physician, occupational health nurse, industrial hygienist, toxicologist, or epidemiologist) who is providing occupational health services to exposed workers for valid reasons described in the OSH Act, a signed confidentiality statement may be required by the manufacturer.

XXXII

Container Labeling and Warning Requirements

A. All chemical containers entering the worksite must be clearly marked with the identity of the chemical, appropriate warnings, and the name of the manufacturer.

B. All chemicals transferred to other containers must be marked with the information listed on the original container.

C. All unmarked containers must be reported to the program coordinator immediately.

D. Generic warning labels are available from U.S. Department of Transportation (DOT) for such chemicals as flammable gas, flammable solid, oxidizer, or corrosive.

XXXIII

Recordkeeping

Although not required by OSHA, keeping records of worker training and education, including the content of the training program and the names and signature of workers, is important to:

A. Assure that all workers have been trained in the handling and storing of products that contain hazardous substances

B. Document HazCom training during an audit for workers' compensation claims

XXXIV

Evaluation

A. Make observations of how chemicals are actually being handled by workers.

B. Solicit feedback from workers and management on how the program is working.

C. Make a checklist of all elements of the program to ensure that the program is working and is in compliance with appropriate standards (see Table 12-8).

Drug and Alcohol Testing Program

It is estimated that substance abuse costs employers billions of dollars each year as a result of increased injuries, fatalities, absenteeism, excessive use of health care benefits, decreased productivity, theft, and alcoholism. Although the worksite is a strategic place for preventing and identifying early substance abuse, many businesses still do not have drug-free worksite programs. The Department of Transportation (DOT) has developed comprehensive federal regulations that mandate

---

TABLE 12-8

Checklist for a Hazard Communication Program

• Obtained a copy of the rule	• Prepared a written program
• Read and understood the requirements	• Made MSDSs available to workers
• Assigned responsibility for tasks	• Conducted training for workers
• Prepared an inventory of chemicals used in the workplace	• Established procedure to maintain current program
• Ensured that containers are properly labeled	• Established procedures to evaluate completeness and effectiveness of the program
• Obtained an MSDS for each chemical	

Source: Adapted from OSHA's *Hazard communication guidelines for compliance.* U.S. Department of Labor, Occupational Safety and Health Administration. OSHA 3111, 1995 (Revised).

drug and alcohol testing for transportation workers. These regulations include an excellent model for employers considering drug and alcohol testing programs; this model serves as the basis of the program described in this chapter.

XXXV

The Purpose of the Program

The purpose of a *drug and alcohol testing program* is to avoid hiring workers who use illegal drugs, to deter workers from abusing drugs and alcohol, and to identify and refer to treatment those workers who are presently abusing drugs and alcohol.

A. Definitions:
   1. A drug is any chemical substance that produces physical, mental, emotional, or behavioral changes in the user.
   2. Drug and alcohol abuse is the use of any drug or alcohol in a medically, socially, or legally unacceptable manner.
   3. Substance abuse occurs whenever an illegal drug is used, when a prescribed drug is misused, when drugs or alcohol are consumed to the point of physical or mental impairment, or when alcohol is used in an amount or at a time prohibited by an employer's policy.

B. Drug-free worksite programs may include:
   1. A company policy
   2. Employee assistance program
   3. Supervisory training
   4. Employee awareness education
   5. Drug and alcohol testing

C. Employers who are federal grantees and contractors receiving awards worth more than $25,000 must comply with the Drug Free Workplace (DFW) Act of 1988, which mandates that they establish and maintain a drug-free worksite. Specifically, these companies must:
   1. Adopt a policy statement prohibiting drugs in the worksite
   2. Require workers to have a copy of the policy statement
   3. Establish a drug awareness program
   4. Notify federal agency of the drug crime conviction of a worker
   5. Impose sanctions on convicted workers or require worker rehabilitation
   6. Make a good-faith effort to maintain a drug-free worksite

XXXVI

Elements of a Drug and Alcohol Testing Program

A. A successful testing program must contract with reliable, professional laboratories.
1. Laboratory certification (and monitoring) by the Substance Abuse and Mental Health Services Administration (SAMHSA) is required for federally mandated testing. (SAMHSA was formerly the National Institute of Drug Abuse [NIDA].)
2. The testing methodology required by the Department of Transportation (DOT) is a two-stage process, starting with an initial screening test, which, if positive for one or more drugs, is followed by a confirmation test.
   a. The very sensitive initial screening test (immunoassay) looks for the presence or absence of drugs.
   b. The confirmation test is performed for each identified drug using state-of-the-art gas chromatography/mass spectrometry (GC/MS) analysis.
3. The testing program must establish testing protocols, such as the specific drugs to be tested and the cutoff levels.
   a. The most common drugs tested for (and required by federal testing) are marijuana (THC metabolite), cocaine, amphetamines, opiates (including heroin), and phencyclidine (PCP).
   b. Other drugs also abused but less commonly tested include barbiturates (including sedatives and tranquilizers), hallucinogens, inhalants, and "designer drugs."
   c. Cutoff (laboratory reporting) levels are established by SAMHSA.

B. The chain-of-custody procedures ensure that the specimen's security, proper identification, and integrity are not compromised.
1. The procedures track the handling and storage from the initial collection to the final disposition.
2. A positive test result must be linked back to the individual whose name appears on the specimen bottle label.
3. All personnel who handle the specimen are documented, no unauthorized access to the specimen is possible, and no adulteration or tampering takes place.

C. The Omnibus Transportation Employee Testing Act of 1991 requires that drug testing procedures for most transportation workers include split specimen procedures.
1. Each urine specimen is subdivided into two bottles labeled as "primary" and "split" specimens; both bottles are sent to the laboratory.
2. Only the primary specimen is opened and used for the urinalysis; the split specimen bottle remains sealed and is stored in the laboratory.
3. If the analysis of the primary specimen confirms the presence of illegal, controlled substances, the worker has 72 hours to request the split specimen be sent to another SAMHSA-certified laboratory for analysis.

D. To protect both the worker and the employer, a medical review officer (MRO) reviews and interprets all drug test results before they are reported to the employer.
1. Federal regulations require the MRO to contact the worker in person or by telephone and conduct an interview to determine if there is an alternative medical explanation for the drugs found in the worker's urine specimen.
2. If the worker provides appropriate documentation and the MRO determines that it is legitimate medical use of the prohibited drug, the drug test result is reported to the employer as negative.

E. As a quality assurance measure for the testing laboratory, employers are required by federal regulations to perform blind sample testing.

F. Types of tests:
1. *Preemployment,* or *applicant, testing* is conducted to prevent hiring workers with drug or alcohol problems; it is the most popular type of drug testing, since it avoids union problems, and potential future problems associated with substance abusing workers.
2. *Post-accident testing* is used to determine if drug or alcohol abuse was a contributing factor in the accident, to identify drug and alcohol abusers, and to deter drug and alcohol abuse.
3. *Reasonable suspicion testing* is conducted when an employer suspects that a worker is using alcohol or drugs in violation of the company's policy, based on "specific, contemporaneous, and articulable observations concerning the appearance, behavior, speech, or body odor" of the worker (U.S. Department of Transportation, 1994b).
4. *Random testing* is conducted without suspicion that any particular worker is using drugs, and it identifies workers who are abusing drugs or alcohol but have been able to use the predictability of other testing methods to escape detection.
   a. Selection should be made by using a simple random sampling method so that all workers eligible for testing are equally likely to be tested.
   b. An excellent deterrent and early intervention tool, random testing is recommended for workers in safety- or security-sensitive positions and for workers in companies in which alcohol and drug abuse problems are common.
   c. Federal regulations require random drug testing of at least 50% and random alcohol testing of at least 25% of the number of safety-sensitive workers (the random testing rate is determined annually based upon the random positive rate for each industry).
   d. Because alcohol is legal, random alcohol testing must be conducted just before, during, or just after a worker's performance of safety-sensitive duties.
5. *Return-to-duty* and *follow-up testing* are conducted when a worker who has tested positive for drugs and has been removed from the worksite returns to work or to performing safety-sensitive duties.
   a. Federal regulations require that follow-up tests must be unannounced and that a minimum of six tests must be conducted in the first twelve months after a worker returns to duty; follow-up testing and monitoring may continue for up to five years.
   b. The frequency of the follow-up tests should depend on the characteristics of the drug of abuse as well as the worker's abuse-related behavior.

G. The federal regulations require that breath testing for alcohol be done with evidential breath testing devices (EBT) approved by the National Highway Traffic Safety Administration (NHTSA).

H. Some federal regulations require certain categories of safety-sensitive workers to report *any* medical use of controlled substances.

I. Federal regulations pertaining to alcohol-related conduct mandate that a worker's performance of safety-sensitive functions is prohibited:
1. If an alcohol breath test indicates an alcohol concentration of 0.04 or greater
2. While using alcohol
3. Within four hours after using alcohol
4. When using alcohol within eight hours after an accident or until tested
5. When refusing to submit to an alcohol test

XXXVII

Consequences of Drug and Alcohol Abuse

A. The consequences of drug and alcohol misuse must be defined prior to beginning the program.

B. Safety-sensitive workers must be immediately removed from safety-sensitive functions. Return to duty requires:
1. Evaluation by a substance-abuse professional (SAP)
2. Compliance with any treatment recommendations to assist them with a drug or alcohol problem
3. A return-to-duty drug and/or alcohol test (with a result less than 0.02)
4. The worker to be subject to unannounced follow-up drug and/or alcohol tests

XXXVIII

Employee Awareness and Education

A. Most employers subject to mandatory federal testing are required to provide workers with detailed information about the effects of drug abuse and alcohol misuse on the individual, including:
1. Signs and symptoms of drug and alcohol abuse
2. The regulation requirements and the employer's policy and procedures
3. How and where workers can get help for drug and alcohol problems

B. Worker training and recordkeeping
1. Keep a record that the workers have been notified and/or trained.
2. Have workers sign a receipt that they received a copy of the policy.
3. Provide information and training well before the program begins.
4. Provide face-to face-training with an opportunity to answer questions (the most effective format).

C. Supervisor training
1. Federal regulations require a minimum of one hour each of training on alcohol misuse and drug abuse symptoms and the behavior and appearance indicators used in making determinations for testing on the basis of reasonable suspicion.
2. Supervisors must feel comfortable with evaluating work performance and understand the procedures.
3. Supervisors also must be able to recognize and manage drug crisis situations.

XXXIX

Employee Assistance Programs, Rehabilitation, and Treatment

A. Employee assistance programs provide a support system and counseling services for workers and for management. (See Chapter 11 for a description of employee assistance programs.)

B. The core activities of employee assistance programs are supervisory training, supervisory consultations, assessment, and referral.

C. The employer is not required under federal regulations to provide rehabilitation, pay for treatment, or to reinstate the worker in a safety-sensitive position; these issues may be negotiated with unions.

XL
Other Considerations for Screening Programs

A. Administrative issues

1. Employers should keep detailed records of their drug and alcohol abuse prevention programs; federal agencies will conduct inspections or audits of employers' programs.
2. Worker's alcohol testing records are confidential and may be released only to the employer and substance abuse professional (and to the DOT, if applicable) without a release.

B. Joining a consortium

1. Consortia are entities, such as groups or associations of employers, that provide testing and other related services.
2. Specific benefits of consortia usually include lower costs, accessibility to greater expertise, reduced administrative burden, and reduced liability.

C. Business analysis

1. Drug abuse in the United States is a severe problem and a factor in business competitiveness.
2. Comparison analysis of costs of drug testing with the costs of accidents, injuries, industrial injury time loss, workers' compensation claims, and productivity before and after initiating a drug testing program can provide helpful information.

D. Considerations in establishing a drug testing policy and program for employers not subject to mandatory federal testing:

1. Studies report a correlation between drug testing and increased safety and productivity.
2. Involve unions in policy development.
3. Include ongoing worker input into policy development.
4. Give workers 30 to 60 days' notice before the testing program starts.

E. Legal and ethical considerations

1. Before establishing a drug testing program, employers must review all laws and regulations applicable to their jurisdiction regarding disabilities, rehabilitation, and discrimination.
2. The National Labor Relations Act requires bargaining with unions before changing work rules and policies.
3. Public employers must consider constitutional rights; unreasonable search and seizure is the most common challenge.

Emergency Preparedness/Disaster Plan

The nature of an emergency-management plan is an attempt to predict the unpredictable. So the best you can do is continue to audit, review, and identify risks associated with the activities at your facility. There is no way you can do it too often (Hans, 1995).

The following basic emergency plan can serve as a framework to use in development of a site-specific emergency preparedness/disaster plan. Some of the suggested actions may not be necessary, but they should be considered to assure a comprehensive program. The program should be tailored to establish regulatory compliance for the applicable region or jurisdiction and to protect workers and the community against the emergency conditions that have the greatest potential for occurring in a given facility.

XLI

The Purposes of the Program

The purposes of an emergency preparedness/disaster plan are to:

A. Prevent, or at least control, harm to people and company property in the event of an emergency or disaster

B. Contain the extent of property loss, only when the safety of all staff and neighbors at risk has been clearly established

C. Prevent harm to the environment and/or the surrounding community

D. Facilitate automatic disaster response by avoiding delays caused by decision making

E. Identify previously unrecognized hazardous conditions that would aggravate an emergency situation and take steps to eliminate them

F. Identify deficiencies, such as lack of resource coordination to handle an emergency

G. Raise safety awareness

H. Demonstrate the company's commitment to the safety of its workers

I. Establish regulatory compliance with OSHA's 29 CFR 1910.38 plans for emergency action and fire response; 29 CFR 1910.119 for process safety management; 29 CFR 1910.120 for "hazwoper" (hazardous waste operations); and 29 CFR 1910.151 for medical services and first aid

J. Provide consistency with and support for local emergency plans and response agencies (Wuorinen, 1986)

XLII

The Scope of the Plan

A. The emergency preparedness/disaster plan is site-specific; it is governed by:
   1. Nature of work performed
   2. Number of workers and contractors at site
   3. Hours of operation (Travers & McDougall, 1995)

B. The plan applies to all persons on site, including workers, contractors, and visitors.

C. Steps in developing the plan include:
   1. A vulnerability assessment, which includes a consideration of required responses and necessary resources
   2. Input from community agencies with responsibilities for emergency response

D. The plan should include regular planning meetings and drills (Travers & McDougall, 1995).

E. Cost considerations: Because major emergencies are low-probability events, they compete with other company financial allocations (Auf der Heide, 1989).

F. A written plan should be available for inspection and copying by workers, their representatives, community emergency response agencies, and OSHA personnel.

XLIII

Program Responsibilities

A. Disaster planning committee
  1. Disaster planning requires the expertise of many people; planners may include company management, occupational health and safety personnel, human resources, risk managers, accounting, security, and union representatives.
  2. The number of people and their functions will depend on the size and complexity of the worksite.
  3. Hazard control, emergency response, legal requirements, and administrative concerns must be addressed in the plan.

B. Safety director
  1. Performs the function of emergency response team coordinator for planning and training
  2. Provides and maintains the inventory of hazard monitoring equipment and personal protective clothing and equipment used for hazardous materials response
  3. In an emergency response, performs the role of safety officer
  4. Conducts post-emergency investigations

C. Management
  1. Encourages and supports emergency response plans, activities, and training
  2. Ensures that workers are familiar with and follow the procedures of the plan
  3. Informs the disaster planning committee of any new conditions or potential problems that warrant planning for emergency responses
  4. Reviews and approves revisions to the plan
  5. Ensures adequate resources for implementation and maintenance of the plan
  6. Supports coordination with local community emergency response programs

D. Supervisors
  1. Encourage and support worker emergency response activities and training
  2. Ensure that workers are familiar with and follow the procedures of this plan
  3. Inform the disaster planning committee of any new conditions or potential problems that warrant planning for emergency responses

E. Human resources director
  1. Acts as public relations officer in an emergency by maintaining communication to the news media
  2. Provides communications between upper management at the site and corporate levels and the emergency response team
  3. Communicates with families that may be affected by the emergency

F. Environmental protection manager
  1. Assures proper reporting of environmental contaminations as required by law and corporate policy
  2. Assures proper disposal of hazardous and medical waste in an emergency

G. Health center manager
  1. Acts as medical officer, as defined in the National Fire Academy Incident Command System, during an emergency
  2. Provides and maintains an inventory of emergency medical equipment and supplies
  3. Supervises on-site medical emergency response team members in caring for victims during an emergency response

4. Directs or provides emergency victim triage, treatment, and transportation
5. Communicates with community rescue and medical emergency responders and with hospital emergency department staff
6. Ensures that current emergency patient care protocols are signed by the appropriate health care professionals and updated regularly
7. Ensures that the on-site training of the medical emergency response team in first aid and cardiopulmonary resuscitation (CPR) is provided and kept current according to criteria of the certifying agency
8. Schedules and arranges respirator user and emergency responder physical examinations according to company protocol and regulatory requirements, such as for hazardous materials (HazMat) technicians outlined in OSHA 29 CFR 1910.120 (See Appendix F for description of the hazardous materials technician.)

H. Emergency response personnel—first-aid team members, hazardous materials response team members, and fire brigade members
1. Provide rapid emergency services within the property boundaries in accordance with the assigned response team
2. Maintain knowledge and skills through participation in on-site training programs and drill exercises
3. Refrain from response activities that are beyond the level of their training and equipment
4. Keep emergency response routine activities from interfering with their normal job responsibilities

I. Workers
1. Know the facility evacuation plans and evacuate as instructed during actual and practice alarms
2. Report all emergency situations, including health, fire, chemical, and intrusion by calling a designated phone number
3. Follow instructions of the evacuation team leaders, emergency response team members, and community emergency response personnel

J. Security personnel
1. During an emergency, rope off the predesignated section of parking lot for emergency response vehicles
2. Prevent site entry of curiosity seekers
3. Prevent removal of company documents and property during the disruptions of a site emergency
4. Escort arrivals to the appropriate company representative, such as escorting the news media to the Human Resources Director, at a predesignated meeting location

K. Switchboard operator
1. Properly handles emergency calls by determining the nature of the emergency and the details outlined on the emergency call form
2. Notifies the on-site emergency response personnel when an employee emergency call is received
3. Summons community emergency response agencies at the direction of the emergency response manager in charge
4. Activates the site alarm system when directed by the emergency response manager in charge
5. Receives all bomb threats telephoned to the switchboard, documents them, and reports them immediately to management

L. Maintenance supervisor

1. Provides, maintains, and ensures monthly inspections of all fire response equipment and supplies, self-contained breathing apparatus (SCBA) equipment and tanks, and rescue hardware/tools stored for emergency response
2. Maintains emergency power-generating capability
3. Directs shutdown, repair, and start-up of utilities involved in site emergencies
4. Provides post-incident assessment of hazards and damage to property and equipment
5. Makes regular rounds, being alert to fire potentials, chemical leaks, and utility failures

M. Technical consultants

1. Respond to the incident command operations center, when requested, to interpret and advise on the current status and potential escalations of a chemical incident
2. Attend annual training on hazardous materials emergency response

XLIV

General Emergency Procedures

A. Strategies for communications include:

1. Notification phone number list (Compose a list of names, site phone extensions, home phone numbers, and pager numbers of everyone whose support your company might need.)
2. Community response agency phone number list (Compose a list of agencies with names, phone numbers and pager numbers of every agency whose support your company might need; possibly include security companies, insurance companies, photographers, attorneys and public relations firms.)
3. Throughout the facility, install bright red manual fire alarm pull stations that are linked to the local fire department alarm console.
4. Locate evacuation alarms throughout the facility that can be activated by the switchboard operator.
5. Set up an internal communication system consisting of a designated emergency telephone number and a pager system.
6. Establish family notification procedures, to be conducted as necessary by the human resources director (or other company official).
7. Utility companies will be contacted as necessary by the maintenance supervisor.
8. Regulatory agencies requiring reporting of hazardous materials release will be notified by the environmental protection manager; the local OSHA office will be notified by the safety director, in accordance with OSHA requirements in the event of a work-related fatality or hospitalization of workers.

B. Organization: Personnel in command will be established according to the nature of the emergency, as follows:

1. Medical emergencies: the occupational health physician or the occupational health nurse is in command.
2. Fire emergencies: the fire brigade captain is in command in incipient level fires; in major structural fires, the local fire department is in command.
3. Hazardous materials releases: the hazardous materials (HazMat) team captain is in command; in major releases involving the community, the local fire department's HazMat technician team is in command.

4. Natural disasters, intrusions, and bomb threats: the human resources and safety directors share command in coordination with security; in events of immediate threat involving bomb threats, violence, and intrusions, the local police authority is in command.
5. Overall coordination of this plan development and implementation is under the direction of the emergency response team coordinator.
6. Design and annual review of this plan are under the direction of the disaster planning committee chairman.

C. Evacuation procedures
1. Assign individuals to assist handicapped workers in emergencies.
2. Identify evacuation routes and alternate means of escape; make these known to all persons at site.
3. Keep the routes unobstructed through regular safety department inspections.
4. Evacuation routes should be clearly posted.
5. Evacuation and fire drills should be held at least annually to practice the documented plans; every drill or actual emergency incident should be followed by an in-depth evaluation to include all levels of responders.

D. Personnel accountability during an evacuation
1. Specify safe locations for staff to gather for head-counts to ensure that everyone has left the danger zone.
2. Each department must assume responsibility for its workers and its visitors.
3. Reenter the building only after being advised to do so by the senior management.
4. Have a designated and an alternate head-counter—one for every 20 workers.
5. Notify the incident command of the results of the count and of any missing persons.

E. Information dissemination
1. Insurers will be notified by the human resources department or site management.
2. Community and media will be advised by the human resources director; a preselected site should be designated for media and press releases.

F. Authority notification/reporting
1. The local emergency planning committee will be notified by the local fire department as required by regulations.
2. The national response center will be notified by the safety director when mandated by regulatory requirements.
3. The local environmental protection agency will be notified, when mandated, by the environmental protection manager.
4. Other notifications may be necessary for your region; company policy may require certain company representative notifications.

G. Recordkeeping
1. All health records will be established and maintained by the occupational health nurse.
2. All fire maintenance and repair records will be maintained by the maintenance supervisor.
3. Boiler records and emergency generator testing records will be maintained by the maintenance supervisor.
4. Incident response records will be established and maintained by an appropriate designee.

5. Hazardous materials release reports will be established and maintained by the environmental protection manager.

6. All other records will be established and maintained by the human resources director and by the safety director, based on the nature of the record and the incident.

XLV

Specific Emergency Procedures

The procedures outlined in this section can be applied to numerous emergency scenarios, including hurricane, flood, major blizzard, bomb threat, fire, medical emergency, and hostile events.

A. A tornado is imminent!

1. Description: If a tornado is imminent, and you have no time to report to the designated tornado shelter:

2. Action plan: Seek safety under a table, desk, or heavy piece of equipment that offers protection from falling debris; use a coat or similar item to protect your face and eyes; put on safety equipment such as safety glasses and hard hat.

3. Post-threat plan: Call the designated numbers for help (if phones are operational); inspect your work area for damage; follow evacuation, cleanup, or other recovery activities as directed.

B. A tornado warning has been issued!

1. Description: If a tornado warning has been issued, and time permits:

2. Action plan: Seek shelter immediately in the auditorium or in restrooms without windows; shut off utilities and processes that will not become hazardous when interrupted; wear any personal safety equipment.

3. Post-threat plan: Call the designated numbers for help if needed (if phones are operational); inspect your work area for damage; follow evacuation, cleanup, or other recovery activities as directed.

C. Hazardous material—a small spill/release has occurred!

1. Description: A small spill that poses no safety, environmental, or health danger and can be handled safely without additional assistance or equipment beyond standard personal safety equipment

2. Action plan: Close valves, right drums or bottles according to your training and the MSDS; prevent the chemical from entering a drain; add neutralizing agents, adsorbents, or pillow.

3. Post-threat plan: Dispose of material according to site hazardous waste procedures. Fill out an accident form.

D. Hazardous material—a large spill/release has occurred!

1. Description: A significant threat to health and safety due to vapors or fume inhalation, skin contact, flammability, environmental contamination, rapid spill proliferation, and loss of site safety control (See Appendix F for summary of OSHA Standard 29 CFR 1910.120: Hazardous Waste Operations and Emergency Response.)

2. Action plan:

   a. Get yourself and others out of the danger zone. Rope off the area to prevent entry, call the designated number immediately and advise on the nature of the spill, the chemical(s) involved, and the exact location; do not attempt to rescue co-workers.

    b. The on-site hazardous materials (HazMat) team will either respond to the incident according to their training and equipment capabilities or will request help from the local fire department's hazardous materials technician team.

    c. Occupational health providers will respond to provide emergency victim care and to monitor the HazMat team members.

    d. Exposure victims will be decontaminated as necessary by the HazMat team prior to release to community emergency response providers. The hospital will be notified.

  3. Post-threat plan: The size of the release may necessitate a report to governmental authorities. Cleanup operations will be arranged according to the nature of the spill, such as via commercial chemical cleanup companies.

XLVI

Recovery Procedures

A. Critical incident stress debriefing: "Reactions to trauma/crisis in the workplace may have far-reaching repercussions on the emotional as well as financial status of an organization. It is imperative to address these issues and situations as they occur" (Lewis, 1993).

  1. Critical incident stress debriefing (CISD) will be offered to all affected employees in the event of an emotionally traumatic emergency response, which can precipitate critical incident stress similar to post-traumatic stress disorder.

  2. This debriefing will be offered between 24 to 48 hours after the event, the time when debriefing is most effective.

  3. Trained CISD leaders will be obtained from the local fire department's CISD resources.

B. Post-incident evaluation

  1. Incident investigation

    a. Its chief purpose is to prevent similar future losses by identifying and evaluating present losses, reporting to OSHA, and assessing insurance claim needs.

    b. Conduct the investigation at the scene of the incident, keeping the site as undisturbed as possible.

    c. Take photos and/or make drawings or measurements.

    d. Interview all witnesses one at a time and privately.

    e. Seek the root causes.

  2. Reports

    a. Provide regulatory reports as required.

    b. Provide company/internal reports according to company policy.

    c. Provide press releases as needed.

C. Damage assessment

  1. Each worker is expected to evaluate the worksite for damages, make a report to supervisors, and complete a maintenance work order.

  2. The occupational health department will provide a report of injuries, fatalities, hospitalizations to the safety and human resources departments and establish follow-up/case management procedures.

  3. Maintenance will evaluate utilities, building structure, and major processing equipment for damages and report to safety and upper management.

4. Section supervisors will evaluate worker reports and departmental damages, including records lost, equipment lost or damaged, and any damages that pose a safety hazard or interrupt the ability to return to normal operations and report these to maintenance, safety and management.

D. Cleanup and restoration
   1. The company's employee assistance program will be contacted for services if applicable.
   2. Cleanup operations will be supervised by the maintenance department, which will use outside contractors as needed, after approval from management.
   3. Accounting will quantify financial losses and restoration costs for management.
   4. Management will establish a priority list for restoration processes to return to normal operations.
   5. Professional services such as legal assistance will be arranged by management as applicable.

XLVII

Program Maintenance

A. Location and upkeep of emergency plan document
   1. Distribution: plant manager, shift supervisors, emergency response team coordinator, safety, occupational health services, human resources, maintenance, switchboard, local fire department, local emergency planning committee.
   2. Plan will be reviewed and updated annually by the disaster planning committee, with changes being implemented by the chairman.

B. Testing and drills
   1. Evacuation drills will be conducted at least annually.
   2. Emergency response team drills will be conducted monthly, using methods such as table-top drills, skills practice, and mock drills.
   3. A mock disaster drill will be conducted annually and should include community emergency response agencies.
   4. Emergency responders will be required to pass annual performance tests of procedures such as CPR, according to their area of response.
   5. Follow-up assessment will include identification of processes that proceeded as planned, areas requiring improvement, and equipment and operating procedures that need to be added, deleted, or modified. Participants will be advised of the findings.

C. Training
   1. The HazMat team training will be conducted by a recognized, qualified training firm with awareness, operations, and technician levels of training in accordance with the requirements of 29 CFR 1910.120 and provided for appropriately designated workers, who will also receive annual refresher training.
   2. Fire brigade members will be trained to the level of incipient fire response in accordance with NFPA 600 and OSHA Standard Subpart L by the local fire department, with refresher training annually.
   3. First-aid and CPR training will be provided by the occupational health nurse with monthly training sessions and annual refresher programs; training curriculum will be in accordance with the standard of the American Heart Association or National Red Cross and with the OSHA Compliance Guideline 2-2.53C, promulgated in October, 1990.

D. Equipment
1. Each emergency response team will maintain its own equipment, with the exception of the fire and self-contained breathing apparatus (SCBA) equipment, which will be maintained by the maintenance department.
2. Equipment inspections will be conducted and recorded monthly; deficiencies will be reported to the emergency response coordinator.
3. The emergency response coordinator will provide annual updated lists of on-site equipment to the disaster planning committee chairman for inclusion in the appendices of this plan as labeled.
4. Medical and first-aid equipment will be located at the occupational health service center, while additional first-aid kits, stocked by the occupational health nurse, will be located at the entrance of each department.

E. Facilities
1. The occupational health service will be the site for client care, if it is not conducted at the scene.
2. A designated meeting location will serve as the media center and will contain a site plot plan, photographs of emergency response drills for reference, telephones, fax machine, podium, and extra tables and chairs.
3. A predesignated location will serve as the incident command post to conduct centralized emergency operations management. This facility will contain two-way radios, site plot plans, telephone, fax machine, set of material safety data sheets (MSDSs), a copy of this plan, and emergency lanterns.

XLVIII

Appendices to Include in a Written Plan

A. Appendix A: Hazardous Materials Inventory with Location (Provide a complete list of all the hazardous substances on site and the department and building where they are located.)

B. Appendix B: Facility/Site Plot Plan (Provide a current map of the entire site. If appropriate, provide building plans for each individual building on site, including locations of fire equipment, emergency exits, evacuation routes, alarm locations, first-aid equipment locations, and other sites as needed.)

C. Appendix C: List of Fire Protection Equipment (Provide a comprehensive list of all fire alarm and response equipment, including fire-fighting foam, fire coats and other protective equipment, fire hoses, etc.)

D. Appendix D: List of Plant Emergency Safety and Rescue Equipment (Provide a comprehensive list of all plant safety and rescue equipment, such as tripods and confined space harnesses, chemical neutralizers, spill blankets, shovels, respirators, etc.)

E. Appendix E: List of Plant Emergency Medical Equipment (Provide a list of all on-site first-aid and professional medical equipment, such as stethoscopes, antidotes, stretchers, splints, etc.)

BIBLIOGRAPHY

International Travel Health and Safety Program

American Public Health Association. (1990). *Control of communicable diseases in man* (15th ed.). Washington, DC: Author.

Bezruchka, S. A. (1992). *The pocket doctor: Your ticket to good health while traveling* (2nd ed.). The Mountaineers, 306 2nd Ave W., Seattle, WA 98111.

Dawood, R. (1994). *Traveler's health: How to stay healthy all over the world*. New York: Random House.

Jong, E. C. (1995). *The travel tropical medicine manual*. Philadelphia: W. B. Saunders Co.

Wolfe, M. S. (Ed.). *Health hints for the tropics* (11th ed.). American Society of Tropical Medicine and Hygiene. Northbrook, IL.

Case Management Program

AAOHN. (1994). Position statement: The occupational health nurse as a case manager. *AAOHN Journal, 42*(4).

American Board for Occupational Health Nurses. (1994, February). Position statement: The certified occupational health nurse as a case manager. Hinsdale, IL: Author.

Burgel, B. J. (1991). Case management: A system of care delivery for the future. *AAOHN Update Series, 4*(13), 2–7.

Henderson, M., & Wallack, S. (1987, January). Evaluating case management for catastrophic illness. *Business and Health*, 7–11.

Martin, K. J. (1995). Workers' compensation case management strategies. *AAOHN Journal, 43*(5), 245–250.

Mazoway, J. (1987, January). Early intervention in high-cost care. *Business and Health*, 12–16.

Rieth, L., Ahrens, A., & Cummings, D. (1995). Integrated disability management: Taking a coordinated approach to managing employee disabilities. *AAOHN Journal, 43*(5), 270–275.

U.S. Department of Health and Human Services. (1994). *Acute low back problems in adults: Assessment and treatment*. AHCPR No. 95-0643, Rockville, MD: Public Health Service, Agency for Health Care, Policy and Research.

Weil, M., & Karls, J. (1985). Historical origins and recent developments. In *Case management in human service practice: A systematic approach to mobilizing resources for clients*. San Francisco: Jossey-Bass Publishers.

Hearing Conservation Program

Gasaway, D. C. (1987, Feb. 26). Thirteen steps to developing an effective hearing conservation program. *Plant Engineering*, 51–53.

Royster, J. D., & Royster, L. H. (1990). *Hearing conservation programs: Practical guidelines for success*. Chelsea, MI: Lewis Publishers.

Suter, A. H. (1993). *Hearing conservation manual* (3rd ed.). Milwaukee: Council for Accreditation in Occupational Hearing Conservation.

U.S. Department of Health & Human Services. (1990). *A practical guide to effective hearing conservation programs in the workplace* (DHHS [NIOSH] publication No. 90-120). Washington, DC: U. S. Government Printing Office.

U.S. Department of Labor, Occupational Safety & Health Administration. (1983). Final Rule. Rules and regulations: OSHA noise standard. 29 CFR 1910.95. *Federal Register, 48*(46).

U.S. Department of Labor, Occupational Safety & Health Administration. (1992). *Hearing conservation*. OSHA Publication No. 3074 (Revised).

U.S. Department of Labor, Occupational Safety & Health Administration. (1991). Occupational noise exposure compliance assistance guideline, 1991-519-701-20406, Washington, DC: U.S. Government Printing Office.

Hazard Communication Program

Daugherty, J. (1995). Hazard communication for small plants. *Occupational Hazards, 57*(2), 37.

LaBar, G. (1992). Hazard communication: A performing art. *Occupational Hazards, 55*(20), 35–38.

Levy, B. S., & Wegman, D. H. (Eds.). (1995). *Occupational health: Recognizing and preventing work-related disease* (3rd ed.). Boston; Little, Brown & Company.

McGill, L. D. (1989, Autumn). OSHA's hazard communication standard: Guidelines for compliance. *Employment Relations Today*, 181–187.

U.S. Department of Labor, Occupational Safety & Health Administration. (1994). *Chemical hazard communication.* (OSHA Publication No. 3084, revised). Washington, DC: U.S. Government Printing Office.

U.S. Department of Labor, Occupational Safety & Health Administration. (1995). *Hazard communication guidelines for compliance* (OSHA Publication No. 3111, revised). Washington DC: U.S. Government Printing Office.

U.S. Department of Labor, Occupational Safety & Health Administration. *OSHA's expanded hazard communication standard* (Fact Sheet No. OSHA 89-26) 1989-242-368/08071. Washington, DC: U.S. Government Printing Office.

U.S. Department of Labor, Occupational Safety and Health Administration. Final Rule. Hazard communication. 29 CFR Part 1910, 1200, *Federal Register, 45*(27). February 9, 1994.

Washington State Department of Labor and Industries, Industrial Safety and Health Division. (1993). *Understanding "Right to Know."* P413-000 (3/93). Olympia, WA: Author.

Weinstock, M. P. (1993). Hazard communication: Clearing up the confusion. *Occupational Hazards, 54*(7), 35–39.

Drug and Alcohol Testing Program

An employer's guide to substance abuse in the workplace. The employer pocket advisor series.

Bernardo, M. A. (1988). *Drug abuse in the workplace: An employer's guide for prevention.* (2nd ed.). Substance Abuse Training Systems, Substance Abuse Awareness Program, Employee Handbook, DPS. Tustin, CA.

How to build a drug-free workplace, Drug-Free Workplace Workshop for the Business Owner and Manager, Washington Drug-Free Business, S/A Tom Pool, Drug Enforcement Administration: Seattle, Field Division.

How to build a drug-free workplace, Drug-Free Workplace Workshop for the Business Owner or Manager, Olympia, WA: Washington Drug-Free Business.

U.S. Department of Transportation. (1994a, February). *Alcohol and drug rules: An overview.* (P.L. 100-690, 41 USF & 701 et seq.).

U.S. Department of Transportation. (1994b, February). *Alcohol and drug rules.* 49 CFR 382 et. al., 49 CFR Part 40, Federal Register.

Washington State Industrial Safety and Health Act, RCW 49.17, Department of Labor, WAC 296.24.073.

Emergency Preparedness/Disaster Plan

American Association of Occupational Health Nurses (1995). Accident investigation. *AAOHN Advisory.* Atlanta: Author.

Auf der Heide, E. (1989). *Disaster response principles of preparation and coordination.* St. Louis: C.V. Mosby.

Fagel, M. J. (1994). Drilling for disaster. *Occupational Hazards, 56*(7), 23–25.

Hans, M., (1995). Are you prepared for a crisis? *Safety + Health, 151*(6), 38.

Hau, M. (1995). Emergency action plans: Is yours just an illusion? *Safety + Health, 151*(9), 156.

Kelly, R. B. (1989). *Industrial emergency preparedness.* New York: Van Nostrand Reinhold.

Lewis, G. W. (1993). Managing crises and trauma in the workplace: How to respond and intervene. *AAOHN Journal, 41*(3), 124–130.

Meyer, M. U., & Graeter, C. J. (1995). Health professional's role in disaster planning: A strategic management approach. *AAOHN Journal, 43*(7), 251–262.

Sarkus, D. J. (1992). A complete written disaster plan helps maintain business as usual. *Occupational Health and Safety, 61*(9), 34–36.

Travers, P. H., & McDougall, C. (1995). *Guidelines for an Occupational Health & Safety Service.* Atlanta, GA: AAOHN Publications.

Wuorinen, V. (1986). *Emergency planning.* Hamilton, Ontario, Canada: Canadian Centre for Occupational Health and Safety.

Section Three:
Advancing Professionalism in Occupational Health Nursing

CHAPTER

13

Research in Occupational Health Nursing

MAJOR TOPICS

- *Purposes of research*
- *Research development*
- *Research dissemination*
- *Research utilization*
- *Ethics in research*
- *Research priorities*
- *Research evaluation*

Research is essential in supporting and expanding the knowledge base for occupational health nursing practice. It contributes to the improvement in workers' health and safety, and thereby to the quality of their lives and work. This chapter focuses on basic elements in the research process, research priorities and funding sources, evaluation criteria, communication of research findings, and the utilization of research findings, which are all critical to advancing occupational health nursing practice.

I

Professional Mandates for Research

A. AAOHN Standards of Occupational Health Nursing Practice, Standard IV Research: The occupational health nurse contributes to the scientific base in occupational health nursing through research, as appropriate, and uses research findings in practice (AAOHN, 1994).

1. The organization supports occupational health nursing research through encouraging participation and/or providing resources to conduct research.
2. The occupational health nurse engages in research through activities such as identifying researchable problems; designing and conducting research; disseminating research findings; writing research grant proposals; and collaborating with other disciplines in research studies.

B. ANA Standards of Clinical Nursing Practice, Standard VII Research: The nurse uses research findings in practice (ANA, 1991).

1. The nurse uses research-based interventions in practice.
2. The nurse participates in research activities that are appropriate to the nurse's education and experience.

II

Research Roles in Occupational Health Nursing by Preparation Level

A. Associate degree/diploma: The occupational health nurse identifies clinical problems for research; assists in the development of the research and the collection of data; and uses research as a basis for clinical practice.

B. Baccalaureate degree: The occupational health nurse evaluates research for its applicability to practice; works with skilled researchers on the development of research projects; uses research to refine and extend the practice; and discusses research findings with colleagues.

C. Master's degree: The occupational health nurse provides clinical expertise related to the research problem, care delivery, and the research process; analyzes the practice problems within the context of the scientific process; facilitates an environment supportive of nursing research; disseminates research findings; collaborates with other disciplines in scientific investigations; and supports the conduct of research and integration of research into practice.

D. Doctoral degree: The occupational health nurse develops and conducts independent and collaborative investigations with other scientists; develops methodology for scientific inquiry of phenomena relevant to nursing; uses analytical methods and integrates findings to explain and extend scientific knowledge to nursing practice; develops and tests interventions to improve worker health and safety; acquires research grant support; and provides leadership for the integration of research findings into practice.

III

Purposes of Research

Research aims to (Polit & Hungler, 1995):

A. Help identify and solve problems relevant to nursing practice.

B. Improve the effectiveness of nursing care through scientific inquiry, using a systematic process.

C. Advance the body of knowledge in the occupational health nursing discipline.

IV

Research Development

A. Identify the problem
  1. The research problem is identified within the context of an existing problem; its intent is to solve the problem and improve practice.
  2. The problem is relevant to contemporary nursing practice and is stated clearly and precisely.
  3. Research of the problem will contribute to the body of nursing knowledge.
  4. Research of the problem will explain, describe, and predict behaviors and will test strategies or interventions to improve outcomes.

B. Significance
  1. The research problem needs to address the "so what?" question.
  2. Rationale for the importance of the problem and/or gaps in the literature that address critical characteristics of or solutions to the problem need to be discussed.

C. Literature review
 1. The literature is discussed to help the researcher critically evaluate prior and current research in order to provide a context or frame of reference for the study.
 2. Literature sources may include previous studies relevant to clinical or substantive articles, conceptual or theoretical understandings, and methodological readings.
 3. When critiquing a research study, the following should be considered:
    a. Clarity, logic, and understandability of the study
    b. Currency of study and applicability to practice
    c. Comprehensiveness and strength of questions and hypotheses in the analysis
    d. Theoretical framework, if used
    e. Appropriate design, sampling, and interpretation of findings
    f. Protection of subjects' rights
    g. Limitations
 4. Literature should be analyzed and synthesized.

D. Problem statement/formulation
 1. The *problem statement* introduces the topic, explains the importance of the problem, and what the research intends to study.
 2. The problem statement may be grounded within a theoretical (links and explains the relationships among different theories) or conceptual framework (building blocks of theories). However, not all research studies may be sufficiently developed to have these frameworks (i.e., descriptive studies).
 3. Several types of research questions exist (Brink & Wood, 1988):
    a. Type I research question: An expression of a single concept with the stem beginning with "what." Little or no knowledge about the topic exists. Example: What are occupational health nurses' attitudes about managed care?
    b. Type II research question: Examines relationships between two or more concepts or variables. Example: What is the relationship between stress and cholesterol?
    c. Type III research question: Builds on type I and II questions and examines a causal relationship using an experimental design. Asks why. Example: Why does an increase in stress result in increased musculoskeletal disorders?

E. Formulation of hypothesis, if appropriate.
 1. A hypothesis requires a theoretical basis and is used to test an idea.
 2. A hypothesis specifies a relationship between two or more variables and is used when the researchers can predict an outcome. Example: Stress-reduction programs are likely to reduce musculoskeletal disorders.

F. Definition of terms
 1. *Conceptual definitions* explain interrelationships between concepts (e.g., between self-esteem and an eating disorder).
 2. *Operational definitions* actualize the variable (e.g,. an occupational health nurse can be defined as a registered nurse who works at least 20 hours per week).

G. Methodology
 1. Designs: There are many types of designs that can be used to answer the research question(s). Designs fall into two major categories (Polit & Hungler, 1995):

a. *Experimental designs* are used to test research hypotheses and are intended to infer causal relationships.

   1) A *true experiment* requires random assignment of subjects, a control group, and manipulation of a treatment or intervention (independent variable) for the experimental group. (e.g., randomly assign subjects to two groups, administer treatment to one group, and measure outcome or effect in both groups).

   2) *Quasi-experimental designs* include manipulation of the treatment or intervention; however, this design lacks either a control group or random assignment of subjects.

   3) *Pre-experimental designs* include only manipulation of the variable or treatment in the one group (i.e., no comparison group or randomization), and measurement of effect.

b. *Nonexperimental designs* are used when the research does not support an experiment (e.g., survey). They fall into two broad categories:

   1) *Descriptive studies* are designed to observe and describe the phenomenon under investigation and are not concerned with relational variables.

   2) *Ex post facto* (sometimes called *correlational*) *research* examines relationships between variables (that have already occurred) and *implies* a correlation (e.g., smoking and lung cancer).

2. Variables

   a. *Dependent* variable: This is the study variable under investigation (i.e., the outcome variable).

   b. *Independent* variable: This is the variable that is presumed to have an effect or influence on the dependent variable. In an experimental design, it is the treatment or intervention.

   c. Example: Is absenteeism higher among workers who work straight shifts than among those who work rotating shifts?

   • Dependent variable: absenteeism
   • Independent variable: shiftwork

3. Research instruments/measurements

   a. Instrumentation

      1) Existing instruments or tools are often available for the researcher to use. The researcher should search the literature carefully for available instruments that can be used or modified to answer the research question(s).

      2) If no instruments/tools are available, the researcher may need to develop and pilot-test a new tool.

   b. Reliability and validity of an instrument

      1) The *reliability* of an instrument is the degree of consistency in the measurement of responses of the attribute under study. Types of reliability measurements include:

         a) *Stability,* which refers to the extent to which the same results are obtained on repeated administrations of the instrument (also referred to as test-retest)

         b) *Internal consistency,* wherein all items included measure a certain attribute, not some other tangential attribute

         c) *Equivalence,* wherein the instrument produces the same (or equivalent) results when administered by two different observers or raters

      2) *Validity* refers to the degree to which an instrument measures what it is supposed to measure. Examples include:

a) *Content validity*, which is concerned with the sampling adequacy of the content area being measured.

b) *Criterion-related validity*, which focuses on the relationship or correlation between the instrument and some outside criterion (e.g., an instrument to measure self-performance would be validated by a manager's ratings).

4. Population and sample
   a. The *target population* includes all persons who fit the characteristics the researcher wants to study and to whom the results can be generalized. When not all individuals can be included in a study, a sample of the population may be used.
   b. The *sample size* needs to be adequate within the context of the design and problem under investigation.
   c. Depending on time, resources, and subject availability, different types of sampling may be used.
      1) *Probability sampling*: all elements or subjects have an equal chance of being included. Types of probability samples include random, stratified random, systematic random, and clusters.
      2) *Nonprobability sampling*: subject selection is not based on chance; for example, the use of volunteers. Types of samples include convenience, quota, purposive, and snowball.
      3) Probability sampling is more representative of the population and usually affords greater generalizability and less bias.

5. Data collection
   The phase of the study wherein the researcher gathers the data specific to the purpose and questions. Several methods can be used, depending on the types of data needed.
   a. *Interview*: can be face-to-face or via the telephone.
   b. *Questionnaire*: involves a written response to survey items, using a structured format or open-ended questions.
   c. *Observation*: involves systematic observation of subjects and recording of data for later analysis.
   d. *Physiologic*: involves methods to measure bio-physiological data, such as blood and urine samples or an electrocardiogram (ECG).

6. Data analysis/interpretation
   The researcher examines the data elements using statistical approaches, addresses the research questions, forms conclusions, and makes recommendations.
   a. *Quantitative data* provide descriptive statistics and comparative analysis about phenomena measured at the nominal, ordinal, interval, or ratio levels. The higher the level of measurement, the more powerful the results.
      1) *Nominal level* measurement (lowest level) is simply the assignment of numbers to classify data into mutually exclusive categories (e.g., 1 = male, 2 = female).
      2) *Ordinal level* measurement involves the sorting of elements on the basis of their relative standing to each other, yielding a rank ordering (e.g., 1 = completely independent to 5 = completely dependent).
      3) *Interval level* measurement yields equivalent distance between numerical values on scales (e.g., temperature scale).
      4) *Ratio level* measurement (highest level) permits numerical calculations and has an absolute zero.

    b. *Qualitative data* provide descriptions about phenomena and are hypothesis generating.

    c. *Descriptive analysis* discusses what was found in the study. Common descriptions include:

        1) Frequency distributions (i.e., counts of the number of times a value was obtained) presented in tables and/or graphs that report the overall summary of group characteristics.

        2) Summary of a group's characteristics about a particular element, such as mean (average), range (highest score minus the lowest score in a given distribution), and the standard deviation (degree to which scores deviate from each other).

    d. *Inferential analysis* begins to specify relationships between variables.

    e. *Interpretation* of findings

        1) Answers to research questions should be clearly provided, and hypotheses supported or not supported. Conclusions and recommendations are made.

        2) Findings are discussed within the context of the practice discipline and future research suggested.

        3) The researcher must be careful in stating to whom the findings are generalized, paying attention to how the sample was selected.

$\overline{\text{V}}$

Research Dissemination

A. It is essential to disseminate research findings in order to build knowledge, improve practice, and share results with colleagues (Mateo & Kirchhoff, 1991).

B. Most original research is published in peer reviewed journals. Articles generally provide an abstract, background information, methodology, findings, and discussion sections. While providing scientific information is critical, research should be reader-friendly and applicable to practice.

C. Research is also disseminated through presentations at scientific meetings and may be discussed in work settings where the research work was conducted.

$\overline{\text{VI}}$

Research Utilization

A. Practice application
Implementation of research into nursing practice is guided by the clinical significance, generalizability of results to populations, and feasibility of implementation, including an analysis of cost-benefit issues.

B. Evaluation
Several factors should be considered prior to practice implementation, including: critical review of the literature, sample representativeness, adequate study design, ethicality, reliability and validity of instruments, consistency with other studies, and cost-effectiveness.

$\overline{\text{VII}}$

Ethics in Research

A. For the protection of all study participants' rights, the research study must provide them with the following:

1. Description of study purpose
2. Discussion of risks and benefits
3. Assurance of confidentiality (and of anonymity, where appropriate)
4. Specification of a contact person

B. Consent to participate in the research must be obtained from each study subject. Consent usually covers an explanation of the study, procedures used, description of risks, invasion of privacy, and methods used to assure confidentiality and anonymity. This is usually done by obtaining a written statement from subjects, or it may be described by the researcher in a cover letter notifying subjects to voluntarily return survey forms.

VIII

Research Priorities

A. Based on guidance from the membership about important research topics to advance the profession and improve the practice, AAOHN has previously published research priorities. These are currently under revision.

B. The National Institute for Occupational Safety and Health (NIOSH) has also published National Occupational Research Priorities, which are grouped into three categories:

1. Disease and Injury
   - Allergic and irritant dermatitis
   - Asthma and chronic obstructive pulmonary disease
   - Fertility and pregnancy abnormalities
   - Hearing loss
   - Infectious diseases
   - Low back disorders
   - Musculoskeletal disorders of the upper extremity
   - Traumatic injuries
2. Work Environment and Workforce
   - Emerging technologies
   - Indoor environment
   - Mixed exposures
   - Organization of work
   - Special populations at risk
3. Research Tools and Approaches
   - Cancer research methods
   - Control technology and personal protective equipment
   - Exposure assessment methods
   - Health services research
   - Intervention effectiveness research
   - Risk assessment methods
   - Social and economic consequences of workplace illness and injury
   - Surveillance research methods

IX

Funding Research

A. Several sources exist to support the conduct of research:
   1. Professional societies (e.g., AAOHN)
   2. Government agencies (e.g., NIOSH)

   3. Foundations (e.g., Macy Foundation)
   4. Voluntary agencies (e.g., American Cancer Society [ACS])
   5. Corporations

B. The researcher should consider the research topic as it relates to the mission of the funding source before applying (Rogers, 1992, 1996). (See Table 13-1 for examples of funding sources.)

$\overline{\text{X}}$

Evaluating Research

The following elements should be addressed when critically evaluating research reports (Rogers, 1995):

A. Title: indicates clearly to the reader the intent and topic of the investigation.

B. Abstract
   1. A clear, but concise statement of purpose is provided.
   2. Data analysis is summarized.
   3. Important findings are described.

C. Problem statement/purpose
   1. An introduction to the study topic, including the importance and need for the study is provided.
   2. Specific variables, basic design, population studied, and data collection methods are identified.

D. Theoretical foundation
   1. The selected framework is relevant to the research and is understandable.
   2. A clear linkage of the problem to the framework exists.

E. Literature review
   1. The literature specific to the problem is reviewed from primary (original) sources in scientific/peer-reviewed journals, whenever possible.
   2. Recent and past empirical studies are progressively presented and provide the context and scope of the problem.
   3. The research reviewed is critically analyzed, gaps identified, and synopsis with implications for the rationale for the study is provided.
   4. The review is clear, concise, and understandable.

F. Methodology
   1. Research questions are clearly stated, and hypotheses show a relationship between variables.
   2. Variables are conceptually and operationally stated and amenable to measurement.
   3. The research design is clearly indicated, providing the overall statement for the conduct of the research.
      a. Experimental
         1) Subjects are randomly assigned, control group is identified and adequate, and the intervention is clear and measurable.
         2) Threats to validity of the design are controlled.
      b. Nonexperimental
         1) The best design method to address the research question(s) is selected and variables are controlled for in the design.
         2) Comparison groups, if used, are equivalent and representative.

TABLE 13-1

Selected Organizations for Research Funding for Health-Related Projects

Organization	Application Deadline
Agency for Health Care Policy and Research Rockville, MD, 301-656-3100	February 1, June 1, October 1; for any grant January 15, May 15, September 15, for small grants
American Association of Occupational Health Nurses Atlanta, GA, 404-262-1162	December 1
American Cancer Society New York, NY, 404-320-3333	April 1, November 1
American Federation on Aging Research New York, NY, 212-752-2327	January 15
American Lung Association New York, NY, 212-315-8700	November 1
American Nurses' Foundation Washington, DC, 202-651-7229	June 1
Association of Occupational Health Professionals Reston, VA, 800-362-4347	July 1
March of Dimes Foundation White Plains, NY, 914-428-7100	Varies
Metropolitan Life Foundation New York, NY, 212-578-7049	None
Ruth Mott Fund Flint, MI, 810-232-3180	March, July, November
National Institute for Nursing Research Bethesda, MD, 301-594-6906	February 1, June 1, October 1
National Institute for Occupational Safety and Health Atlanta, GA, 1-800-35-NIOSH	February 1, June 1, October 1
National Institutes of Health Bethesda, MD (Cancer; Eye; Heart, Lung & Blood; Allergy/Infectious Diseases; Arthritis/Musculoskeletal/Skin; Child Health; Diabetes/Digestive/Kidney; Environmental Health; General Medical; Drug Abuse; Mental Health; Alcohol; Neuro/Communicative Disorders) 301-496-4000—Inquire for contact for individual institute	February 1, June 1, October 1
National Science Foundation Washington, DC, 703-306-1243	None
PPG Industries Foundation Pittsburgh, PA, 412-434-2970	September
Prudential Foundation Newark, NJ, 1-800-289-9558	None
Robert Wood Johnson Foundation Princeton, NJ, 609-452-8701	None
Sigma Theta Tau International Indianapolis, IN, 317-634-8171	March 1

4. Subjects and sample
   a. The target population is defined, subjects ascertained, and solution prescribed.
   b. The sample should be representative of the population and the sample size adequate for the statistical analysis and scientific rigor.
5. Instrumentation
   a. Instruments or tools used should be clearly described and the questions asked should be pertinent to the research questions or hypotheses.
   b. Validity and reliability data are provided.
   c. Newly developed instruments or tools should have adequate testing and description.
6. Data collection procedures
   a. Methods used to collect the data (e.g., reviews, questionnaires, physiological measurements) are clearly described.
   b. Data collection procedures are internally consistent.
   c. The setting for data collection is described.
   d. Subject's rights are protected.
7. Data analysis
   a. Demographics of the sample are provided and described.
   b. A description of statistical procedures used for data analysis is provided, including levels of measurement appropriate to the questions.
   c. Research questions or hypotheses are addressed with appropriate descriptive and inferential statistics.
   d. Results are reported and interpreted correctly.
   e. Tables and graphs are used to clarify results and are reported in such a way that the reader can evaluate the results.
8. Interpretation and conclusions
   a. Findings that address the research questions are discussed along with statistical significance and what that means. Other findings are addressed.
   b. Findings are discussed within the context of existing knowledge, and any gaps are identified.
   c. Application of the findings to nursing practice and a discussion of practical strategies are given.
   d. Methodological problems and limitations are discussed.
   e. Generalizability of the findings are addressed.
   f. Suggestions for further research are made.

BIBLIOGRAPHY

American Association of Occupational Health Nurses. (1994). *Standards of occupational health nursing practice.* Atlanta: Author.

American Nurses Association. (1991). *Standards of clinical nursing practice.* Washington, DC: Author.

Brink, P. J., & Wood, M. J. (1988). *Basic steps in planning nursing research.* Boston: Jones and Bartlett.

Mateo, M. A., & Kirchhoff, K. T. (1991). *Conducting and using nursing research in the clinical setting.* Baltimore, Williams and Wilkins.

Polit, D., & Hungler, B. (1995). *Nursing research: principles and methods.* Philadelphia: J.B. Lippincott.

Rogers, B. (1992). Research funding. *AAOHN Journal, 39,* 485–486.

Rogers, B. (1995). Critically evaluating research studies. *AAOHN Journal, 43,* 54–55.

Rogers, B. (1996). Researchability and feasibility issues in conducting research. *AAOHN Journal, 44,* 58–59.

CHAPTER

14

Professional Issues: Advancing the Specialty

MAJOR TOPICS

- *Professional associations*
- *Professional credentialing*
- *Strategies for advancing practice*
- *Partnerships*
- *Future directions*

Professional development is the process by which the occupational health nurse assumes the responsibility to maintain professional competency and to contribute to the professional growth of self and others. The purpose of this chapter is to provide an overview of issues and activities that are related to professionalism in occupational health nursing.

I̲

Professional Associations

A. The American Association of Occupational Health Nurses (AAOHN) is the professional association of nurses engaged in the practice of occupational health nursing.

1. Some of the major roles and responsibilities of AAOHN are:
   a. AAOHN defines the scope of practice and sets standards for occupational health nursing practice.
   b. AAOHN develops standards of professional conduct for the occupational health nurse as described in the AAOHN Code of Ethics (see Appendix B).
   c. AAOHN promotes the health and safety of workers.
   d. AAOHN promotes and provides continuing education for occupational health nurses and professionals.
   e. AAOHN advances the profession by encouraging and facilitating research.
   f. AAOHN is an advocate for occupational health nursing in business, government, and other professional areas.
   g. AAOHN responds to issues critical to the practice of occupational health nursing; examples include:
      1) Governmental affairs action alerts
      2) Position statements and advisories, such as Entry into Professional Practice, Occupational Health Surveillance (see Appendix G)
      3) Examination of competency levels in occupational health nursing practice

2. The *AAOHN Journal* is the official Journal of the American Association of Occupational Health Nursing. It provides information related to occupational health nursing practice, advisories, continuing education modules, and research literature.

B. AAOHN collaborates with other professional associations to advance the specialty; these associations include:
1. The American Nurses Association (ANA)
2. The American Industrial Hygiene Association (AIHA)
3. The American College of Occupational and Environmental Medicine (ACOEM)
4. The American Society of Safety Engineers (ASSE)

II

Professional Credentialing in Nursing

Obtaining and maintaining high-quality nursing care for the public good is the basis of any process used in credentialing nurses, nursing education, and nursing services (ANA, 1979); credentialing is a complex process intended to define levels of practice and associated knowledge, skills, abilities, and competencies.

A. Major credentialing processes include:
1. *Accreditation* is the process by which an agency or organization evaluates and recognizes an institution or program of study as meeting certain predetermined criteria or standards (Joel & Young, 1995).
2. An *academic degree* is awarded to an individual who has successfully taken an officially recognized, predetermined series of steps in a particular branch of learning.
   a. The designation of the academic degree signifies the level of education and indicates an arts or sciences area.
   b. The professional degree is similar, but the designation is an indication of the specific field of study (ANA, 1979).
3. *Licensure* is the process by which an agency of government grants permission to persons to engage in a given profession or occupation by certifying that those licensed have attained the minimal degree of competency.
   a. This process is intended to ensure that the public health, safety, and welfare will be reasonably well protected (Joel & Young, 1995).
   b. Licensure also authorizes the use of a particular title.
4. *Certification* in nursing is a process by which a nongovernmental agency or association validates, based on predetermined standards of nursing practice, an individual registered nurse's qualifications, knowledge, and practice in a defined functional or clinical area of nursing (National Specialty Nursing Certifying Organization [NSNCO], 1987).

B. The American Board for Occupational Health Nursing is the organization recognized for certifying individuals in the specialty of occupational health nursing.

III

Strategies for Advancing the Discipline and Practice

Occupational health nursing is advanced through education, research, continuing education, practice, and other professional activities.

A. Academic education in safety and health

    1. Occupational Safety and Health Educational Resource Centers (ERCs), funded by the National Institute for Occupational Safety and Health (NIOSH), are the primary vehicles for the training and education of occupational health and safety professionals, including occupational health nurses, industrial hygienists, occupational physicians, and occupational safety professionals. (See Table 14-1 for list of NIOSH-funded occupational health nursing programs.)

    2. These ERCs provide academic, research, continuing education, and outreach programs.

    3. Other schools of nursing offer academic degrees and coursework related to occupational health and safety.

B. Research (described in detail in Chapter 13)

    1. The occupational health nurse participates in research activities at levels appropriate to the individual's education and experience, which may include problem identification, critical analysis of reported research, research project participation, acting as a resource person, and collaborating with colleagues.

TABLE 14-1

Listing of Occupational Health Nursing Programs at
Educational Resource Centers and Other Graduate Schools

Organization	Address	Phone/Fax
University of Alabama in Birmingham	School of Nursing University Station Birmingham, AL 35294-1210	(205) 934-6858
University of California, Los Angeles	School of Nursing 10833 LeConte Avenue Los Angeles, CA 90024-6919	(310) 206-3858
University of California, San Francisco	School of Nursing, N505 San Francisco CA 94143-0608	(415) 476-3221 (415) 476-6042 (fax)
University of South Florida	College of Nursing, Health Science Center Box 22, 12901 Bruce B. Downs Blvd. Tampa, FL 33612-4799	(813) 974-9160
University of Illinois at Chicago	College of Nursing 845 South Damen Street, M/C 802 Chicago, IL 60612-7350	(312) 996-7974 (312) 996-7725 (fax)
Simmons College (part of Harvard ERC)	Graduate School for Health Studies 300 The Fenway Boston, MA 02215	(617) 521-2135
The Johns Hopkins University	School of Hygiene & Public Health 615 Wolfe Street Baltimore, MD 21205	(410) 955-4082 (410) 955-1811 (fax)
The University of Michigan	School of Nursing 400 N. Ingalls, Room 3340 Ann Arbor, MI 48109	(313) 747-0347 (313) 747-0351 (fax)

(continued)

TABLE 14-1

Listing of Occupational Health Nursing Programs at Educational Resource Centers and Other Graduate Schools (continued)

Organization	Address	Phone/Fax
The University of Minnesota	School of Public Health 420 Delaware St. SE, Box 197 Minneapolis, MN 55455	(612) 625-7429 (612) 626-0650 (fax)
University of North Carolina at Chapel Hill	School of Public Health Rosenau Hall Chapel Hill, NC 27559-7400	(919) 966-1030
University of Medicine and Dentistry of New Jersey (Part of New York/New Jersey ERC)	Department of Nursing Education School of Health Related Professions 65 Bergen St. Newark, NJ 07107-3006	(201) 982-4322
University of Cincinnati	College of Nursing & Health 200 Proctor Hall Cincinnati, OH 45219-0038	(513) 558-5280
University of Pennsylvania	School of Nursing 420 Service Drive Philadelphia, PA 19104	(215) 898-4725
University of Texas	The Univ. of Texas Houston Health Science Center PO Box 20186 Houston, TX 77225-0186	(713) 792-4670 (713) 792-4407 (fax)
University of Utah	RMCOEH, Building 512 Salt Lake City, UT 84112	(801) 581-3291 (801) 581-7224 (fax)
University of Washington	School of Nursing Box 357262 Seattle, WA 98195-7262	(206) 685-0857 (206) 543-8147 (fax)

2. The occupational health nurse develops grant proposals commensurate with education and experience.
3. The occupational health nurse uses research findings in the development of policies, procedures, and guidelines.

C. Continuing education

AAOHN Standards of Occupational Health Practice (1994), Professional Practice Standards, Standard I: Professional Development/Evaluation: The occupational health nurse assumes responsibility for professional development and continuing education and evaluates personal professional performance in relation to practice standards.

1. Organizational resources are allocated for professional growth activities.
2. The occupational health nurse determines continuing education needs, initiates independent learning opportunities, seeks additional academic/continuing education, and evaluates learning for effectiveness.
3. The occupational health nurse acts as role model and student mentor.

4. The occupational health nurse facilitates learning of colleagues through discussion, demonstration, and quality improvement techniques; the occupational health nurse incorporates new knowledge into practice, based on scientific research.

5. The occupational health nurse meets continuing education requirements for certification, licensure, etc.

D. Practice

1. Occupational health nursing practice is characterized by professionalism and professional commitment.
   a. Professionalism describes the conduct or qualities that characterize a practitioner in a particular field or occupation.
   b. Professional commitment is carried out in accordance with the occupational health nursing standards, scope of nursing practice, and an ethical code.
   c. The occupational health nurse maintains professional image and exhibits a high level of respect and dignity for the profession.

2. All nurses are accountable to the client and society for actions taken in nursing practice.

3. The occupational health nurse demonstrates practice accountability through validations of desired outcomes.

4. The occupational health nurse facilitates the leadership role by recognizing the value of and utilizing professional resources.

E. Growth of the profession

1. The occupational health nurse supports the growth of the profession through:
   a. Membership in professional associations
   b. Serving on association committees and/or boards
   c. Assuming leadership positions in elected capacity

2. The occupational health nurse acts as a role model.
   a. Applies concepts of autonomy, influence, fairness, and risk-taking in the professional role
   b. Supports education to increase one's knowledge and expertise
   c. Supports research as the foundation for professional practice
   d. Precepts students regarding the professional role and knowledge enhancement

IV

Partnerships in Occupational Health

A. Advocacy: The occupational health nurse:
1. Respects the right of employees to question recommendations and treatments
2. Encourages the employee to ask questions and participate in decision making
3. Provides support for workers and the profession in regulatory and legislative arenas

B. Collaboration

The occupational health nurse collaborates with a multidisciplinary team in assessing, diagnosing, planning, implementing, and evaluating care of workers.

1. Collaboration often occurs with physicians, industrial hyginists, toxicologists, safety professionals, and ergonomists to identify, monitor and control workplace hazards and promote a healthy workplace.

2. Collaboration among professionals and others is essential to providing appropriate interventions and treatments of high quality.

3. Collaboration with external agencies supports a safe and healthful work environment.
   - Governmental agencies (i.e., Occupational Safety and Health Administration, National Institute for Occupational Safety and Health, Environmental Protection Agency, Agency for Toxic Substance and Disease Registry) and governmental programs
   - Voluntary agencies (i.e., American Heart Association, American Cancer Society, American Diabetes Association)
   - Nursing organizations (i.e. the American Nurses' Association)
   - Other specialty organizations (i.e., National Safety Council) and professional associations (i.e., American Industrial Hygiene Association)

C. Mentoring: The occupational health nurse assumes a leadership role and serves as a role model for the professional development of peers, colleagues, and others.

$\overline{\text{V}}$

Role Expansion

The role of the occupational health nurse will continue to expand. In collaboration with other professionals, the occupational health nurse will assume new responsibilities (Rogers, 1994).

A. *Case management* will require conducting job analyses and functional capacity job assessments as well as working with community agencies to provide the most appropriate and cost-effective services for employees and family members with complex illnesses and injuries.

B. *Environmental health* responsibilities will include analyzing aggregate data relative to incidence/prevalence, epidemiological trends and patterns, and work practices related to injury/illness events (O'Brien, 1995; Rogers, 1994).

C. *Management* responsibilities/opportunities will include conducting cost-benefit analyses of available internal/external health care services, participating in selection and design of benefits and benefit programs, and providing expertise in program design, implementation, management, and outcome measurement.

D. *Primary care* responsibilities/opportunities will be in consumer education relative to health promotion, disease prevention, self-care, and appropriate access to a reformed health care system, nurse-managed primary care delivery at the worksite for employees and their families, and provision of international health care services to traveling employees (O'Brien, 1995; Rogers, 1994).

E. *Consulting* opportunities will be to provide expertise in occupational health to colleagues, government, and private sector for the purpose of improving workers' health.

BIBLIOGRAPHY

American Association of Occupational Health Nurses (1994). *Standards of occupational health nursing practice.* Atlanta: Author.

American Nurses Association. "By-laws," Article 1, Section 2, 1995.

American Nurses Association. (1979). *The study of credentialing in nursing: A new approach. VI*(12) 82–92.

Burgel, B. (1993). *Innovations at the worksite: Delivery of nurse-managed primary health care services.* Washington, DC: American Nurses Publishing.

Joel, L. A., & Young, L. K. (1995). *Dimensions of professional nursing.* McGraw-Hill Inc., *20:* 457–490.

National Specialty Nursing Certifying Organizations. (1987). "Statement of Purpose."

O'Brien, S., Occupational health nursing roles: Future challenges and opportunities. *AAOHN Journal, 43,* 148–152.

Rogers, B. (1994). *Occupational health nursing: Concepts and practice.* Philadelphia: W.B. Saunders Co.

Standards of Occupational Health Nursing Practice

American Association of Occupational Health Nurses

This publication was developed by the American Association of Occupational Health Nurses (AAOHN) Standards of Practice Task Force, a committee comprised of members of AAOHN. The committee worked under the direction of the AAOHN Board of Directors. These standards have been approved and adopted by the AAOHN Board of Directors.

AAOHN Standards of Practice Task Force:

Janie Spicer-Stailey, BS, RN, COHN
Chairman

Elizabeth Lawhorn, MSN, RN, COHN
Bonnie Rogers, DrPH, COHN, FAAN
Betty Winslow, BSN, COHN

AAOHN also recognizes the following for their contributions:

Annette B. Haag, BA, RN, COHN
President

Ann R. Cox, CAE
Executive Director

Geraldine C. Williamson, MN, RN
Director of Communications and Governmental Affairs

Mary Lou Wassel, MEd, RN, COHN
Director of Professional Affairs

Published by:
American Association of Occupational Health Nurses
50 Lenox Pointe
Atlanta, GA 30324-3176

INTRODUCTION

Standards of nursing practice are developed by the profession to guide practice and provide practitioners with a framework for evaluating practice. They are the means by which a profession maintains accountability to the public.

The American Association of Occupational Health Nurses, the professional association for occupational health nurses, promulgates standards for this nursing specialty, based on the scope of members' practice.

Standards of practice are dynamic and evolve over time to reflect the changing scope of practice and development of new knowledge. This document represents the current scope and knowledge base in occupational health nursing practice.

Framework

The Standards of Occupational Health Nursing Practice consist of Standards of Clinical Nursing Practice and Professional Practice Standards. Criteria developed for each standard permit occupational health nurses to evaluate their practice related to each standard.

Structure criteria describe the resources necessary to deliver care or perform the professional role. Employers have a responsibility to provide the resources and create the environment for achieving the standards; at times, achievement of structure criteria may not be within the control of the nurse. Process criteria describe the nurse's actions in delivering care. Outcome criteria describe the results of the nursing care.

The Standards of Clinical Nursing Practice describe components of care provided to all clients. Clients receiving occupational health nursing care may be individual workers, workers' families, the worker population in a workplace or company, and/or employers.

Professional practice standards describe components of the professional role, that is, behaviors nurses are expected to exhibit in fulfilling their professional responsibilities. The measurement criteria for these standards are broadly written to reflect the different levels of education and different practice environments for occupational health nurses. However, all occupational health nurses are expected to demonstrate professional role responsibilities.

Definition and Scope of Occupational Health Nursing Practice

Occupational health nursing is the specialty practice that provides for and delivers health care services to workers and worker populations. The practice focuses on promotion, protection, and restoration of workers' health within the context of a safe and healthy work environment. Occupational health nursing practice is autonomous, and occupational health nurses make independent nursing judgments in providing occupational health services.

The foundation for occupational health nursing practice is research-based with an emphasis on optimizing health, preventing illness and injury, and reducing health hazards. This specialty practice derives its theoretical, conceptual, and factual framework from a multidisciplinary base including, but not limited to:

- nursing science;
- medical science;
- public health sciences such as epidemiology and environmental health;
- occupational health sciences such as toxicology, safety, industrial hygiene, and ergonomics;
- social and behavioral sciences; and
- management and administration principles.

Guided by an ethical framework made explicit in the AAOHN Code of Ethics, occupational health nurses encourage and enable individuals to make informed decisions about health care concerns. Confidentiality of health information is integral and central to the practice base. Occupational health nurses are advocates for workers, fostering equitable and quality health care services and safe and healthy work environments.

Occupational health nurses collaborate with workers, employers, and other professionals to: identify health needs; prioritize interventions; develop and implement interventions and programs; and evaluate care and service delivery. The nurse is the key to the coordination of this holistic approach to delivery of quality, comprehensive occupational health services which include:

- health promotion and primary, secondary, and tertiary prevention strategies;
- health hazard assessment and surveillance of the worker population and workplace;
- investigation, monitoring and analysis of illness and injury episodes and trends and methods to promote and protect worker health and safety;
- primary care including clinical nursing diagnosis and management of occupational and non-occupational illness and injury;
- case management for occupational and non-occupational illnesses and injuries;
- counseling interventions and programs;

- management and administration of occupational health services, including program planning, policy development and analysis, and cost-containment measures; and
- compliance with regulations and laws governing safety and health for workers and the work environment.

   Occupational health nursing practice is dynamic and recognizes socio-cultural, community, economic, political, technological, and ecological influences and the impact of larger policy issues. Consequently, occupational health nurses must know the legal parameters of practice and respond to legislative mandates which govern worker health and safety. Occupational health nurses are professionally accountable primarily to workers and worker populations and also to the employer, the profession, and self.

Standards of Clinical Nursing Practice

Standard I. Assessment

THE OCCUPATIONAL HEALTH NURSE SYSTEMATICALLY
ASSESSES THE HEALTH STATUS OF THE CLIENT.

Rationale

Assessment of the individual, the workforce, and the environment
provides information that enables the occupational health nurse, through
appropriate planning and intervention, to deliver effective comprehensive
care and programs.

Structure Criteria

A system for collecting, recording, analyzing and retrieving data in a
confidential manner is available in the occupational health care setting.

Process Criteria

1. The occupational health nurse systematically collects subjective and
   objective data pertinent to the client (see Appendix A).
2. The client's immediate condition or needs determine the priority of
   data collection.
3. Appropriate data collection techniques are used, and information is
   obtained from the worker, other health care providers, and significant
   others when appropriate. The data collection process is systematic and
   ongoing.

Outcome Criteria

1. The assessment lays the foundation and provides:
   a. baseline and ongoing data for future comparative purposes.
   b. a database to formulate a nursing diagnosis.
2. Data are current.
3. Data are documented in retrievable form.

Standard II. Diagnosis

THE OCCUPATIONAL HEALTH NURSE ANALYZES DATA
COLLECTED TO FORMULATE A NURSING DIAGNOSIS.

Rationale

Nursing diagnoses are derived from the health status and trend data and guide planning for interventions related to health promotion and all levels of prevention and care.

Structure Criteria

1. Resources to validate nursing diagnoses are available.
2. Written policies specify who has access to information about the nursing diagnoses.

Process Criteria

The occupational health nurse:
1. gathers, interprets, and analyzes data to formulate nursing diagnoses.
2. establishes priorities for interventions.
3. records nursing diagnoses.

Outcome Criteria

1. Diagnoses are derived from the assessment data.
2. Diagnoses are validated with the client, and when appropriate, with significant others and health care providers.
3. Diagnoses are documented in a manner that facilitates the determination of expected outcomes and the clinical/programmatic plan of care, choice of interventions, and evaluation.
4. Diagnoses provide data for research.

Standard III. Outcome Identification

THE OCCUPATIONAL HEALTH NURSE IDENTIFIES EXPECTED
OUTCOMES SPECIFIC TO THE CLIENT.

Rationale

The occupational health nurse identifies an outcome-oriented plan based
on the nursing diagnoses.

Structure Criteria

1. Identification of the problem enables the occupational health nurse to
   make nursing judgments in the provision and delivery of occupational
   health services.
2. Opportunities and resources are available for the occupational health
   nurse to achieve the desired outcomes.

Process Criteria

The occupational health nurse:
1. establishes outcomes derived from diagnoses.
2. identifies outcomes that are measurable.
3. collaborates with both internal and external members of the
   multidisciplinary team, when appropriate, to provide competent care.
4. formulates outcomes with the client and other health care providers
   when appropriate.

Outcome Criteria

1. The occupational health nurse identifies appropriate care from
   assessment and nursing diagnoses.
2. The occupational health nurse provides for continuity of care.
3. Clients are informed of the nursing diagnoses.
4. Outcomes are realistic in relation to the worker's present and potential
   capabilities and the requirements of the job.
5. Outcomes are attainable in relation to resources available to the worker.

Standard IV. Planning

THE OCCUPATIONAL HEALTH NURSE DEVELOPS A PLAN OF CARE THAT IS COMPREHENSIVE AND FORMULATES INTERVENTIONS FOR EACH LEVEL OF PREVENTION AND FOR THERAPEUTIC MODALITIES TO ACHIEVE EXPECTED OUTCOMES.

Rationale

Planning is goal directed and guides occupational health nursing interventions toward achievement of desired outcomes.

Structure Criteria

1. Established scope and standards of practice are available in the occupational health setting.
2. Resources are available for the development of occupational health nursing care plans derived from nursing diagnoses.
3. The practice setting provides the occupational health nurse with the opportunity to collaborate with others to develop a plan of care that optimizes worker health.
4. The practice setting provides a recordkeeping system for client care plans to be documented, communicated to others as appropriate, revised, and updated as worker health status changes.
5. The practice setting allows for health and safety promotion program planning, development, and referral.

Process Criteria

1. The occupational health nurse develops plans of care for workers and worker populations based on current knowledge of nursing, medical, public health, occupational health, social and behavioral sciences, management and administration principles, and laws and regulations governing practice.
2. The occupational health nurse documents the plan of care in record systems.
3. Individual and population care plans:
   - are developed with the client(s).
   - prioritize nursing interventions and assign time frames for achievement of desired outcomes.
   - are congruent with other treatment modalities.
   - identify strategies to foster self-care capabilities.
   - identify interventions that emphasize health promotion and prevention strategies.
   - incorporate workplace surveillance activities to monitor health hazard risks.
   - address employees' fitness for work.

4. The occupational health nurse collaborates with appropriate members of the multidisciplinary team, as needed, to foster cost effective health care outcomes.
5. The occupational health nurse identifies health and safety education needs and includes specific teaching plans and/or referrals.
6. The occupational health nurse establishes realistic and measurable outcomes with the client to maximize functional capabilities and comply with government regulations.

Outcome Criteria

1. The plan reflects nursing diagnoses.
2. The client participates in the decision-making process pertaining to the plan of care and life activities.
3. Specific measurable care objectives are developed for each problem or need identified (see Appendix B).
4. The plan is written and retrievable.
5. The plan documents achievement and revision of goals and objectives.

Standard V. Implementation

THE OCCUPATIONAL HEALTH NURSE IMPLEMENTS INTERVENTIONS TO PROMOTE HEALTH, PREVENT ILLNESS AND INJURY, AND FACILITATE REHABILITATION, GUIDED BY THE PLAN OF CARE.

Rationale

Implementation of nursing interventions is essential to effect desired outcomes.

Structure Criteria

1. Independent nursing actions are promoted in the occupational health setting.
2. Resources, including qualified and appropriate personnel, are provided to meet intervention needs.
3. Implementation strategies are identified in client care plans.

Process Criteria

1. The occupational health nurse integrates current scientific, research, and regulatory information in designing and implementing interventions.
2. The occupational health nurse implements the plan of care in a professional manner with accurate documentation and the understanding, consent, and participation of the client.
3. Appropriate health promotion and prevention strategies are incorporated as a component of care.
4. Interventions are consistent with the care plan. Episodic emergency care treatment and follow-up are provided as needed.
5. Interventions may be delegated to ancillary personnel with appropriate supervision.
6. The occupational health nurse initiates investigative interventions such as worksite walk throughs or job hazard analyses as needed.

Outcome Criteria

1. Interventions are recorded in a systematic, retrievable manner.
2. Evidence of client progress toward outcome achievement is apparent.
3. Interventions are re-examined based on client responses.

Standard VI. Evaluation

THE OCCUPATIONAL HEALTH NURSE SYSTEMATICALLY AND CONTINUOUSLY EVALUATES THE CLIENT'S RESPONSES TO INTERVENTIONS AND PROGRESS TOWARD THE ACHIEVEMENT OF EXPECTED OUTCOMES.

Rationale

Occupational health nursing is a dynamic process that requires ongoing evaluation to reflect state-of-the-art care and service and revision of the plan of care accordingly.

Structure Criteria

1. The practice setting provides access to resources that will allow the nurse to coordinate care and evaluate the care delivered.
2. The occupational health nurse has access to changes in client health information that would influence alteration of the care plan.
3. The practice setting provides opportunity for consultation and guidance to evaluate the results of nursing interventions and to develop alternative plans when appropriate.
4. Appropriate staff participate in the evaluation process.
5. A written plan for progress evaluation is in place.

Process Criteria

1. The occupational health nurse conducts follow up and collects and analyzes pertinent data from all available sources.
2. Evaluation data are compared to expected outcomes.
3. The occupational health nurse collaborates with the client and members of the occupational health team and external providers in the evaluation process.
4. The occupational health nurse revises the client's plan of care to reflect alterations in the client's health status or working conditions and achievement of desired outcomes.
5. The occupational health nurse documents evaluation results and revision of the plan of care which are part of the permanent record.
6. The occupational health nurse conducts and documents program evaluation which includes measurement of immediate and long term outcomes, quality of intervention, and cost benefit analysis.

Outcome Criteria

1. Evaluation of nursing intervention is documented with respect to effectiveness and potential for research.
2. If expected outcomes are not attained, reasons are documented and the plan of care or interaction is revised accordingly.
3. Client participation in the evaluation process is documented.
4. Results of program evaluation are used in the decision-making processes.

PROFESSIONAL PRACTICE STANDARDS

Standard I.
Professional Development/Evaluation

THE OCCUPATIONAL HEALTH NURSE ASSUMES RESPONSIBILITY FOR
PROFESSIONAL DEVELOPMENT AND CONTINUING EDUCATION AND
EVALUATES PERSONAL PROFESSIONAL PERFORMANCE IN RELATION TO
PRACTICE STANDARDS.

Rationale

The occupational health nurse pursues knowledge to enhance professional
growth and thereby maintain professional competency. Overall evaluation
of the occupational health nurse's work is accomplished through ongoing
self-evaluation and analysis of data from quality improvement/quality
assurance mechanisms.

Structure Criteria

1. Opportunities are available to develop performance based goals and
   objectives. The occupational health nurse is evaluated on these goals
   and objectives and participates in the process.
2. A mechanism is in place to provide for staff development and
   continuing education opportunities.
3. Resources and opportunities are provided for the nurse's participation
   in professional organizations' activities and educational activities
   designed to enhance professional growth and leadership development.

Process Criteria

The occupational health nurse:
1. initiates independent learning activities to increase knowledge of
   occupational health nursing concepts and skills.
2. seeks additional academic and continuing education activities to
   increase professional and specialty knowledge and skills.
3. demonstrates professional responsibility by participation in appropriate
   professional organizations.
4. evaluates occupational health nursing interventions to determine the
   effectiveness of professional and nursing activities.
5. serves as a role model and mentor to nursing students and other
   nurses.
6. participates in performance evaluation processes.
7. provides guidance to other health care professionals and students, as
   appropriate, to facilitate learning.
8. communicates new knowledge to colleagues.

9. continually examines and evaluates individual performance to improve and enhance self-competency.

Outcome Criteria

The occupational health nurse:
1. incorporates new information and methods into practice.
2. maintains and updates professional and specialty knowledge and skills.
3. meets continuing education requirements necessary for credentialing.
4. participates in performance evaluation processes and professional development activities.
5. takes action to achieve or modify goals/objectives identified in the evaluation process.

Standard II. Quality Improvement/Quality Assurance

THE OCCUPATIONAL HEALTH NURSE MONITORS AND EVALUATES THE QUALITY AND EFFECTIVENESS OF OCCUPATIONAL HEALTH PRACTICE.

Rationale

The occupational health nurse has an obligation to follow professional practice standards, guidelines, and relevant statutes and regulations while providing care.

Structure Criteria

1. An organized mechanism is in place for monitoring and evaluating the quality of care provided to the workforce.

Process Criteria

The occupational health nurse:
1. participates in the design and implementation of methods for quality improvement/quality assurance and interpretation of data related to quality of care and health care outcomes.
2. develops and evaluates guidelines for practice.
3. evaluates effectiveness of nursing care.
4. recommends changes to improve quality of care.

Outcome Criteria

1. The occupational health nurse maintains quality of care by correcting deficits identified through quality improvement/quality assurance activities.
2. Changes in care are documented and monitored for effectiveness.

Standard III. Collaboration

THE OCCUPATIONAL HEALTH NURSE COLLABORATES WITH EMPLOYEES, MANAGEMENT, OTHER HEALTH CARE PROVIDERS, PROFESSIONALS, AND COMMUNITY REPRESENTATIVES IN ASSESSING, PLANNING, IMPLEMENTING, AND EVALUATING CARE AND OCCUPATIONAL HEALTH SERVICES.

Rationale

The complex demands of the occupational health environment necessitate multidisciplinary collaboration to promote employee health, a safe and healthy working environment, and effective and efficient health care services.

Structure Criteria

1. Opportunities for internal and external multidisciplinary collaboration are provided.
2. Opportunities for participation with other colleagues in decision making and policy setting are encouraged within the practice setting.
3. The team process is supported.

Process Criteria

The occupational health nurse:
1. consults with colleagues as needed to provide optimum care to the client.
2. participates in the formulation of goals, plans, and decisions.
3. collaborates with other disciplines in teaching, continuing education, and research.
4. recognizes and respects colleagues and their contributions.
5. involves clients in decisions about their health care.
6. articulates nursing knowledge and science related to appropriate interventions.

Outcome Criteria

The occupational health nurse:
1. is a member of the interdisciplinary team and participates in occupational health and safety committees, team meetings, and workplace walk throughs.
2. brings the expertise of the multidisciplinary team to client care.
3. engages team members in problem solving activities and planning new services as appropriate.
4. works toward continuity of care.
5. collaborates with others to facilitate change in complex systems.
6. utilizes community resources.
7. manages clients' care from onset of injury/illness to safe return to work or an optimal alternative.

Standard IV. Research

THE OCCUPATIONAL HEALTH NURSE CONTRIBUTES TO THE SCIENTIFIC BASE IN OCCUPATIONAL HEALTH NURSING THROUGH RESEARCH, AS APPROPRIATE, AND USES RESEARCH FINDINGS IN PRACTICE.

Rationale

Improvement in occupational health nursing practice and health care outcomes depends upon the continued development of knowledge through research. The occupational health nurse's commitment to develop knowledge and disseminate and utilize research findings is essential to practice advancement.

Structure Criteria

1. The organization supports occupational health nursing research by encouraging participation in research initiatives and providing necessary resources and materials.
2. Opportunities are provided to gain access to research participants and/or data.
3. Safeguards are in place to protect the rights of research participants.
4. Mechanisms exist to support the dissemination of research results and the integration of research findings into occupational health nursing practice.

Process Criteria

The occupational health nurse participates in research activities at levels appropriate to the individual's education and experience such as:

1. identifying researchable problems related to practice.
2. critically reviewing and evaluating reported research for applicability of findings to practice.
3. initiating or participating in research according to research skills.
4. reporting and disseminating research findings.
5. preparing proposals for support of research projects (internal & external).
6. acting as a resource person for identifying researchable problems, conducting research investigations, and interpreting and evaluating research findings.
7. collaborating with other disciplines in the development of research studies and the dissemination of research findings.

Outcome Criteria

1. The occupational health nurse's practice reflects the integration of currently validated findings from research.
2. Clients receive care based on current knowledge.

Standard V. Ethics

THE OCCUPATIONAL HEALTH NURSE USES AN ETHICAL FRAMEWORK AS A GUIDE FOR DECISION MAKING IN PRACTICE.

Rationale

Occupational health nurses are confronted with complex ethical dilemmas that require careful communication with both the recipients of care and management. An ethical framework provides parameters within which the nurse makes ethical judgments. The occupational health nurse is an advocate for clients to receive accessible, equitable, and quality health care services, including a safe and healthful work environment.

Structure Criteria

1. A structure exists to provide and maintain care within ethical guidelines and legal parameters, such as a policy for safeguarding confidentiality of employee health information.
2. A mechanism exists for identifying and resolving ethical dilemmas, and occupational health nursing is involved in the decision-making process.
3. The AAOHN Code of Ethics and Interpretive Statements are available to occupational health nurses, employers, and employees in the practice setting.
4. Ethical decision-making is facilitated through encouraging participation in educational programs regarding ethical issues.

Process Criteria

1. The occupational health nurse's practice is guided by an ethical framework.
2. The occupational health nurse maintains client confidentiality.
3. The occupational health nurse delivers care to the client respectful of self-determination, diverse cultural preferences, and capabilities for self-care, and acts as a client advocate.
4. The occupational health nurse obtains and uses resources to facilitate ethical decision-making.

Outcome Criteria

1. The rights of the client and the occupational health nurse are protected.
2. Mechanisms are in place for documentation of ethical issues and their resolution such as in the client's health record and/or minutes of appropriate committee meetings.

Standard VI. Resource Management

THE OCCUPATIONAL HEALTH NURSE COLLABORATES WITH MANAGEMENT TO PROVIDE RESOURCES THAT SUPPORT AN OCCUPATIONAL HEALTH PROGRAM THAT MEETS THE NEEDS OF THE WORKER POPULATION.

Rationale

The corporate goals and objectives, number of clients, client health needs, the health hazards of the specific industry, and associated costs determine the elements of a multi-dimensional health and safety program. Policies and practices must be in place to address equality and continuity, for cost-effective service delivery within a safe and healthful work environment. Occupational health nurses are empowered and enabled to apply their expertise in an interactive role in the determination of the organization's resources relevant to occupational health and safety. Authority and accountability are commensurate with resource management responsibility.

Structure Criteria

1. A mechanism exists for strategic, long-range planning within the organization.
2. The organizational structure provides for occupational health nursing representation at administrative and policy-making levels.
3. Personnel and operational and capital resources are provided for the adequate development and maintenance of occupational health nursing services and unit functions.
4. A mechanism exists for managing human or operational resources needed to adequately implement occupational health services.
5. An environment is provided for occupational health nursing staff to participate in decision-making regarding occupational health nursing practice and personnel and material resources.
6. Resources are provided for participation in educational programs to meet the continuing learning needs of occupational health nurses.
7. Support services and equipment are available to facilitate nursing practice.

Process Criteria

The occupational health nurse, at levels appropriate to personal education, experience, and position:

1. participates in the strategic and long-range planning related to occupational health and safety.
2. maintains knowledge of current technology, laws, and trends in health care and occupational health and safety.

3. participates in decisions regarding acquisition, allocation, and utilization of occupational health unit resources.
4. demonstrates managerial skills and implements managerial functions using knowledge of organizational theory, business principles, and dimensions of professional practice.
5. collaborates with all appropriate staff and other health care professionals to develop occupational health unit services.
6. determines and prioritizes clinical and administrative occupational health nursing goals and objectives with input from occupational health nursing staff.
7. prepares, administers, and monitors the budget.
8. provides for ongoing programmatic evaluations of organized services.
9. meets professional and regulatory standards to promote efficient, effective, and safe care delivery as well as safe working conditions.
10. provides leadership in human resource development and management.
11. supports and facilitates occupational health nursing research.
12. reviews alternative approaches to occupational health care and administers quality, cost-effective occupational health service delivery.
13. fosters interdisciplinary team functioning for the provision of optimal occupational health services.

Outcome Criteria

1. Occupational health nursing contributes to the strategic and operational management of the organization.
2. Occupational health nursing strategies and practice models evolve to deliver the most cost-effective occupational health services.
3. Occupational health nursing performance is recorded, recognized, and compensated appropriately.

APPENDIX A
Assessment Data

Data which occupational health nurses may use as part of assessment include:

a. physical and mental requirements of the job.
b. complete health history, including present problems, past illnesses, occupational history, and lifestyle assessment.
c. physical assessment.
d. screening and baseline laboratory tests.
e. identification of high risk worker populations.
f. identification of high risk environmental areas.

g. programs for determining health status which include screening, physical examinations (job placement, periodic health surveillance), and epidemiological studies.
h. periodic review of the health care needs of workers.
i. health promotion and primary, secondary, and tertiary prevention strategies.
j. health hazards and data from surveillance of the worker population and workplace:
   - morbidity and mortality trends.
   - cluster events.
   - exposure data.
   - MSDS.
   - risk perception.
   - knowledge/satisfaction/motivation.
   - risk factors for work-related situations.
   - use of personal protective equipment.
k. communication of information to others.
l. documentation of pertinent client information.

APPENDIX B
Occupational Health Problems or Needs

Examples of problems or needs which occupational health nurses may identify include:

a. improvement in health status of the worker/workforce.
b. reduction in morbidity and mortality.
c. increase in knowledge of associated risk factors.
d. elimination or reduction in risk or hazards related to the work environment, work processes, and work practices.
e. initiation, improvement, or utilization of control strategies changes in policies/procedures related to improvements in worker health and safety.
f. increase in knowledge related to health promotion, preventive health, and therapeutic strategies.
g. reduction in health care costs/premiums.
h. identification of appropriate community and personal resources.
i. use of appropriate resources to enhance coping skills.
j. identification and alteration of conditions or situations which potentiate risk.
k. inability to meet job requirements.

GLOSSARY

Case Management—process of coordinating an individual client's total health care services to achieve optimal, quality care delivered in a cost effective manner. The process integrates assessment, planning, implementation, and evaluation components (AAOHN, 1994). The goal of case management is to provide the right care at the right time—by the most appropriate provider—and in the right setting at the right price (Burgel, 1993).

Client—recipient of the health care services. For the occupational health nurse this may include individual workers, workers' families, the worker population in a workplace or company, and/or employer(s).

Criteria—attributes or measures for evaluating nursing care provided in a particular setting. Three approaches or types of criteria may be used:

- **Structure criteria**—measures of the organizational characteristics of nursing services, facilities, equipment, resources and policy.
- **Process criteria**—measures of the nursing care, what the nurse actually does.
- **Outcome criteria**—measures of the end result or change in status of the client that results from the care provided (Migliozzi, 1990).

Independent Nursing Actions—interventions or strategies implemented by the nurse, based on the nursing diagnoses and/or clinical judgment, to achieve desired client outcomes. Nurses are empowered through education and professional licensure to take appropriate independent actions. However, the complex nature of the work environment at times requires the expertise of other disciplines, and the occupational health nurse initiates or participates in multidisciplinary collaboration, consultation, or referral as necessary (Rogers, 1992).

Levels of Prevention—three levels of prevention conceptualized by Leavell and Clark, using principles of epidemiology; that is, for prevention to be possible, one must know the natural life history of a disease or condition, including how host, agent, and environment interact to produce a disease or condition. The prevention strategies apply to individuals and groups of individuals, families, and communities.

- **Primary prevention** takes place before disease or injury occurs. Its purpose is to prevent illness or injury from occurring. Interventions are directed to general health promotion as well as specific protections from disease or injury.

- **Secondary prevention** begins after a disease or condition is present, and the purpose is to lessen the complications and disability. Emphasis is on early detection and intervention.
- **Tertiary prevention** begins when a condition stabilizes. The goal is to return to the highest possible level of function (Leavell, 1965; Moore, 1984).

Nursing Diagnosis—clinical judgment about a client's response to actual or potential health and safety conditions or needs. Nursing diagnoses provide the basis for planning and implementing care. Occupational health nursing diagnoses include, but are not limited to:

- client health status.
- workforce morbidity.
- populations at risk.
- workplace hazards.

Quality Care—care which:

- conforms to standards or guidelines for appropriate and necessary care.
- meets client requirements.
- offers value at an affordable price.

Health care quality is assessed through measurement of structures, processes, and outcomes of care (Widtfeldt, 1992a; Widtfeldt, 1992b).

Quality Assurance—process for measuring the quality of care delivered. It is internally focused on standards of care. Problems or deficits are identified retrospectively, i.e., after the fact. The focus is on correcting problems or deficits through peer review. A program of systematic evaluation of the care provided is established to ensure that the care meets the established standards and that actions to improve the care are taken as appropriate (Migliozzi, 1990).

Quality Improvement—defined as "what we can do to more effectively and efficiently exceed expectations and/or meet requirements" (Crosby, 1979).

It is internally and externally focused on standards of care and the process of delivery. Problems are identified prospectively, i.e. in advance. The focus is on anticipating potential problems in health care delivery systems, and it involves eliciting the input of consumers, suppliers, and other professionals (Widtfeldt, 1992a).

Resource—personnel, money and/or equipment necessary to achieve the desired outcomes or goals of the nursing services.

Strategic Planning—a special kind of organizational planning which pertains primarily to the future relationship or "goodness of fit" between the organization and its environment (Smith, 1980).

It results in a long-range plan which provides future direction to the organization. It is a process which includes: identification of needs, issues and trends; evaluation of the mission; and formulation of strategies for achieving the long range plan (Cox, 1989).

REFERENCES

AAOHN (1994). *Occupational Health Nurse as a Case Manager,* Position Statement.

Burgel, B. (1993). *Innovation at the Work Site,* American Nurses Association.

Crosby, P.B. (1979). *Quality is Free.* New York: New American Library.

Cox, A. (1989). Planning for the Future of Occupational Health Nursing, Part I. *AAOHN Journal,* Vol.37 (9), 352–355.

Leavell, H.R. and Clark, E.G. (1965). *Preventive Medicine for the Doctor in His Community.* New York: McGraw-Hill.

Migliozzi, A. (1990). Developing Quality Assurance Programs in the Occupational Health Setting. *AAOHN Journal,* Vol. 38 (3), 101–104.

Moore, P. and Williamson, G. (1984). Health Promotion, Evolution of a Concept. *Nursing Clinics of North America.* Philadelphia: WB Saunders Company.

Rogers, B., Mastroianni, K., and Randolph, S. (1992). *Occupational Health Nursing Guidelines for Primary Clinical Conditions.* Boston: OEM Press.

Smith, H.R., Carroll, A.B., Kefalas, A.G. and Watson, H.J. (1980). *Management: Making Organizations Perform.* New York: Macmillan Publishing Co. Inc.

Widtfeldt, A. (1992a). Quality and Quality Improvement in Occupational Health Nursing, *AAOHN Journal,* Vol. 40 (7), 326–332.

Widtfeldt, A. (1992b). Total Quality Management in American Industry, *AAOHN Journal,* Vol. 40 (7), 311–318.

APPENDIX B

AAOHN
Code of Ethics and
Interpretive Statements

Preamble

The AAOHN Code of Ethics has been developed in response to the nursing profession's acceptance of its goals and values, and the trust conferred upon it by society to guide the conduct and practices of the profession. As a professional, the occupational health nurse accepts the responsibility and inherent obligation to uphold these values.

The Code of Ethics is based on the belief that the goal of the occupational health nurse is to promote worker health and safety. This specialized practice is devoted to health promotion, prevention, and management of illness and injury at the worksite. The client can be both an individual worker or an aggregate worker population. The purpose of the AAOHN Code of Ethics is to serve as a guide for the registered professional nurse to maintain and pursue professionally recognized ethical behavior in providing occupational health services.

Ethics is synonymous with moral reasoning. Ethics is not law, but a guide for moral action. Universal moral principles are utilized by the professional nurse when making judgements related to the health and welfare of the worker or worker population.

The most significant principle for the occupational health nurse is autonomy, or the right to self-determination, which encompasses respect for an individual's right to privacy and refusal of care. Confidentiality and truth-telling are related concepts. Other key principles are beneficence (doing or producing good); nonmaleficence (avoiding harm); and justice (fair and nondiscriminatory treatment of all individuals).

Occupational health nurses recognize that dilemmas may develop that do not have guidelines, data, or statutes to assist with problem resolution; thus, the occupational health nurse may use problem-solving, collaboration, and appropriate resources to resolve dilemmas.

The Code is not intended to establish nor replace standards of care or minimal levels of practice. In summary, the Code of Ethics and Interpretive Statements provide a guiding ethical framework for decision-making and evaluation of nursing actions as occupational health nurses fulfill their professional responsibilities to society and the profession.

---

1. The occupational health nurse provides health care in the work environment with regard for human dignity and client rights, unrestricted by considerations of social or economic status, personal attributes, or the nature of the health status.

The profession of occupational health nursing is dedicated to the promotion, protection, and preservation of the life and health of every client. Occupational health nurses render nonprejudicial and nondiscriminatory care to clients.

Occupational health nurses have an obligation to treat clients fairly, respecting their dignity and worth. While recognizing the existence of a vast diversity of cultural beliefs and values in society, occupational health nurses demonstrate respect for these beliefs and values inherent in their clients and themselves, and plan health care services for and with that client accordingly.

The occupational health nurse respects the client's right to autonomy. Clients are encouraged to participate in planning their own health care and occupational health nurses are truthful in providing clients with necessary information to make an informed judgement. While respecting the client's interest and well-being, the nurse examines the short-term and long-term outcomes of the decision-making process. As client advocates, occupational health nurses have the responsibility to be knowledgeable about the client's rights. These rights include acceptance or refusal of care and are acknowledged by the professional nurse. When personal convictions of the occupational health nurse prohibit participation in providing health services and/or when the client refuses care, the nurse may not be exempt from protecting the client's health and safety. The occupational health nurse avoids abandonment and refers clients to available, alternative sources of care.

---

2. *The occupational health nurse promotes collaboration with other health professionals and community health agencies in order to meet the health needs of the workforce.*

The occupational health nurse is a member of the occupational health and safety team. The occupational health nurse functions both interdependently and independently in promoting the welfare of clients. Providing health services to clients requires a commitment to collaborative planning with other health professionals and members of the occupational health team. The occupational health nurse makes referrals to appropriate community resources and seeks assistance and expertise from other recognized health professionals in the provision of services, as appropriate. The occupational health nurse functions within the scope of nursing practice and delegates responsibility to members of the health and safety team as necessary. Occupational health nurses have an obligation to promote adequate distribution of health care and nursing resources to meet clients' needs. The occupational health nurse is responsible to management as an employee. As a professional, the occupational health nurse is an advocate for the workers. The occupational health nurse recognizes situations in which the interests of management and workers may conflict.

As a professional, the occupational health nurse has a responsibility to observe professional codes and uphold practice standards. The occupational health nurse demonstrates fairness in conflict resolution. The promotion of health and safety and prevention of injury and illness at the worksite requires occupational health nursing representation and participation in the decision making process within the institutional and political arenas. Occupational health nurses are encouraged to become and remain participants in decision-making processes that define or pertain to occupational health nursing functions or activities.

---

3. *The occupational health nurse strives to safeguard the employee's right to privacy by protecting confidential information and releasing information only upon written consent of the employee or as required or permitted by law.*

Occupational health nurses have an obligation to maintain the trust bestowed upon them by the client and to protect the client's right to privacy. Public trust is ensured by maintaining the confidentiality of health information through prevention of unauthorized access. Written policies and procedures should guide the access, release, transmittal, and storage of health information, including computerized records.

Occupational health nurses are encouraged to use current professional literature and resources for guidance. The occupational health nurse is knowledgeable about and adheres to the organizational, local, state, and federal policies and laws governing access to confidential information. Employees are then protected from unauthorized and indiscriminate access and disclosure of health and/or personal information. Confidentiality is crucial to the effectiveness of the occupational health program.

---

4. *The occupational health nurse strives to provide quality care and to safeguard clients from unethical and illegal actions.*

Occupational health nurses are dedicated to providing quality, competent, and professional services to their clients. Each occupational health nurse is a representative of the profession and demonstrates competent, ethical, and professional conduct and accountability. The profession's primary commitment is to the health, safety, and welfare of clients. The occupational health nurse strives to protect the client and the profession from incompetent professionals and individuals who misrepresent themselves and the profession. Any person or persons who exhibit incompetence or engage in unethical or illegal activities may be reported to licensing, accrediting, or certifying authorities, as may be appropriate. The occupational health nurse should participate in the development of policies to promote competent, ethical, and legal nursing practice. Occupational health nurses have a commitment to comply with the laws and regulations that govern the workplace in an effort to provide workers with a safe and healthful workplace.

---

5. *The occupational health nurse, licensed to provide health care services, accepts obligations to society as a professional and responsible member of the community.*

As a licensed health professional, the occupational health nurse has an obligation to the client, employer, community, society, and profession to demonstrate credibility and competence. The occupational health nurse is a responsible citizen in the community adhering to all laws and statutes (local, state, and federal), including those governing occupational health practice. As a professional, the occupational health nurse respects the client's and society's right to know and to receive factual information about potential and actual job and environmental hazards. The occupational health nurse is knowledgeable of community issues and dilemmas affecting health, safety, and the welfare of society, and participates in appropriate resolution when able.

---

6. *The occupational health nurse maintains individual competence in health nursing practice, based on scientific knowledge, and recognizes and accepts responsibility for individual judgements and actions, while complying with appropriaite laws and regulations (local, state, and federal) that impact the delivery of occupational health services.*

The profession of occupational health nursing is dedicated to promoting competent professional practice. Occupational health nurses have the responsibility to strive for excellence and maintain a level of knowledge, judgement, technical skills, and professional values necessary for delivering health services. Individual professional licensure provides for protection of the public to ensure that basic professional competencies have been achieved. The occupational health nurse utilizes professional and educational activities to improve professional practice.

Occupational health nurses may engage in professional, educational, and quality improvement activities, such as peer review. The occupational health nurse acknowledges the importance of continued and advanced educational activities beyond the basic level of nursing education. As professionals, occupational health nurses have a personal and professional responsibility to maintain competence in practice. All occupational health nurses are professionally and morally accountable for their actions and compliance with nurse practice acts, standards of practice, and other laws/regulations governing occupational health practice. In a situation where the occupational health nurse does not have the necessary skills or knowledge or is unable to render services personally, the nurse has a moral responsibility to refer the client to appropriate services.

---

7. *The occupational health nurse participates, as appropriate, in activities such as research that contribute to the ongoing development of the profession's body of knowledge while protecting the rights of subjects.*

Research is an integral part of occupational health nursing practice. Research provides new information to improve and validate the tenets underlying the profession's scope of practice. This validation can be accomplished by designing studies, testing theories to guide nursing practice, utilizing and applying research findings, or participating in the research process. Occupational health nursing, as an applied discipline, engages in scholarly inquiry to build upon the body of knowledge that serves as the foundation for practice. Occupational health nurses must strive to create and expand this body of knowledge, both empirically and theoretically, through research activities.

Research activities are usually approved by appropriate bodies, such as institutional review boards. Occupational health nurse researchers should respect and protect the autonomy, rights, and privacy of the subjects. One mechanism to ensure this respect and protect subjects is by voluntary informed consent. The occupational health nurse has a moral obligation to self, the client, the profession, and society to conduct sound ethical research. Occupational health nurses have the responsibility to communicate and disseminate research findings to other occupational health nurses and professionals and to appropriately utilize research findings within their practice.

AAIN: American Association of Industrial Nurses (AAOHN's name until 1977)

AAOHN: American Association of Occupational Health Nurses

ABOHN: American Board of Occupational Health Nurses

ACGIH: American Conference of Governmental Industrial Hygienists

ACOEM: American College of Occupational and Environmental Medicine

ADA: Americans with Disabilities Act

AIDS: acquired immunodeficiency syndrome

AIHA: American Industrial Hygiene Association

ALS: advanced life support

ANA: American Nurses Association

ANSI: American National Standards Institute

ASSE: American Society of Safety Engineers

ATSDR: Agency for Toxic Substances and Disease Registry

BBE: blood-borne pathogen

CAOHC: Council for Accreditation in Occupational Hearing Conservation

CARF: Commission on Accreditation of Rehabilitation Facilities

CCM: Certified Case Manager

CDC: Centers for Disease Control and Prevention

CDL: commercial driver's license

CFR: Code of federal regulations

CISD: critical incident stress debriefing

COBRA: Consolidated Omnibus Budget Reconciliation Act

COHC: Certified Occupational Hearing Conservationist

COHN: Certified Occupational Health Nurse

COHN-S: Certified Occupational Health Nurse—Specialist

CPI: consumer price index

CQI: continuous quality improvement

CTD: cumulative trauma disorder

dB: decibel

dB (A): decibel, "A-weighted"

dB (C): decibel, "C-weighted"

DFW: Drug-Free Workplace Act (1988)

DI: disposable income

DLS: Division of Labor Standards

DOT: Department of Transportation

EAP: employee assistance program

EBRI: Employee Benefit Research Institute

EBD: evidential breathing device

EBT: evidential breath testing

EEOC: Equal Employment Opportunity Commission

EPA: Environmental Protection Agency

ERC: Educational Resource Center

ERISA: Employment Retirement Income Security Act

FAA: Federal Aviation Administration

FDA: Food and Drug Administration

FFDCA: Federal Food, Drug and Cosmetic Act

FHWA: Federal Highway Administration

FMEA: failure mode and effect analysis

FMLA: Family and Medical Leave Act

FRA: Federal Railroad Administration

FTA: Federal Transit Administration

FTE: full-time equivalents

GATT: General Agreement for Trade and Tariffs

GNP: gross national product

HAZOP: hazard and operability

HCFA: health care financing organization

HCP: hearing conservation program

HCS: Hazard Communication Standard (29 CFR 1910, 1915, 1917, 1918, 1926, 1928)

HCW: health care worker

HEDIS: health plan employer data information set

HEPA: high efficiency particle air

HIV: human immunovirus

HMO: health maintenance organization

HPD: hearing protection device

ICOH: International Commission on Occupational Health

IH: industrial hygienist

ILO: International Labor Organization

IMS: information management system

INS: informatics nurse specialist

IPA: independent practice association

JCAHO: Joint Commission for Accreditation of Health Care Organizations

LC50: lethal concentration 50%

LD50: lethal dose 50%

LSS: lumbosacral strain

MCS: multiple chemical sensitivity

MRO: medical review officer

MSDS: material safety data sheet

NAFTA: North American Free Trade Act

NCQA: National Committee for Quality Assurance

NGO: nongovernmental organization

NHTSA: National Highway Traffic Safety Administration

NIDA: National Institute of Drug Abuse

NIHL: noise-induced hearing loss

NINR: National Institute for Nursing Research

NIOSH: National Institute for Occupational Safety and Health

NRR: noise reduction rating

OHN: occupational health nurse

OHNAC: occupational health nurses in agricultural communities

OSH Act: Occupational Safety and Health Act (1970)

OSHA: Occupational Safety and Health Administration

OSHRC: Occupational Safety and Health Review Commission

OTC: over-the-counter

PEL: Permissible Exposure Limits (OSHA exposure limits)

PPE: personal protective equipment

PPI: producer price index

POS: point of service

PPO: preferred provider organization

PTS: permanent threshold shift

REL: recommended exposure levels

RSPA: Research and Special Programs Administration

SAMHSA: Substance Abuse and Mental Health Services Administration

SAP: substance abuse professional

SARA: Superfund Amendments and Reauthorization Act

SHE-O: sentinel health event—occupational

SIC: standard industrial classification

STD: sexually transmitted diseases

STEL: short-term exposure levels

STS: standard threshold shift (also referred to as significant threshold shift)

TLD: thermal luminescent dosimeter

TLV: threshold limit value (ACGIH recommended exposure limit)

TPA: third-party administration

TQM: total quality management

TSCA: Toxic Substances Control Act

TTS: temporary threshold shift

TWA: time-weighted average

USCG: United States Coast Guard

USDHHS: United States Department of Health and Human Services

USDL: United States Department of Labor

USDL, BLS: United States Department of Labor, Bureau of Labor Statistics

USDLWB: United States Department of Labor, Women's Bureau

USPHS: United States Public Health Services

WHO: World Health Organization

WTO: World Trade Organization

APPENDIX D

Glossary

Accident: An undesired event in which harm to people, property, and/or the environment occurs, and which may cause the interruption of business, incurring losses.

Accident investigation: A fact-finding procedure to identify the pertinent factors that allow accidents to occur, with the aim of preventing similar future accidents.

Administrative controls: Supervisory and management practices that promote safe work behaviors in order to eliminate or limit exposure to hazards.

Aggregates at risk: Workers who engage in similar work activities or who have similar exposures that increase their potential for contracting a particular health problem.

Air-purifying respirator: A type of personal protective equipment (PPE) that uses filters or adsorbents to remove toxic materials from inhaled air.

Area sample: A sample most commonly collected when doing environmental monitoring to detect where contaminants are most likely to be generated, creating a "map" of levels present.

Assigned protection factor (APF): The minimum anticipated protection provided by a properly functioning respirator or class of respirators to a given percentage of properly fitted and trained users.

Atmospheric monitoring: The testing of air over a period of time to detect the presence and measure the concentration of airborne contaminants to which a worker is being exposed.

Atmosphere-supply respirator: A type of PPE that uses bottled or compressed air via an air-line or a tank worn by the worker to protect against inhalation of toxic or oxygen-deficient atmospheres.

Benchmarking: The "process of measuring a company's products, services, and practices against industry-leading competitors" (Collins, 1995, p. 50) or "against industry's best practices" (Landwehr, 1995, p. 120).

Bias: Systematic error in an epidemiologic study that results in an incorrect estimate of the association between exposure and risk of disease.

Budgeting: The process by which programs and activities are quantified into monetary terms for the purpose of planning and managing resources for a given time period.

Capitalism: An economic system that allows private ownership of property. Income from property or capital accrues to the individual or firms that accumulated it and own it; individual firms are relatively free to compete with others for their own economic gain; and the profit motive is basic to economic life.

Case management: A process of coordinating an individual client's health care services to achieve optimal, quality care delivered in a cost-effective manner (AAOHN, 1994).

Common law: The legal precedents that have been established as a result of decisions handed down in past cases within a given jurisdiction.

Communism: An economic system in which production systems are government- or state-owned, and production decisions are made by official policy and not directed by market action.

Co-employment: A "relationship between two or more employers in which each has actual or potential legal rights and duties with respect to the same employee or group of employees" (Lenz, 1994, p. 13).

Confidentiality: The implicit promise that information divulged to another will be respected and not released or repeated.

Confined space: An area not designed for human occupancy that has limited entry and egress and often has a lack of ventilation, thus presenting an existing and potential hazard to a worker inside it.

Consensus standard: A standard accepted among professional organizations and individuals to be regarded as a guideline representative of general opinion; it is, however, not legally enforceable unless quoted in a regulation of a legislative body.

Consumer price index (CPI): An index measuring the price changes of goods and services consumed by an urban family of four on a moderate income; CPI is also known as cost-of-living index.

Containment: Enclosure of a hazardous unit or container inside another container in the event of a leak or release of a contaminant or toxin.

Contingent workers: A category of workers also known as floaters, regular part-time, formal intermittents, limited duration hires, informal intermittents, casuals, contract labor services, independent contractors, leased workers, or temporary help services workers.

Dilution ventilation: The circulation of fresh air into the worksite to dilute to an acceptable exposure level a contaminant that is emitted into worksite air.

Direct-reading instrument: An instrument that provides immediate data on the contents of the surrounding atmosphere.

Disposable income (DI): The gross national product (GNP) minus depreciation, business and personal taxes, and transfer payments (such as social security, welfare payments, and so on); "the money in people's pockets" to spend as they want.

Documentation: The written communication of information that is the basis of the legal occupational health record.

Engineering controls: Devices or methods that stop hazards at their source or in the pathway of transmission before they can reach the worker and that do not depend on the worker to control their effectiveness.

Environmental health: The "freedom from illness or injury related to exposure to toxic agents and other environmental conditions that are potentially detrimental to health" (Institute of Medicine, 1995, p. 15).

Epidemiology (from *epi,* meaning "upon," *demos,* or "people," and *logos,* which means "science") The study of the distribution and determinants of health-related states or events in specified populations, and the application of this study to the control of health problems.

Ergonomics: The study of the interaction between humans and their work; ergonomics is concerned with the design of the worksite, equipment, physical environment, and organization of work in order to fit them to the worker.

Exposure monitoring: Often done by or with the aid of an industrial hygienist, it is the quantitative assessment of worksite exposures to hazards that are recognized, suspected, or reasonably predictable, based on other preliminary hazard-identification methods.

Federal Reserve discount rate: The rate at which the Federal Reserve Bank lends funds to its member banks.

Focused inspections: Inspections of a workplace that are conducted periodically to target specific processes, equipment, or work areas; to investigate an accident; to evaluate a reported health or safety hazard; or in response to complaints about such things as a strange odor or loud noise.

Grab sample: An air sample collected over a short period of time, which may range from a few seconds to less than two minutes.

Gross national product (GNP): The total final value of domestic goods and services produced in a national economy over a particular period of time, usually one year.

Hazard: The potential for harm or damage to people, property, or the environment. Hazards are classified as physical, chemical, biological, psychological, or mechanical.

Hazard analysis: Procedure performed to identify potential hazards and evaluate data relating to the probability of their occurrence, the severity of their consequences, and the vulnerability of workers to potential exposures.

Hazardous energy control: A device or method that prevents contact between the worker and the source(s) of hazardous energy.

Hazardous energy source: These can be electrical energy, chemical reactivity, thermal extremes, mechanical energy, and physical energy.

Health promotion: The "science and art of helping people change their lifestyle to move towards a state of optimal health" (O'Donnell, 1989).

Incidence rate: An epidemiological term that describes the rate of disease development among persons at risk.

Incident historical review: The compilation and analysis of accidents and near misses that have occurred over a selected period of time.

Industrial hygiene: That "science and art devoted to the anticipation, recognition, evaluation, and control of those environmental factors arising in or from the workplace that may result in injury, illness, impairment, or affect the well-being of workers and members of the community" (American Industrial Hygiene Association, 1996).

Informatics: The "specialty that integrates nursing science, computer science, and information science in identifying, collecting, processing, and managing data and information to support nursing practice, administration, education, and research, and to expand nursing knowledge" (ANA, 1992).

Informatics nurse specialists: The "nurses who practice in the field of nursing informatics, which includes the development and evaluation of applications, tools, processes, and structures intended to assist nurses to manage data in taking care of patients or in supporting the practice of nursing . . . in all sites and settings of care, whether at the basic or advanced practice level" (ANA, 1994)

Informed consent: A decision made with a complete understanding of a treatment or action including risks, benefits, and alternative treatments; informed consent must be obtained without coercion or deception.

Integrated, or long-term, sample: A sample that consists of a known volume of air drawn through an appropriate medium for a sampling period of less than one hour to a full eight hours, reflecting the length of time of a worker's overall exposure.

Integrated disability management: A comprehensive approach to integrating all disability benefits, programs, and services to help control the employer's disability costs while returning the employee to work as soon as possible and maximizing the employee's maximal functional capacity.

Information management systems: A means to collect, access, and apply large amounts of information from many sources in order to effectively manage all aspects of the occupational health unit.

Isolation: Interposition of a barrier between a hazard and those who might be affected by that hazard.

Job hazard analysis, also known as **job safety analysis (JSA):** The process of carefully studying and recording each step of a job in order to identify existing or potential safety and health job hazards and to determine the best way to perform the job to reduce or eliminate those hazards.

Leadership: The "process of influencing the activities of an individual or a group in efforts toward the achievement of goals" (Adams, 1991, p. 22).

Local exhaust: Removal of contaminated air from the point of origin, away from the worker's breathing zone, through a scrubber or cleaning system to the outside atmosphere.

Machine safeguarding: Eliminating hazards of pinch-, nip-, or shear-points at which it is possible to be caught between the moving parts of a machine or between the materials and the moving part(s) of a machine.

Macroeconomics: A study of economics concerned with the behavior of economic aggregates such as the gross national (domestic) product (national income), consumption, the level of employment, investment, money supply, inflation, and international trade and production relationships.

Malpractice: A type of negligence that involves professional misconduct or unreasonable lack of skill.

Managed care: Any form of health plan that initiates selective contracting between providers, employers, and/or insurers to channel employees/patients to a specified set of cost-effective providers (a provider network); these providers have procedures in place to ensure that only medically necessary and appropriate use of health care services occurs.

Microeconomics: A study of economics that deals with the economic behavior of individual units, such as consumers, firms, and resource owners.

Multiple chemical sensitivity: A condition that has been described as a chemically-induced immune system dysfunction, a low-grade yeast infection, a psychological response to low-level chemical exposures, antioxidant vitamin deficiencies, and various other causes.

Negligence: The failure to perform one's duties according to acceptable standards.

Net national product: The GNP less capital consumption allowance (allocated costs for depreciation of capital equipment).

Noise exposure assessment: Measurements of sound-pressure levels, expressed in terms of decibels (dB).

Occupational health nursing: The "specialty practice that provides for and delivers health care services to workers and worker populations" (AAOHN).

Occupational illness: Any abnormal condition or disorder, other than one resulting from an occupational injury, caused by exposure to environmental factors associated with employment.

Occupational injury: Any injury, such as a cut, fracture, sprain, or amputation, that results from a single incident in the work environment.

Occupational health surveillance: The "process of monitoring the health status of worker populations to gather data on the effects of workplace exposures and using data to prevent injury and illness" (AAOHN, 1996).

Organizational climate: Set of employee perceptions, environmental properties, or relatively enduring characteristics of an organization that describe how an organization operates, what is important to an organization, and what ultimately influences worker behavior (Butcher, 1994; Al-Shammari, 1992; Moran & Volkwein, 1992).

Organizational culture: set of assumptions about the organization, based on explicit and implicit patterns of behavior of the members of an organization, that guide the collective organization in dealing with internal and external situations and challenges (Moran & Volkwein, 1992).

Permissible exposure limits: Standards promulgated by the Occupational Safety and Health Administration that refer to 8-hour, time-weighted averages of airborne exposure to a hazard over 5 working days per week.

Personal protective equipment (PPE): Devices, such as respirators, gloves, or special clothing and shoes, that are worn by workers to protect against hazards in the workplace.

Political economy: A term used to describe macroeconomics as it is influenced by political and social institutions.

Prevalence rate: An epidemiological term that describes the proportion of the population that has a particular condition at a given time or during a given time period.

Primary care: The provision of integrated, accessible health care services by clinicians who are accountable for addressing a large majority of personal health care needs, developing a sustained partnership with patients, and practicing in the context of family and community (Donaldson, Yordy, & Vanselow, 1994, pg. 15).

Primary prevention: Those health promotion and health protection measures that prevent the occurrence of disease.

Prime rate: The rate that banks charge their commercial customers (those with good credit ratings and lowest risk) for short-term loans.

Producer price index: A measurement of the wholesale price of goods.

Privatization: A system in which government services are sold or transferred to private businesses and corporations.

Process safety review: A careful evaluation of what could go wrong and what safeguards must be implemented to prevent hazardous chemical releases, explosions, or other process accidents.

Quantity reduction: A measure used to reduce the potential hazard in the event of a leak, spill, or release by keeping only enough hazardous substance on hand which will actually be needed and consumed in a reasonable time, rather than storing large amounts of material over long periods of time.

Risk: The possibility of loss or injury.

Screening: The application of a test to people who are as yet asymptomatic for the purpose of classifying them with respect to their likelihood of having a particular disease.

Secondary prevention: Early detection and treatment of disease so that its progression is slowed or its complications limited; *screening* is a secondary prevention measure.

Self-contained breathing apparatus (SCBA): Respirable air carried in a tank on the back of the wearer.

Sentinel health event—occupational (SHE-O): A preventable disease, disability, or untimely death that is occupationally related and whose occurrence may: 1) provide the impetus for epidemiologic or industrial hygiene studies; or 2) serve as a warning signal that materials substitution, engineering control, personal protection, or health care may be required.

Site survey/walk-through: A worksite inspection not related to any particular incident, area, or piece of equipment.

Socialism: An economic system in which government owns or controls many major industries but may allow markets to set prices in many areas.

Standards of care: Actions that the average, reasonable, and prudent health care provider would perform in similar circumstances; also known as "reasonable and customary care."

Standard industrial classification: Reference to a four-digit number used by the Bureau of Labor Statistics to classify industries according to type.

Standards of nursing practice: Standards developed by nursing professions to guide practice and provide practitioners with a framework for evaluating practice.

Statutes: Laws that have been drafted through state or federal legislative processes.

Tertiary prevention: The prevention of disability; includes rehabilitative efforts.

Threshold Limit Values: Guidelines for rating exposure to hazardous substances that are developed by the American Conference of Governmental Industrial Hygienists (ACGIH); they are published annually by that organization and generally refer to 8 hours of time-weighted average exposure in a 5-day week.

Tort: A legal wrong against the person or property of another; examples include assault, battery, and defamation.

Toxic Substances Control Act (TSCA): A law that requires documentation of worker allegations of previously unrecognized adverse health effects from new chemicals, mixtures, or processes.

Toxicology: The study of adverse effects of chemicals on biologic systems.

Work-conditioning, or work-hardening, program: A "highly structured, goal-oriented, individualized treatment program designed to maximize the person's ability to return to work" (Commission on Accreditation of Rehabilitation Facilities [CARF]).

Workers' compensation: A publicly funded insurance system that provides for lost wages, medical costs, and rehabilitation for persons who experience an occupational injury or illness.

Workplace violence: Harassment, threats, and actual physical assaults in the worksite.

APPENDIX E

Resources

Professional Associations

American Association of Occupational Health Nurses, 50 Lenox Pointe, Atlanta, GA 30324, (404) 262-1162

American College of Occupational and Environmental Medicine, 55 West Seegers Road, Arlington Heights, IL 60005, (847) 228-6850

American Conference of Governmental Industrial Hygienists, 6500 Glenway Avenue, Cincinnati, OH 45211, (513) 742-2020

American Industrial Hygiene Association, 2700 Prosperity Avenue, Suite 250, Fairfax, VA 22031, (703) 849-8888

American Public Health Association (APHA), Occupational Safety and Health Section, 1015 15th Street NW, Washington, DC 20005, (202) 789-5600

American Society for Safety Engineers (ASSE), 1800 East Oakton, Des Plaines, IL 60018, (847) 699-2929

National Safety Council (NSC), 1121 Spring Lake Drive, Itasca, IL 60143-3201, (630) 285-1121

Certifying Organization

American Board of Occupational Health Nurses, Inc., Concorde Building, Suite 205, 9944 South Roberts Road, Palos Hills, IL 60465, (708) 598-6368, FAX (708) 598-6245

Journals and Books

AAOHN Journal, the official journal of the American Association of Occupational Health Nurses, published monthly by SLACK, Inc., 6900 Grove Road, Thorofare, NJ 08086-9447

Journal of Occupational and Environmental Medicine, the official journal of the American College of Occupational and Environmental Medicine, published monthly by Williams & Wilkins, 428 East Preston Street, Baltimore, MD 21202-3993

American Industrial Hygiene Association Journal, the official journal of the American Hygiene Association, published monthly by the American Industrial Hygiene Association, 2700 Prosperity Avenue, Suite 250, Fairfax, VA 22031

Safety and Health, published monthly by the National Safety Council, 1121 Spring Lake Drive, Itasca, IL 60143

Source of Internet/Computer Information

AAOHN Home Page: www.aaohn.org—provides information on association products and services and links to practice resources, including topic discussion forums, on the Internet.

Computers in Nursing Journal, Lippincott Company Publishing, 12107 Insurance Way, Suite 114, Hagerstown, MD 21740

Directory of Occupational Health and Safety Software, Computers in Occupational Medicine (section of ACOEM), 55 West Seegers Road, Arlington Heights, IL 60005, (708) 228-6850

Informatics Issues and Strategies for the 21st Century Health Care Executive, American Organization of Nurse Executives, AHA Services, Inc., P.O. Box 92683, Chicago, IL 60675-2683

The Nurse Executive's Guide to Directing and Managing Information Systems, The Center for Health Care Information Management (CHIM), 900 Victors Way, Suite 124, Ann Arbor, MI 48108

Menzel, Nancy N. (1994) *Occupational health software: Selecting the right program.* AAOHN.

OSHA Computerized Information System (OCIS), U.S. Government Printing Office, Washington, DC 20402-9325, (202) 783-3238. Contains agency documents, technical information, and training materials on CD-ROM.

Sources of Technical Information

CHEMTREC: 24-hour hotline to provide information about chemicals, 1-800-424-9300

TOXNET: Comprehensive database that provides toxicity data on chemicals, available though Melars Management Section, National Library of Medicine, Building 38, Room 4N421, 8600 Rockville Pike, Bethesda, MD 20894, (800) 638-8480

Poison Control Centers: These centers are located in every state. Each has a 24-hour hotline to provide emergency information and referrals. Information about centers can be found on the inside covers of local phone directories.

Government Resources

National Institute for Occupational Safety and Health (NIOSH) Headquarters, 1600 Clifton Road, NE, Atlanta, GA 30033. NIOSH Technical Information Service provides information and technical assistance on workplace hazards; phone (800) 35-NIOSH or (800) 356-4674

Occupational Safety and Health Administration (OSHA), U.S. Department of Labor, 200 Constitution Avenue, NW, Washington DC 20210. Films and printed material available through regional OSHA offices, or through OSHA Publications Office, 200 Constitution Avenue NW, Washington DC, (202) 219-4667 or (FAX) (202) 219-9266.

Office of Occupational Health Nursing, Occupational Safety and Health Administration, Directorate of Technical Support, Room N-3653, 200 Constitution Avenue NW, Washington, DC 20210.

Environmental Protection Agency (EPA), Public Information Center, PM-211B, 401 M Street, SW, Washington, DC 20460

Agency for Toxic Substances and Disease Registry (ATSDR), ATSDR-Chamblee, 1600 Clifton Road, NE, Atlanta, GA 30033

National Institute of Nursing Research, National Institutes of Health, Building 45, Room AN-12, 45 Center Drive MSC 6300, Bethesda, MD 20892-6300

National Institute of Environmental Health Sciences (NIEHS), National Institutes of Health, Public Health Service, U.S. Department of Health and Human Services, P.O. Box 12233, Research Triangle Park, NC 27709

Clearinghouse on Health Indexes, Office of Epidemiology and Health Promotion, National Center for Health Statistics, Centers for Disease Control, 6525 Belcrest Road, Room 1070, Hyattville, MD 20782, (301) 436-7035

International Agencies and Organizations

International Labour Office—Occupational Safety and Health Branch (ILO-SHB), Bureau International de Travail—Service de la securité et de l'hygiène du travail (BIT-Sec-Hyg), 4 route des Morillons, CH-1211 Geneva 22 (Switzerland)

International Occupational Safety and Health Information Centre, Centre international d'information de securité et d'hygiène du travail (CIS). ILO, 4 route des Morillons, CH-121 Geneva 22 (Switzerland)

International Organization for Standardization (ISO), Organization internationale de normalization. 1 rue de Varembe, CH-1211 Geneva 20 (Switzerland)

Regional Office for Europe of the World Health Organization (WHO-EURO—Environmental Health Service). Scherfigvej 8, DK-2100 Copenhagen (Denmark).

World Health Organization—Office of Occupational Health (WHO-OCH). Organization Mondials de la Sante—Office de la medicine du travail (OMS-OCH). 20 rue Appia, CH-1211 Geneva 27 (Switzerland)

Pan American Health Organization and Regional Office for the Americas of the World Health Organization (PAHO). 525 Twenty-third Street NW, Washington DC 20037 (USA)

Additional References on International Occupational Health

ILO (1997). *Encyclopedia of Occupational Health and Safety,* Fourth Edition. Geneva: International Labour Office

Lehtinen, S., & Mikheev, M. (1994). *WHO Worker's Health Programme and Collaborating Centers in Occupational Health.* Geneva: World Health Organization

Sources for Inspection Checklists

Travers, P.H., & McDougall, C. (1995). *Guidelines for an Occupational Health and Safety Service,* AAOHN Publication, Appendix J, Conducting a Safety Walkthrough

National Institute of Occupational Safety and Health, *Self evaluation of Safety and Health Programs,* U.S. Government Printing Office, Washington, DC 20212

Sources for Accident Investigation

Travers, P.H., & McDougall, C. (1995). *Guidelines for an Occupational Health and Safety Service,* AAOHN Publication, Appendix K. Sample Corporate Accident Investigation Policy and Procedure and Appendix L, Sample Supervisor Accident Investigation Form.

The U.S. Department of Labor, Bureau of Labor Statistics, *Evaluating Your Firm's Injury and Illness Record,* Reports 813 and 814, available from regional OSHA offices.

Further Information on Process Safety Reviews

OSHA 3133 *Process Safety Management—Guidelines for Compliance,* OSHA Publications Office 200 Constitution Avenue NW, Washington, DC (202) 219-4667

Mullan R. J., & Murthy, L.I. (1991). Occupational sentinel health events: an updated list for physician recognition and public health surveillance. *American Journal of Industrial Medicine.* 1991 (19), 775-799

Guidelines for Respirator PPE Health Clearance

American National Standards Institute (ANSI) 88.6, *Respirator Use Physical Qualifications for Personnel,* ANSI, 11 West 42nd Street, New York, NY 10036

APPENDIX F

U.S.C.G.—United States Coast Guard OSHA Standard 1910.120— Hazardous Waste Operations and Emergency Response

The OSHA Standard 1910.120, Hazardous waste operations and emergency response, requires hazardous materials emergency response capability for hazardous waste sites, Environmental Protection Agency–permitted treatment, storage, and disposal (TSD) facilities, and any emergency response operations for releases of, or substantial threats of releases of, hazardous materials. Components of this standard include:

- Site-specific safety and health plan
- Personal protective equipment
- Exposure monitoring equipment and procedures
- Decontamination procedures
- Medical surveillance
- Use of the Incident Command System
- Emergency Response Plan
- Training according to the following requirements:

1. *First responder awareness level.* First responders at the awareness level are individuals who are likely to witness or discover a hazardous substance release and who have been trained to initiate an emergency response sequence by notifying the proper authorities of the release. They would take no further action beyond notifying the authorities of the release. First responders at the awareness level shall have sufficient training or have had sufficient experience to objectively demonstrate competency in the following areas:
   a. An understanding of what hazardous materials are, and the risks associated with them in an incident.
   b. An understanding of the potential outcomes associated with an emergency created when hazardous materials are present.
   c. The ability to recognize the presence of hazardous materials in an emergency.
   d. The ability to identify the hazardous materials, if possible.
   e. An understanding of the role of the first responder awareness individual in the employer's emergency response plan including site security and control and the U.S. Department of Transportation's Emergency Response Guidebook.
   f. The ability to realize the need for additional resources and to make appropriate notifications to the communication center.

2. *First responder, operations level.* First responders at the operations level are individuals who respond to releases or potential releases of hazardous substances as part of the initial response to the site for the purpose of protecting nearby persons, property, or the environment from the effects of the release. They are trained to respond in a defensive fashion without actually trying to stop the release. Their function is to contain the release from a safe distance, keep it from spreading, and prevent exposures. First responders at the operational level shall have received at least eight hours of training or have had sufficient experience to objectively demonstrate competency in the following areas in addition to these listed for the awareness level, and the employer shall so certify:
   a. Knowledge of the basic hazard and risk assessment techniques.
   b. Know how to select and use proper personal protective equipment provided to the first responder operational level.
   c. An understanding of basic hazardous materials terms.
   d. Know how to perform basic control, containment, and/or confinement operations within the capabilities of the resources and personal protective equipment available with their unit.
   e. Know how to implement basic decontamination procedures.
   f. An understanding of the relevant standard operating procedures and termination procedures.

3. *Hazardous materials technician.* Hazardous materials technicians are individuals who respond to releases or potential releases for the purpose of stopping the release. They assume a more aggressive role than a first responder at the operations level in that they will approach the point of release in order to plug, patch, or otherwise stop the release of a hazardous substance. Hazardous materials technicians shall have received at least 24 hours of training equal to the first responder operations level and in addition have competency in the following areas, and the employer shall so certify:
   a. Know how to implement the employer's emergency response plan.
   b. Know the classification, identification, and verification of known and unknown materials by using field survey instruments and equipment.
   c. Be able to function within the assigned role in the Incident Command System.
   d. Know how to select and use proper specialized chemical personal protective equipment provided to the hazardous materials technician.
   e. Understand hazard and risk assessment techniques.
   f. Be able to perform advance control, containment, and/or confinement operations within the capabilities of the resources and personal protective equipment available with the unit.
   g. Understand and implement decontamination procedures.
   h. Understand termination procedures.
   i. Understand basic chemical and toxicological terminology and behavior.

APPENDIX G

American Association of Occupational Health Nurses Publication List

Informative

- Compensation & Benefits Study
- Answer to Health Care Cost Containment

Codes

- Code of Ethics and Interpretive Statements

Standards

- Standards of Occupational Health Nursing Practice

Guidelines

- Developing Job Descriptions
- Implementation of a Respiratory Surveillance System
- Guidelines for an Occupational Health & Safety Service

Position Statements (Set of 10)

- Delivery of Occupational Health Services
- Confidentiality of Health Information
- Education Preparation/Entry into Professional Practice
- Occupational Health Nurse: A Manager
- Respiratory Surveillance in the Workplace
- Impaired Nurses
- The LPN in Occupational Health
- Paramedics and EMTs in the Workplace
- The Occupational Health Nurse as a Case Manager
- Occupational Health Surveillance

Monthly Association Subscriptions

- AAOHN News
- AAOHN Journal

Advisories

- Bloodborne / Airborne Pathogens
- Ergonomics
- Americans with Disabilities Act
- Case Management
- Confidentiality

- Tuberculosis
- Over-the-Counter Medications
- Accident Investigation
- Department of Transportation / Drug & Alcohol Testing
- The Family Medical Leave Act
- Cost-Benefits and Cost-Effectiveness Analyses
- Employee Health Records: Requirements Retention, Access
- Adult Immunizations

Videos

- Ergonomics . . . Creating a Healthier Workplace for a Healthier Bottom Line
- The Occupational Health Nurse . . . Your Key to Managing Health Care Costs
- AAOHN History and Membership Promotion Video

To obtain a current copy of the AAOHN Publication Order Form and pricing information, contact: AAOHN, Inc., 50 Lenox Pointe, Atlanta GA 30324–3176; phone (404) 262-1162; fax (404) 262-1165; e-mail www.aaohn.org

INDEX

Note: Page numbers in *italics* refer to illustrations; page numbers followed by t refer to tables.